DEVELOPMENTAL NEUROPSYCHOLOGY, *13*(3), 2
Copyright © 1997, Lawrence Erlbaum Associates, Inc.

Origins of Language Disorders

Donna J. Thal
San Diego State University
University of California, San Diego

Judith S. Reilly
San Diego State University

This special issue represents the initial products of the first 5 years of a multiproject center titled Origins of Communicative Disorders. The center is part of the Project in Cognitive and Neural Development at the University of California, San Diego. As the title implies, the common goal of investigators involved in this project is to describe the development of communicative skills from their earliest measurable points so that factors that characterize the earliest stages of communicative disorders can be teased apart from those that lead to the development of typical language ability in later childhood.

To meet this goal our studies were designed to obtain information about change over time, to compare individuals, and to compare groups of subjects. Many of our studies are prospective in nature, beginning when the children are at prelinguistic stages and following them through the period during which most basic language skills are acquired. This labor-intensive longitudinal design is combined with cross-sectional studies to increase the numbers of subjects at each datapoint. Together, these research designs provide a powerful means of identifying critical factors related to change over time.

The research in this center also focuses on cross-population comparisons of populations known to be at risk for communicative disorders. The populations studied in the first 5 years of the center included children with late onset of language ("late talkers"), children with pre- or perinatal focal brain injury, children with syndromes that create cognitive impairments (Williams syndrome and Down

---

Requests for reprints should be sent to Donna J. Thal, Department of Communicative Disorders, San Diego State University, 6330 Alvarado Court, Suite 231, San Diego, CA 92120. E-mail: dthal@mail.sdsu.edu

syndrome), and children with prenatal exposure to the stimulant drugs cocaine or methamphetamine.

The articles in this issue illustrate three themes that characterize our research with these populations. First, some of the studies are designed to search for patterns of selective impairment or selective sparing; that is, patterns of association and dissociation within populations and across populations in aspects of language together with those aspects of cognition that may be related to language. Second, these studies emphasize the way communicative ability changes over time in these at-risk and typically developing populations. Third, we are able to pursue questions about brain–behavior relations using new technologies (i.e., event-related brain potentials associated with linguistic and nonlinguistic stimuli), specific populations (e.g., children with well-defined focal brain injury), or both.

In addition to these themes, the five studies that follow share a common methodology: a parent report instrument called the MacArthur Communicative Development Inventory (CDI). The instrument, which has been described in detail in several publications (see especially Fenson et al., 1993; Fenson et al., 1994), was developed over a 20-year period by several of the investigators in our San Diego group, working closely with colleagues in Seattle, New Haven, and Rome. One of the most striking results reported in those studies was the wide range of individual variability present in all aspects of language measured by the CDIs. In fact, the authors concluded that variation is the rule in early language development, and there is no such thing as a "modal child." This makes an endeavor to identify the origins of language disorders not only more challenging but also more urgent, given federal mandates to identify and treat infants and toddlers with communicative disorders (Education of Handicapped Act Amendment, 1986).

Each of the articles in this issue includes a description of those aspects of the CDI that are particularly important for that study. However, two general points are important enough to warrant mention here. First, the reliability and validity of the CDI are both well documented. As reported by Fenson et al. (1994), all the scales on the CDI (which include vocabulary comprehension and production, gesture production, and grammatical complexity) showed strong internal consistency, and longitudinal samples across a 6-month period demonstrated good test–retest reliability as well. Studies of concurrent validity included comparisons of the CDI to standardized and experimental measures of language, including the language tasks on the Bayley Scales of Infant Development, standardized tests of language such as the Expressive One-Word Picture Vocabulary Test (EOWPVT) and the Preschool Language Scale, and various measures from spontaneous language samples (Bates, Bretherton, & Snyder, 1988; Beeghly, Jernberg, & Burrows, 1989; Dale, 1991; Dale, Bates, Reznick, & Morisset, 1989; O'Hanlon & Thal, 1991). Because a number of measures were used in these studies of concurrent validity, it was possible to get some estimates of the range of items sampled through each methodology. Dale, for example, carried out a multiple correlation between children's scores on the CDI and the EOWPVT and a type-token ratio derived from language samples from the same children. The multiple correlation between the children's scores on the vocabulary measure from the CDI and the two vocabulary measures obtained in the laboratory was higher than either of the simple correlations of the single tests to the CDI. In addition, a multiple regression analysis showed that each was related to a distinct proportion of the variance in the CDI vocabulary. The author concluded that the toddler CDI vocabulary checklist assesses a broader vocabulary range than does either the direct observational measure obtained from language samples or the standardized test. Similarly, the sentence complexity subscale and the mean length of the three longest utterances are correlated strongly with the mean length of utterance obtained from a spontaneous language sample. Thus, all the measures obtained from the MacArthur CDI are strongly predictive of the actual behaviors measured in spontaneous communicative situations, and they may provide a more representative sample of children's early language than do other means of sampling early language.

A second important point to make about the CDI is that it provides a method that is comparable across different populations and different laboratories. In the past, research on language acquisition was hampered by the need for different methodologies for children with different handicapping conditions, and by the fact that methodologies were not easy to replicate across laboratories. Within the age range for which the CDIs are normed we finally have a methodology that allows us to make more valid and reliable cross-population and cross-laboratory comparisons.

What follows are four articles, each focused on one or two populations known to be at risk for communicative disorders, and one article concerning changes in brain activity associated with changes in language ability in typically developing children. In the first article, Thal, Bates, Goodman, and Jahn-Samilo examine the continuity of development in children at the extremes of the normal continuum and attempt to determine whether children who start out late or early continue to be late or early 6 months later. They show that there is significant continuity at the group level, and that we do not yet possess the means to predict trajectories of development for individual children.

Bates et al. focus on children with pre- and perinatal focal brain injury, in three cross-sectional studies of communication and language across the period in which typical children progress from first words to grammar. The authors explore the effect of lesion location on language and find effects different from those reported for adults with similar lesions. In the age range between 10 and 17 months, children with right-hemisphere damage are at greater risk for delay in comprehension and use of symbolic gestures than are children with left-hemisphere damage. In addition, throughout the period from 10 to 44 months, children with left-temporal-lobe damage are at risk for greater delay in expressive vocabulary and grammar than are children with damage in other areas.

Singer Harris, Bellugi, Bates, Jones, and Rossen explore the different trajectories and associated patterns of gesture use, vocabulary, and grammar in children with Williams syndrome and Down syndrome. They report that both groups of children are equally and seriously delayed in the early stages of language development. However, the patterns of development differ. In the earliest stages children with Down syndrome use significantly more gestures than do children with Williams syndrome. At a later point, when the vocabulary levels of both groups were high enough to support the development of grammar, children with Williams syndrome began to develop grammatical structure in a manner similar to normally developing children. By contrast, children with Down syndrome demonstrate an atypical dissociation between vocabulary size and the development of grammatical structure.

Dixon, Thal, Potrykus, Bullock Dickson, and Jacoby describe an exploratory study of two groups of children with prenatal exposure to stimulant drugs. One group comprises a large clinical sample of children in a wide range of home settings. The second is a smaller experimental group living in stable, middle-class adoptive homes. Dixon et al. report significant delay in all aspects of language for a large proportion of these children. However, there is also a wide range of variability in this population, with some children falling well within the normal range. In both groups, older children performed more poorly than did younger children. Dixon et al. suggest that this "delayed impact" could reflect damage to frontal lobe structures that develop relatively late, compared with other parts of the cerebral cortex.

Finally, Mills, Coffey-Corina, and Neville describe developmental changes in the brain activity of typically developing children that are linked to comprehension of single words at 13 and 20 months of age. They show that brain activity changes from bilateral activity that is broadly distributed over anterior and posterior portions of the brain at 13 to 17 months, to more specifically localized activity in the temporal and parietal regions of the left hemisphere at 20 months of age. However, this is not a simple age-related phenomenon: Children with higher levels of comprehension are reported to have more localized brain activity in both groups than do those with lower levels of comprehension.

Taken together, the articles in this issue provide a comprehensive picture of early language development and its neural correlates, across a range of typical and atypical populations. By looking at language abilities from their point of origin, that is, from the very first signs of word comprehension to the emergence of grammar, the authors hope to lay the foundation for future research on the nature and etiology of communication disorders.

REFERENCES

Bates, E., Bretherton, I., & Snyder, L. (1988). *From first words to grammar: Individual differences and dissociable mechanisms.* New York: Cambridge University Press.

Beeghly, M., Jernberg, E., & Burrows, E. (1989, April). *Validity of the Early Language Inventory (ELI) for use with 25-month-olds.* Paper presented at the biennial meeting of the Society for Research in Child Development, Kansas City, MO.

Dale, P. (1991). The validity of a parent report measure of vocabulary and syntax at 24 months. *Journal of Speech and Hearing Sciences, 34,* 565–571.

Dale, P., Bates, E., Reznick, J. S., & Morisett, C. (1989). The validity of a parent report instrument of child language at 20 months. *Journal of Child Language, 16,* 239–250.

Education of Handicapped Act Amendment, 100 Fed. Reg. 1145 (1986).

Fenson, L., Dale, P., Reznick, J. S., Bates, E., Thal, D., & Pethick, S. (1994). Variability in early communicative development. *Monographs of the Society for Research in Child Development, Serial, 59*(5, Serial No. 242).

Fenson, L., Dale, P., Reznick, J. S., Thal, D., Bates, E., Hartung, J., Pethick, S., & Reilly, J. (1993). *MacArthur Communicative Development Inventories: User's guide and manual.* San Diego, CA: Singular Publishing Group.

O'Hanlon, L. & Thal, D. (1991, November). *MacArthur CDI/Toddlers: Validation for language impaired children.* Paper presented at the annual convention of the American Speech–Language–Hearing Association, Atlanta, GA.

DEVELOPMENTAL NEUROPSYCHOLOGY, *13*(3), 239–273

Continuity of Language Abilities: An Exploratory Study of Late- and Early-Talking Toddlers

Donna J. Thal
San Diego State University
University of California, San Diego

Elizabeth Bates
University of California, San Diego

Judith Goodman
University of Missouri

Jennifer Jahn-Samilo
University of California, San Diego

Three exploratory studies were carried out to determine if there was continuity in the development of language in young children at the upper and lower extremes of the normal continuum, and if it was possible to use variables from an early assessment to predict their language status at a later date. Studies 1 and 2 examined continuity over 6-month periods (from approximately 20 to 26 months and 13 to 20 months of age, respectively); Study 3 examined continuity from 8 to 30 months of age. Results provided solid evidence for continuity at the group level but no evidence of an ability to predict outcome for individual children using the vocabulary production, vocabulary comprehension, and gesture production variables included in this study.

Requests for reprints should be sent to Donna J. Thal, Department of Communicative Disorders, San Diego State University, 6330 Alvarado Court, Suite 231, San Diego, CA 92120. E-mail: dthal@mail.sdsu.edu

Many parents wonder about their child's early development. They wonder whether he or she is abnormally slow to develop, or so precocious that early celebration is warranted. During their child's 1st year of life, most parents worry about such issues as sleeping, eating, and attainment of motor milestones (especially crawling and walking). During the 2nd year, the focus switches to communication and language. This also is true for physicians and other health care professionals because disorders of higher cognitive functions in toddlers and preschoolers often are manifested as language disorders (Tuchman, Rapin, & Shinnar, 1991).

Until recently, developmental psychologists and psycholinguists have had little to say in response to these concerns, beyond some relatively limited norms established early in the 20th century (Gesell, 1925; McCarthy, 1954). This is true in part because modern developmental research has focused on the universal characteristics of language learning, based on an idealized *modal child* who acquires his or her native language in a standard sequence, on a standard schedule, with a single set of mechanisms (i.e., the Language Acquisition Device; for discussions of this point, see Fenson et al., 1994; Hardy-Brown, 1983; Plomin, 1989). In the absence of more systematic information concerning normal variability, a folk wisdom emerged among many health professionals, including an exaggerated belief in gender differences ("Boys are usually late.") coupled with an optimistic view of the outcomes associated with language delays before 3 or 4 years of age ("Don't worry, he'll catch up.").

Fortunately, variability in early language development has become an active topic of research in recent years, rendering the notion of a modal child less tenable. Large variations in vocabulary size and rate of growth were reported by a number of researchers (Bates, Bretherton, & Snyder, 1988; Fenson et al., 1994; Goldfield, 1987; Hampson & Nelson, 1993; Huttenlocher, Haight, Bryk, Seltzer, & Lyons, 1991). In most cases, these variations were too large to explain with traditional biological variables (e.g., gender or rate of sensorimotor development) or social variables (e.g., birth order, social class, maternal style, or quality of mother–child attachment). For example, Fenson et al. looked at variability in the rate of development among more than 1,800 infants between 8 and 30 months of age, the largest study of early language development to date. Among other things, they reported girls were ahead of boys on most measures of language and communication. However, this difference was far smaller than one might expect based on the conventional wisdom. Gender differences accounted for less than 2% of the variance on any single measure of language and communication, with girls averaging about 1 month ahead of boys across the period from 8 to 30 months. Rate is not the only type of variability in language development. Qualitative differences in the "style" of development also have been observed, leading to the suggestion that there may be qualitative differences among normal children in the mechanisms used to acquire language (Bates et al., 1988; Bates, Dale, & Thal, 1995; Plunkett, 1993; Shore, 1995; Vihman & Miller, 1988).

The problems that such variability presents for theories of normal language development were discussed at length by Fenson et al. (1994). This variability also poses significant problems for professionals charged with determining whether a child who is under 3 or 4 years of age is exceptional, either precocious or delayed. If there are no clear criteria for identifying what is "normal," then it is especially difficult to be certain that a child is truly delayed or precocious. Given that professionals who serve young children are now charged by Public Law 99–457 (Education of Handicapped Act Amendment, 1986) to evaluate communicative abilities and provide appropriate treatment for children from birth to 3 years of age, this creates a serious dilemma.

Although tremendous variability in rate and style of language acquisition has been documented, it remains unclear whether individual differences during the early period of language acquisition have any consequences for language abilities at a later point in time. We need to assess whether children who are delayed or accelerated in their language acquisition at one point in development remain so at a later time and whether variability of this sort has long-term consequences for the child's ability to function successfully. There is still no answer to the second question, but there is evidence for short-term stability in the rate of development in early language and communication, across the normal range. As part of their large norming study of more than 1,800 infants, Fenson et al. (1994) obtained 6-month follow-up data from approximately a third of the sample, including children whose parents filled out the 8- to 16-month MacArthur Communicative Development Inventory (CDI) Infant scale at two time points (infant–infant sample), children whose parents filled out the 16- to 30-month Toddler scale at two time points (toddler–toddler sample), and another group whose parents filled out the Infant scale at Time 1 and the Toddler scale at Time 2 (infant–toddler sample). Results indicated clearly that the individual differences in language comprehension and production observed in the larger cross-sectional study were relatively stable across a 6-month period. Because the Fenson et al. study used the same methodology as did the study of extreme groups discussed in this article, it is useful to consider their longitudinal results in a bit more detail.

In the first study, Fenson et al. (1994) used the CDI Infant scale at both datapoints. The CDI: Words and Gestures (Infant form) is normed for vocabulary comprehension, vocabulary production, and gesture production in children from 8 to 16 months of age. The Infant form has two parts: One samples language, and the other samples gestures. The major portion of Part 1 consists of a 396-item vocabulary checklist organized into 19 semantic categories. Ten of those categories are composed of nouns, (animals, vehicles, toys, food and drink, clothing, body parts, furniture and rooms, small household items, outside things and places to go, and people). The remaining sections include sound effects and animal sounds, games and routines, action words (i.e., verbs), words about time, descriptive words (i.e., adjectives), pronouns, question words, prepositions and locations, and quantifiers.

Parents are asked to mark the appropriate space if their child comprehends or comprehends and produces each word. They are asked to leave the space blank if their child does not yet comprehend or produce each word. Part 2 samples actions and gestures, examples of early communicative and representational skills that are not dependent on verbal expression. The gestures are divided into five subscales as follows: first communicative gestures (those that signal the onset of intentional communication such as giving, showing, and pointing), games and routines (early social interactive gestures such as "pat-a-cake"), actions with objects (e.g., sniffing a flower, pretending to stir), pretending to be a parent (among the first types of symbolic actions, such as brushing a doll's hair, pretending to feed a doll), and imitating other adult actions (pretending to drive, pretend to sweep with a broom). These are behaviors that have been described as predecessors, correlates, or both predecessors and correlates of early language (Bates, Benigni, Bretherton, Camaioni, & Volterra, 1979) and as potential predictors of risk for language delay (Thal & Tobias, 1994; Thal, Tobias, & Morrison, 1991).

The Fenson et al. (1994) infant–infant sample demonstrated continuity in vocabulary comprehension, vocabulary production, and gesture production in 62 children with a mean age of 9.61 months ($SD = 0.72$) at Time 1, and a mean age of 16.34 months ($SD = 0.81$) at Time 2. To identify the independent stability of each of these three dependent variables over time, multiple regression analyses were conducted in which the relation between that variable at Time 1 and its equivalent at Time 2 was tested after variance due to age, sex, birth order, and socioeconomic status (SES) was removed. In the longitudinal analysis of word comprehension, Time 1 comprehension scores accounted for 21.8% of the variance in Time 2 comprehension after other factors were controlled (all the Time 1 variables together accounted for 32.9% of the variance at Time 2). In a similar regression analysis using gesture production as the dependent variable, Time 1 gesture accounted for an additional 16.7% of the variance in Time 2 gesture (out of a total of 36.7% for all predictors together). In a third regression analysis, Time 1 word production accounted for an additional 8.1% of the variance in Time 2 production (out of a total of only 12.0% for all variables together on the final step). All these unique contributions were highly reliable ($p < .001$). As Fenson et al. pointed out, the weaker longitudinal stability for vocabulary production in the infant dataset probably reflects the fact that many of the infants in this subsample did not produce any language at the first datapoint (i.e., a statistical floor effect).

The second study used the CDI: Words and Sentences (Toddler form) at the second datapoint. It is normed for vocabulary production, utterance length, and grammatical complexity in children from 16 to 30 months of age. Part 1 of the Toddler form contains a 680-word vocabulary production checklist organized into 22 semantic categories. In this inventory parents are only asked about the words a child produces. Part 2 contains five sections designed to assess morphological and syntactic development. Two of those, utterance length and grammatical complexity, were used in this study. The utterance length section provides an upper-limit measure. Parents are asked to provide examples of the three longest utterances they have heard their child produce, and the mean number of morphemes (as distinguished from the more familiar mean length of utterance) is calculated. The grammatical complexity section contains 37 sentence pairs in which one represents typical immature grammatical structures and the other represents more mature forms. Three levels of grammatical ability are represented within the 37 pairs: bound morphemes (e.g., "Daddy car" vs. "Daddy's car"), functor words (e.g., "Doggie table" vs. "Doggie on table"), and early emerging complex sentence forms (e.g., "I sing song" vs. "I sing song for you"). Parents are asked to choose the exemplar in each of the pairs that reflects the child's current level of speech.

In the Fenson et al. (1994) infant–toddler sample, mean age at Time 1 was 13.45 months (SD = 1.71), whereas mean age at Time 2 was 20.15 months (SD = 1.86). In this particular dataset, word production was the only measure with equivalents at both time points. Using the same regression strategy previously described, Time 1 vocabulary production alone accounted for a highly reliable 24.5% of the variance in Time 2 production after other factors were controlled (bringing the total for all Time 1 predictors to 54.1%). In other words, parent reports of vocabulary production have substantial predictive value from 13 to 20 months of age.

Finally, the Fenson et al. (1994) toddler–toddler sample yielded more evidence for short-term stability of individual differences in early language development. In this dataset, the mean age of children at Time 1 was 20.26 months (SD = 2.40), and the mean age at Time 2 was 26.88 months (SD = 0.62). Regression analyses comparable to those just described for the infant–infant and infant–toddler samples were conducted for two key measures: total vocabulary and grammatical complexity. Vocabulary production at Time 1 added 32.3% to the variance in Time 2 vocabulary, out of a total of 60.5% from all the predictors together on the final step. Grammatical complexity at Time 1 added 19.2% to complexity at Time 2, out of a total 47.8% of the variance from all predictors. All predictions were highly reliable (p < .001).

To summarize, although there are large individual differences in the timing of early language milestones, the Fenson et al. (1994) longitudinal data suggest that these differences are relatively stable across a 6-month period. Is this also true for children at the extreme end of the distribution? Do groups of children who are significantly delayed or very precocious in early language and communication maintain their standing across time? Perhaps more important from an applied perspective, can we use variables from an early assessment to predict whether individual children will remain "late talkers" or "early talkers" at a later point in time? These three questions are explored in the studies reported next.

We used the CDIs described earlier to examine the value of parental reports of vocabulary and gesture production for predicting precocity or delay. Experiments 1 and 2 used the same database and group design used by Fenson et al. (1994), but they focused on children in the upper and lower 10% of the normal distribution rather than on mean or modal developmental trends. These were exploratory studies designed to use data already gathered to help formulate hypotheses for further work. Our emphasis on late talkers is easy to justify on clinical grounds. However, early talkers are equally interesting. Their development is relevant to theoretical questions such as whether late and early status are equally stable, and whether the same factors that predict late status also predict continued precocity. They also provide useful information for the interpretation of language delay (e.g., as a control for psychometric factors like regression toward the mean). We chose a working definition of late talkers as children who fall at or below the 10th percentile. A working definition of early talkers was established as children who fall at or above the 90th percentile. These definitions were adopted because the 10th and the 90th percentiles are the cutoff points adopted in several previous studies of children with atypical profiles (Robinson, Dale, & Landesman, 1990; Thal & Bates, 1988; Thal & Tobias, 1994).

Experiment 3 reports on developmental trajectories of individual children from a new longitudinal study of 34 children who were followed monthly across the period from 8 to 30 months of age. Here we focused on children who were late or early talkers at any point across the period from 18 to 24 months—the time window used by Thal and Bates (1988), Thal and Tobias (1994), and Thal, Tobias, and Morrison (1991) to identify late and early talkers in previous studies. We look at where these children end up at 30 months of age (the end of the study) and how they fared on the infant measures in the months prior to their identification as late or early talkers. These three studies provide further evidence for stability of individual differences across the period from first words to grammar, but they also show that our ability to predict outcomes for individual children is still quite limited.

EXPERIMENT 1

Method

Participants

The subsample from the complete cross-sectional norming study of the CDIs analyzed in Experiment 1 included 185 children whose parents completed the CDI Toddler form twice, once when they were between 16 and 25 months of age ($M = 19.73$ months, $SD = 2.08$) and again when they were between 22 and 31 months of age ($M = 26.39$ months, $SD = 2.12$ months). The average time between completing the two toddler CDIs was 6.65 months ($SD = 0.34$ months). The samples were collected at three sites: New Haven, Connecticut; Seattle, Washington; and San Diego, California. Together the subsample contained 24.3% of the original CDI: Toddler norming sample.

Children were excluded from the study if they were 6 or more weeks premature, had a genetic disorder such as Down or Williams syndrome, had extended illnesses or were subjected to serious medical or surgical procedures, or had other serious medical problems. Repeated ear infections were not an exclusionary criterion as they had not been for the normative sample. In the original sample 4.3% of the children were reported to have had repeated ear infections.

The ethnic and educational characteristics of the whole sample were described in detail by Fenson et al. (1993, 1994). These were representative of the subsample used in this study. In comparison to the 1990 census figures (Bureau of the Census, 1991), the educational level of the parents in this study was above the national average. The ethnic diversity was not significantly different from the 1991 Bureau of the Census figures.

The sample was restricted to children for whom English was the primary language. However, children with exposure to a second language were not eliminated from the normative study because bilingual environments are common for many children in the United States. A total of 12.2% of the families in the normative sample reported their children had some exposure to a second language.

Children were placed into late-talker or early-talker categories based on percentile norms from Fenson et al. (1994). Although (as we noted earlier) gender differences are relatively small in this sample, they were significant, and Fenson et al. recommended assignment of percentile scores based on separate norms for boys and girls. These recommendations were followed in this study, so that late-talker status always meant the child obtained a vocabulary score at or below the 10th percentile for his or her age and sex; similarly, early-talker status always meant the child obtained a vocabulary score at or above the 90th percentile for his or her age and sex.

Procedure

As noted, the CDI Toddler form was used for Experiment 1. Because of the exploratory nature of this work, we examined stability of extreme scores in this sample with a number of statistical analyses, some of which are mathematically redundant. However, each analysis has an advantage for a different kind of question. The kinds of questions and the statistical analyses used to examine them follow.

Breakdown of late and early talkers. Based on cross-sectional norms for the CDI, we determined how many longitudinal participants fell at or below the 10th percentile (i.e., late talkers) and how many fell at or above the 90th percentile (i.e., early talkers), at both Time 1 and Time 2. Binomial tests were used to determine whether late or early talkers were under- or overrepresented in the longitudinal dataset, compared with the cross-sectional norms.

Participant and family variables. One-way analyses of variance (ANO-VAs) were conducted to compare late talkers, early talkers, and children who fell between the two extremes for age in days at both Time 1 and Time 2, birth order, SES, maternal and paternal education, and maternal and paternal vocation. Chi-square tests were used to compare the same three groups on four categorical variables: sex, ethnicity, presence or absence of limited exposure to a second language, and presence or absence of mild medical complications.

Stability of late or early status. Binomial tests were used to determine if children who were delayed (or early) at the first datapoint were likely to be delayed (or early) at the second datapoint. After determining whether and to what extent children maintained their extreme group status, we checked to see if those who stayed late (or early) differed from those who changed status on the participant and family variables.

Factors that predict Time 2 status. We then asked whether any of the Time 1 language measures predicted late- or early-talker status at Time 2, first across the sample as a whole, and then only for those children who fell into extreme groups at Time 1. ANOVA comparing late talkers and early talkers with middle-range children at Time 2 on the major language variables at Time 1 were carried out, followed by post hoc tests to determine which pairwise comparisons were significant when the ANOVA was significant. Regression analyses were used to explore whether any of the major language variables at Time 1 contributed unique variance to Time 2 status (for the group as a whole, and for those who fell in the extremes at Time 1).

Predicting individual cases. Finally, we conducted discriminant analyses using the same Time 1 predictors to classify children into late or early status at Time 2. Whereas the first four analyses examined continuity at the group level, these discriminant analyses told us how successful we were in predicting the short-term future for individual children.

Results

Breakdown of late and early talkers. At Time 1, when the children averaged just under 20 months of age, 24 of the 185 participants (13.0%) fell at or below the 10th percentile according to the MacArthur cross-sectional norms. A binomial test indicated this was no more than would be expected if the longitudinal sample had been drawn randomly from the cross-sectional population. Similarly, 25 of the 185 children (13.5%) fell at or above the 90th percentile, again no more than would be expected by chance on a binomial test. At Time 2, 17 of these 185 children (9.2%) qualified as late talkers, slightly below 10% but still no more than would be expected by chance on a binomial test. By contrast, 30 out of 185 children (16.2%) qualified as early talkers at Time 2, which is significantly more than would be expected by chance ($p < .007$) if children were drawn randomly from the cross-sectional norms. There are at least two possible explanations for the over-representation of early talkers in this longitudinal sample at Time 2, and they are not mutually exclusive: (a) Parents who are willing to participate in a longitudinal study tend to be more attuned and attentive to language, and such individuals are more likely to have precocious children; and (b) parents of precocious children are particularly proud of their offspring and are more motivated to continue at the second datapoint.

Participant and family variables. We used the percentile rankings previously described to divide the children into three groups (i.e., late talkers, middle-range talkers, and early talkers), one for each of the two time points. One-way ANOVAs were then conducted on all the participant and family variables that form an interval or ordinal scale (Time 1 age in days, Time 2 age in days, birth order, SES, maternal education, paternal education, maternal occupation, and paternal occupation). Chi-square tests were conducted to compare the three groups on categorical variables, including sex, presence or absence of mild medical complications, presence or absence of exposure to a second language, and ethnicity (White, African American, Hispanic, Asian, other).

The three groups identified at Time 1 differed significantly on three measures: Time 1 age, $F(2, 182) = 3.42$, $p < .04$; Time 2 age, $F(2, 182) = 3.11$, $p < .05$; and SES, $F(2, 182) = 3.43$, $p < .04$. Post hoc Tukey tests ($p < .05$) indicated that early talkers were older than children in the middle range at both time points. Late talkers were younger than children in the middle range at Time 1, but they were not significantly different at Time 2 (Time 1: late = 19.38, mid = 19.62, early = 20.71; Time 2: late = 26.08, mid = 26.26, early = 27.35). It is possible that some of the early talkers crept to the 90th percentile or above because they were closer to the border for the next age-in-month bracket (where they might have received somewhat lower percentile scores). A similar (but reverse) phenomenon may have produced the effect for late talkers. The Tukey post hoc test for SES was not significant. Early talkers tended to come from families with slightly higher SES, and late talkers tended to come from families with slightly lower SES (late = 43.1, mid = 44.0, early = 50.9; Hollingshead, 1965).

The three groups identified at Time 2 also differed on age, including their age at the earlier time period, $F(2, 182) = 3.85$, $p < .023$, and their age at Time 2, $F(2, 182) = 3.20$, $p < .05$. Again, post hoc Tukey tests ($p < .05$) indicated that early talkers were older than children in the middle range at both time points. However, late talkers were also significantly older than children in the middle range at both time points (Time 1: late = 20.24, mid = 19.49, early = 20.55; Time 2: late = 26.82, mid = 26.17, early = 27.26). Once again, some of the variance in the early talker group may be an artifact of age brackets, as noted for the previous set of analyses. This cannot explain the late talker findings, however. None of the other effects reached significance in the Time 2 analyses, including the SES variable. This suggests that the weak SES advantage for early talkers at Time 1 was probably a transient phenomenon, or of little significance in both the statistical and the practical sense of the term.

Stability of late- and early-talking status. For children who were early or late at Time 1, binomial tests were conducted to determine whether more of them retained that status at Time 2 than would be expected by chance (i.e., more than would be expected if there were no continuity of status across the 6-month period). A complementary set of analyses was conducted to determine if children who were early or late at Time 2 had the same status at Time 1. Of the 24 children who were late talkers at Time 1, 12 (50%) retained that status at Time 2, far more than would be expected by chance ($p < .00001$). Of the 25 children who were early talkers at Time 1, 15 (60%) were also early talkers at Time 2 ($p < .0001$). Hence it was the case that children who fell in the extremes around 20 months of age had a higher-than-chance probability of retaining that status 6 months later. It is also true, however, that 50% of the late talkers and 40% of the early talkers regressed back into the middle range. Looking back in the opposite direction, we found that 12 of 17 (70.6%) children who were late talkers at Time 2 came from the same extreme group at Time 1 ($p < .00001$). Of the children who were early talkers at Time 2, 15 of 30 (50%) were also early talkers at Time 1 ($p < .00001$). It is clear that there is some stability in language status across this 6-month period, although between 30% and 60% of the children migrated in or out of the extremes across this period of rapid development.

Can we distinguish between late talkers who "stay late" and those who move into the middle range, or between early talkers who "stay early" and those who move back toward the mean? In a first attempt to answer this critical diagnostic question, we conducted analyses comparing late talkers who stayed late with those who did not, and early talkers who stayed early with those who did not, on all the participant and family variables reviewed in the previous section. *T* tests were used for the continuous or interval variables (i.e., age, birth order, and various measures of family status), and chi-square tests were used for categorical variables (i.e., sex, ethnicity, presence or absence of mild medical problems, and presence or absence of second-language exposure).

For Time 1 late talkers, we found no significant differences on any of the participant or family variables between children who stayed late and children who moved into the middle, with two exceptions. First, children who stayed late tended to have more mild medical complications than did children who moved into the middle (i.e., 4 of the 12 children who stayed late had some kind of reported complication, compared with 0 of the 12 children who regressed toward the mean, chi-square likelihood ratio, $p < .02$). Second, there was a tendency for children who stayed late to be slightly older at Time 1 than children who regressed toward the mean; stay late, Time 1 mean age = 20.23; regress, Time 1 mean age = 18.52, $t(22)$ = −1.79, $p < .09$. This latter finding may reflect outcome for children who were having more serious difficulty. That is, the older late talkers had a longer time to regress toward the mean (into the middle range) but had not done so. Alternatively, it may be an artifact of assigning percentile scores based on age-in-month brackets. That is, some of the children may have been classified as late talkers at Time 1 because they were particularly old for their age bracket and would not have fallen below the 10th percentile if they were just a few days younger.

For Time 1 early talkers, we found only one reliable difference between those who stayed early and those who regressed toward the mean. Specifically, children who remained precocious across this 6-month period had mothers with significantly lower rankings on an occupational scale, $t(23) = 3.69$, $p < .001$; stay high = 4.67; regress = 7.50.

Predicting Time 2 status from Time 1 language measures. In this section, we consider whether children who were late or early at Time 2 differed on specific language measures at Time 1. Five variables were used: (a) ability to combine words (scored as *never, sometimes,* or *often*), (b) sentence complexity, (c) mean length (in morphemes) of the three longest utterances, (d) percentile score (based on vocabulary size rather than age) for the proportion of words in their vocabulary that were grammatical function words (an attempt to assess "closed-class style"; Bates et al., 1994; Shore, 1995), and (e) total number of words (i.e., the measure used to assign late- and early-talker status at each time point). One-way ANOVAs were conducted comparing the late, early, and middle-range groups at Time 2 on each of these Time 1 language variables, followed by Tukey tests ($p < .05$) to identify significant pairwise differences. Results are summarized in Table 1. We then carried out regression analyses to determine whether any of the individual variables contributed unique variance to late or early status when other variables were controlled.

There was a significant main effect for all of the language variables except closed-class percentile score (see Table 1). For children who were late talkers at Time 2, post hoc tests demonstrated significant differences for all Time 1 language measures for which there was a main effect in the ANOVA (Table 1). Similarly, for children who were early talkers at Time 2, significant differences also were observed for the same Time 1 language measures (Table 1). Hence children who were late or early talkers around 26 months were (as a group) already well behind or ahead of their peers, respectively, at 20 months in vocabulary and grammar.

Our next question pertains to the unique contribution of individual Time 1 measures to extreme group status at Time 2. Regression analyses were used because they allowed us to evaluate the separate contributions that each of the correlated variables made. Two separate regression analyses were conducted, one for late

TABLE 1
Comparison of Children Who Were Delayed, Precocious, or Average in Language at the
Second Datapoint on Measures of Language at the First Datapoint

Time 1 Variables	Late Talkers	Middle Level	Early Talkers	F value	p value	Post hoc results
Total production	37.50	186.00	357.00	40.58	< .001	LT < M < ET
Combining	0.35	1.03	1.63	18.06	< .001	LT < M < ET
Complexity	0.17	3.36	8.67	22.26	< .001	LT < M < ET
Mean of the three longest utterances	1.67	2.80	4.57	25.66	< .001	LT < M < ET
Closed-class percentile score	6.00	8.10	7.17	1.74	ns	na

Note. LT = later talker; M = middle level; ET = early talker; ns = not significant; na = not applicable.

talker status and the other for early talker status at Time 2. In both of the analyses we evaluated the joint and unique variance of the following eight predictor variables: Time 1 age, Time 2 age, SES, and five Time 1 language variables (viz., total number of words produced, level of word combinations, sentence complexity, mean length of the three longest utterances, and closed-class scores). Unique variance was determined by running eight separate stepwise regressions with the same variables but changing the variable that was added last for each analysis.

In the analysis for Time 2 late talkers, the eight predictors together accounted for 14.6% of the variance, a highly reliable prediction ($p < .001$). However, only one of the eight predictors added significant unique variance when it was entered into the equation last. Specifically, total vocabulary increased the prediction by an additional 3.7% ($p < .01$). This reflects a partial correlation of $-.20$, indicating that late talkers had smaller vocabularies than did other children in the sample, even after all the age, SES, and grammar measures were controlled on the first step. However, age, SES, and grammatical abilities did not add to the prediction when vocabulary size was controlled.

In the analysis for Time 2 early talkers, the eight predictors together accounted for a robust 30.9% of the variance ($p < .001$). Note that this is more than twice the variance accounted for when the same variables are used to predict late-talker status, suggesting that it is easier to predict who will stay ahead than who will stay behind. Once again, however, the only variable that made a significant unique contribution on the final step was total vocabulary size at Time 1 (7.3%, $p < .001$), with a partial correlation of $+.31$, indicating that early talkers at Time 2 were ahead of their peers in vocabulary size at Time 1 even after all the age, SES, and grammatical predictors were controlled. Grammatical measures did not add significantly to the prediction, although there was a trend in that direction (with Time 1 utterance length contributing 1.2% on the last step, $p < .10$).

This brings us to our most important question: Can we use Time 1 language variables to predict whether children will maintain their status across a 6-month period? To answer this question, we began with t tests on the five language variables comparing Time 1 late talkers who stayed late with those who moved toward the mean, and Time 1 early talkers who stayed early with those who moved into the middle range. Results are summarized in Table 2.

In the late-talker analyses, none of the t tests reached significance. There was a trend in the t test on Time 1 production, but it was in the opposite direction from what might be predicted if persistence and severity of delay were related. Specifically, children who stayed late had slightly larger vocabularies at Time 1 ($M = 25.08$), compared with children who caught up later, $M = 11.91$, $t(22) = -2.02$, $p < .065$.

In the early-talker analyses, there was no significant difference between those who stayed early and those who regressed toward the mean on vocabulary size, combining, or closed-class proportion scores at Time 1. However, there was a significant difference on grammatical complexity (although the difference just missed significance when the Bonferroni correction was applied), and the difference for utterance length approached significance in the direction that would be predicted if persistence and precocity were related. Specifically, children who stayed precocious across this 6-month period had higher complexity scores at Time 1, $t(23) = -2.25$, $p < .04$, stay early, $M = 13.87$, regress, $M = 6.90$; and they were reported to produce longer utterances, $t(23) = -1.79$, $p < .09$, stay early, $M = 5.69$ morphemes, regress, $M = 6.55$ morphemes.

Finally, we conducted regression analyses using the same eight predictors previously described to determine which factors jointly or uniquely predicted staying late, staying early, or both.

In the analysis of late talkers, the eight predictors together accounted for 32.2% of the variance. However, the prediction as a whole did not reach significance. Furthermore, none of the individual variables made a unique prediction when it was entered on the final step. We repeated the regression using only two language measures: total vocabulary and grammatical complexity. Taken together, the two measures accounted for 21.0% of the variance in staying late, but this prediction also failed to reach significance ($p < .09$). When it was entered on the last step, total vocabulary size did make a significant contribution (16.7%, $p < .05$), but the partial correlation was positive (+.42), indicating that children who stayed late actually had slightly larger vocabularies at Time 1, in line with the previous report using simple t tests. We also conducted a regression using nothing but age and social class as predictors and captured a nonsignificant 29.2% of the variance in staying late ($p < .07$). Social class and Time 2 age did not make significant contributions on the last step, but Time 1 age did increase the prediction by a reliable 17.6% ($p < .04$). The partial correlation was +.45, which meant that children who stayed late were somewhat older at Time 1. As we already noted, this may reflect greater risk for

TABLE 2

Comparison of Children Who Stayed Late or Early Over the Two Time Points to Those Who Regressed Toward the Mean on Language Variables at the First Datapoint

Time 1 Variables	Late at Both Datapoints	Average at Follow-up	t value	p value	Early at Both Datapoints	Average at Follow-up	t value	p value
Total production	25.08	11.91	-2.02	.065	474.70	427.70	-1.54	ns
Combining	.02	0.00	na	—	1.87	1.90	0.25	ns
Complexity	0.83	0.00	na	—	13.87	6.90	-2.25	.04
Mean of the three longest utterances	1.52	1.00	na	—	5.69	4.39	-1.79	.09
Closed-class percentile score	8.62	7.03	-.41	ns	8.55	6.55	-1.52	ns

Note. ns = not significant; na = not applicable.

continued language delay with increasing age as was suggested by Rescorla and Schwartz (1990), or it may be nothing more than an artifact of age bracketing in the assignment of percentile scores. That is, some children were given lower scores because they were only a few days from the age boundary, and those children were more likely to "catch up" at the next time point.

Analogous regressions were conducted on staying early. When all eight predictors were used together, the total variance accounted for was 36.4%, a figure that was not significant. None of the predictors made a reliable contribution on the final step. We also repeated the regression using only two language predictors: total vocabulary and grammatical complexity. The total prediction was only 15.4% ($p < .16$), and neither of these language variables made a unique contribution when the other was controlled. Hence, there was no evidence to suggest that grammar made a reliable contribution to persistence of early-talker status above and beyond the variance shared by grammar and vocabulary around 20 months of age (see also Bates et al., 1988). Finally, we conducted a regression using age and SES as our only predictors. This equation accounted for a nonsignificant 14.5% of the variance in staying early, with no significant contribution from SES or age. There was a trend for SES, which added 12.5% to the prediction after Time 1 and Time 2 age were controlled ($p < .10$), but the partial correlation was negative, indicating that the families of children who stayed early tended to have slightly lower SES scores.

To summarize, we found evidence for continuity at the group level in late-talker and early-talker status from 20 to 26 months of age. However, we were not yet in a position to predict which late talkers would stay delayed, nor could we predict which early talkers would stay precocious. We attempted to partially resolve this problem by using discriminant analysis to determine whether the eight variables described earlier formed a factor that distinguished between late talkers and middle-level children, and between early talkers and middle-level children. By determining whether such a factor could predict group membership we would get a clearer picture of our ability to make short-term predictions for individual children with the participant, family, and language variables at hand (Munro & Page, 1993).

Discriminant analysis and classification.   We began by attempting to predict late-talker status at Time 2 from a factor composed of the same eight variables employed for the regression analyses described earlier. A chi-square analysis indicated that the prediction of late-talker status at Time 2 for the group as a whole was statistically reliable, $\chi^2(3, N = 164) = 26.60$, $p < .008$, as would be expected from the regression analyses. The critical contribution of discriminant analysis, however, comes from the classification tables because they provide information about the success of predicting outcomes for individual members of the group. Table 3 shows the classification data for prediction of late-talker status at Time 2.

TABLE 3
Prediction of Late-Talker Status From Eight Predictor Variables

		Predicted Group Membership (Time 2)	
Actual Group (Time 2)	Number of Cases	Late Talker	Average Talker
Late talker	16	11	5
		(68.8%)	(31.2%)
Average talker	158	39	119
		(24.7%)	(75.3%)

The number of children actually classified as late talkers or middle-level producers at Time 2 is listed on the left. The two columns on the right indicate the number (and percentage) of those actually classified in either category that were predicted from our SES and language factor.

For the group as a whole, 74.7% of the cases were classified correctly. Of the children who actually qualified as late talkers at Time 2, 68.8% were correctly identified, but 31.2% were misassigned to the normal range by the variables used in the analysis. Of the children who should have been classified in the normal range, 75.3% were correctly assigned, but 24.7% were misdiagnosed as late talkers. In short, we did not have good specificity or sensitivity for the prediction of late-talker status with the variables we have at hand, even though there was significant continuity over time at the group level.

In the early-talker analysis using the same factor, 79.9% of the cases were classified correctly for the group as a whole, significant by a chi-square statistic, $\chi^2(3, N = 174) = 62.21, p < .001$, and this was compatible with the regression analyses, reported earlier. For those children who should have been identified as early talkers, 66.7% were correctly classified, but 33.3% were misassigned to the normal range (see Table 4). For those children who should have been assigned to the normal range, 82.6% were correctly placed, and 17.4% were assigned incorrectly to the early-talker group. Once again, even though we had evidence for continuity at the group level, the sensitivity and specificity of our prediction was not very good.

Finally, we used the same combination of variables in discriminant analyses of children who were late or early at Time 1 to see how many cases of staying late or staying early we could predict. In the staying-late analysis, 76.2% of the cases were classified correctly. However, the chi-square analysis evaluating this prediction was not reliable, analogous to our findings with regression, $\chi^2(3, N = 21) = 5.83, ns$. The classification table for this analysis is presented in Table 5. Among the children who really did maintain late-talker status, 72.7% were classified correctly, but

TABLE 4
Prediction of Early-Talker Status From Eight Predictor Variables

		Predicted Group Membership (Time 2)	
Actual Group (Time 2)	Number of Cases	Early Talker	Average Talker
Early talker	30	20 (66.7%)	10 (33.3%)
Average talker	144	25 (17.4%)	119 (82.6%)

TABLE 5
Prediction of Continuity of Late-Talker Status Using Eight Predictor Variables

		Predicted Group Membership	
Actual Group	Number of Cases	Late Talker Times 1 and 2	Late Talker Time 1, Average Time 2
Late talker Times 1 and 2	11	8 (72.7%)	3 (27.3%)
Late talker Time 1, average Time 2	10	2 (20.0%)	8 (80.0%)

27.3% were misassigned to the normal range. Among the children who had moved into the normal range, 80.0% were correctly placed, but 20.0% were classified as late talkers.

In the staying-early analysis, 76.0% of all cases were classified correctly. However, in line with our regression results, a chi-square statistic evaluating this prediction failed to reach significance, $\chi^2(3, N = 25) = 8.61$, *ns*. Among the children who maintained early-talker status (Table 6), 66.7% were classified correctly, but 33.3% were misassigned to the normal range. Among the children who moved from early-talker status back toward the mean, 90.0% were correctly classified, but 10.0% were assigned to the early-talker group.

We conclude that there is significant stability in late and early-talker status from 20 to 26 months at the group level. However, these predictions are not very sensitive at the level of individual children. Above all, we are not yet in a position to predict which late talkers will stay late or which early talkers will stay early across this period of development. We turn now to our findings for a sample of younger children in Experiment 2, children in an age range during which measures of language production may not be available for use as predictors.

TABLE 6
Prediction of Continuity of Early-Talker Status From Eight Predictor Variables

| | | Predicted Group Membership | |
Actual Group	Number of Cases	Early Talker Times 1 and 2	Early Talker Time 1, Average Time 2
Early talker Times 1 and 2	15	10 (66.7%)	5 (33.3%)
Early talker Time 1, average Time 2	10	1 (10.0%)	9 (90.0%)

EXPERIMENT 2

Method

Participants

The subsample from the complete cross-sectional norming study of the CDI analyzed in Experiment 2 included 217 children whose parents completed the CDI Infant form when their children were between 10 and 16 months of age ($M = 13.45$ months, $SD = 1.71$) and the CDI: Words and Sentences when they were between 16 and 25 months of age ($M = 20.15$ months, $SD = 1.86$). The average time between completing the two CDIs was 6.71 months ($SD = .07$ months).

Procedure

We used the data from the two CDIs to look backward in the Infant–Toddler sample to see what kinds of stability and predictive validity could be obtained using infant measures around 13 months of age to forecast late- and early-talker status around 20 months.

The same analytic procedures used in Experiment 1 were followed for the Infant–Toddler dataset, with one important exception. Because so many children produced little or no speech at the first datapoint (mean age = 13 months), there was no reliable way to assign late-talker status at Time 1, and hence no way to determine whether late-talker status is stable over time. Thus, we looked only at the stability of early-talker status from 13 to 20 months of age.

Results

Breakdown of late and early talkers. At Time 1, when children average 13 months of age, 44 of 217 children in the sample were at or above the 90th percentile

(20%), exactly twice the number that would be expected by chance ($p < .00001$). At the second time point, when we could use the cross-sectional norms to identify both late and early talkers, 30 of the 217 of children (14%) qualified as late talkers, slightly (but not reliably) more than would be expected by chance on a binomial test ($p < .08$). In the same group, 23 of 217 (11%) qualified as early talkers, no more than would be expected if children had been drawn randomly from the cross-sectional norms.

Participant and family variables.   Similar to our procedure for the Toddler–Toddler sample, we constructed a single variable at Time 2 representing extreme group status. Because late-talker status could not be assigned at Time 1, analyses at that datapoint were restricted to t tests and chi-square tests comparing only early talkers with the rest of the sample. The full extreme group variable established for the Time 2 datapoint was used in one-way ANOVAs on interval and ordinal variables (i.e., birth order, SES, and maternal and paternal education and occupation), and in chi-square analyses with categorical variables (i.e., sex, ethnicity, presence or absence of mild medication complications, and presence or absence of exposure to a second language).

In the analyses of groups identified at Time 2, the only significant main effect was that for age at Time 1, $F(2, 214) = 4.07$, $p < .018$. However, Tukey post hoc tests ($p < .05$) were not significant. The main effect for age at Time 2 approached significance, $F(2, 214) = 2.466$, $p < .087$. None of the other effects was reliable.

In the analyses of groups identified at Time 1 (which were restricted to early talkers compared with the rest of the sample), t tests revealed significant effects of birth order, $t(42) = 2.86$, $p < .005$, early = 1.32, not early = 1.63; SES, $t(42) = 2.04$, $p < .05$, early = 38.48, not early = 43.23; and maternal vocation, $t(42) = 2.24$, $p < .03$, early = 3.11, not early = 4.39. However, only the birth order effect remained significant after applying a Bonferroni correction. The birth order effect was in the direction that might be predicted based on literature concerning language development in firstborns versus laterborns. That is, more firstborns than laterborns were early talkers at 13 months of age. The SES effects, however, were in the opposite direction from what might be predicted based on the literature concerning SES factors in language development; early talkers at 13 months came from families with lower SES.

Stability of late- and early-talking status.   Of the 44 children who qualified for early-talker status at Time 1, binomial tests were conducted to see if more than would be expected by chance retained that status at Time 2. Sixteen cases (36%) were still at or above the 90th percentile at Time 2, far more than would be expected by chance ($p < .00001$). Conversely, of the 23 children who qualified as early talkers at Time 2, a total of 16 (70% of the sample) were also early talkers at Time 1 ($p < .00001$). In other words, linguistic precocity often was maintained between 13 and 20 months of age, and children who were well ahead at 20 months usually had a very early start.

What factors differentiated those children who stayed ahead from those who regressed toward the mean? *T* tests and chi-square tests were used to compare children who stayed early with those who fell behind on all our participant and family variables. Significant differences were found on a number of variables, including age at Time 1, $t(42)= -2.11$, $p < .043$, stay early = 14.2, regress = 13.1; paternal occupation, $t(42) = -2.21$, $p < .034$, stay early = 6.69, regress = 5.17; presence of mild medical complications (somewhat more likely in children who stayed early, $p < .02$ by a chi-square likelihood ratio); and some exposure to a second language (also somewhat more likely in children who stayed early, $p < .04$ by a chi-square likelihood ratio). However, none of the *t* tests remained significant after application of the Bonferroni correction. There were also trends favoring the children who remained precocious on other family variables, including maternal education, $t(42) = -1.86$, $p < .08$, stay early = 15.37, regress = 14.25; and paternal education, $t(42) = -1.94$, $p < .06$, stay early = 15.81, regress = 13.86. Because we obtained such conflicting findings on the effects of social class, a two-tailed test was used in every case. We conclude that demographic factors may have some influence on the likelihood that children will retain their precocity across the period from 13 to 20 months, but the effects, if present, are very small.

Predicting Time 2 status from Time 1 language measures.
Analogous to our procedure for the Toddler–Toddler sample, we used measures of language and gesture at Time 1 to compare children classified as late and early talkers at Time 2 with children in the middle range of vocabulary production. We performed ANOVAs followed by Tukey tests ($p < .05$) for pairwise comparisons where appropriate. Four Time 1 language measures were used: total word comprehension, total word production, total gesture production, and the percentage of all words in the child's receptive vocabulary that she or he also produced. These are the four measures used by Bates et al. (this issue) to evaluate language and communication in infants with focal brain injury, and they are related to measures used in previous studies of development in late talkers (Thal & Bates, 1988; Thal & Tobias, 1994; Thal, Tobias, & Morrison, 1991). Results are summarized in Table 7. After these simple group comparisons on individual measures, we carried out regression analyses using the same four language variables as predictors, together with Time 1 age, Time 2 age, and SES, to determine whether any of the individual measures contributed unique variance to early- or late-talker status when the others are controlled.

There was a significant main effect for all the language variables measured. For children who were late talkers at Time 2, post hoc Tukey tests demonstrated significant differences for all Time 1 language measures except total comprehension (for which there was a trend toward significance, $p < .07$). For children who

TABLE 7
Comparison of Children Who Were Delayed, Precocious, or Average in Language at the Second Datapoint on Measures of Language at the First Datapoint and on Demographic Variables

Time 1 Variables	Late Talkers	Middle Level	Early Talkers	F value	p value	Post hoc Results
Total comprehension	79.70	103.73	230.96	33.52	< .0001	LT = M < ET
Total production	4.13	17.72	102.65	60.48	< .0001	LT < M < ET
Total gesture production	23.33	31.25	43.74	25.17	< .0001	LT < M < ET
% of comprehension vocabulary produced	7.69	16.47	41.41	34.91	< .0001	LT < M < ET

Note. LT = later talker; M = middle level; ET = early talker.

were early talkers at Time 2, significant differences also were observed for the same Time 1 language measures (see Table 7). Hence, children who were late or early talkers around 20 months were (as a group) already well behind or ahead of their peers, respectively, at 13 months in vocabulary comprehension, vocabulary production, gesture production, and the percentage of their comprehension vocabulary that they produced.

We also used t tests (with the Bonferroni correction) to determine whether children who stayed precocious from 13 to 20 months differed from those who regressed toward the mean at 20 months in their initial status on language and gesture variables. Results indicated that this was indeed the case; that is, the children who stayed precocious were already significantly ahead at the first time point, on all four measures (see Table 8).

Turning now to the regression analyses, an equation with seven predictors (Time 1 age, Time 2 age, SES, and the Time 1 language and gesture variables) accounted together for 15.2% of the variance in late-talker status at 20 months of age ($p <$ .001). Analyses were repeated so that there was an opportunity to enter each variable into the equation last. No unique variance was contributed by age, SES, total comprehension, or total production. However, there were significant unique contributions on the last step by total gesture (6.0%, $p <$ .0002, partial correlation = −.26) and by the percentage of receptive vocabulary that also was produced (3.4%, $p <$ .004, partial correlation = −.20). The negative partial correlations meant that children who became late talkers were lower at 13 months in gesture, and in the proportion of words they knew that they also said, even after the other five variables were controlled. As we point out in more detail in the discussion, these findings are particularly interesting in view of independent evidence that infants with right-hemisphere lesions are particularly poor at production of gestures, whereas infants

TABLE 8
Comparison of Children Who Stayed Early Over the Two Time Points to Those Who
Regressed Toward the Mean on Language Variables at the First Datapoint

Time 1 Variables	Early at Both Datapoints	Average at Follow-up	t value	p value
Total comprehension	230.13	138.32	−2.94	< .007
Total production	131.00	40.07	−3.69	< .002
Total gesture production	42.69	33.75	−3.15	< .004
% of comprehension vocabulary produced	51.93	30.18	−3.70	< .001

with left-hemisphere lesions find it difficult to produce the words that they understand (Bates et al., this issue).

Rather different findings were obtained in the regressions predicting early-talker status at Time 2. The seven predictors together accounted for 39.8% of the variance in early-talker status at 20 months ($p < .001$). Overall, this was a much better prediction than we obtained for late-talker status. However, when each of the variables was entered into the equation last, the only unique contributions came from total production (2.1%, $p < .008$, partial correlation = +.18) and total comprehension (1.8%, $p < .02$, partial correlation = +.17). Although these contributions were quite small, it is interesting that they were very different from the results for late talkers.

Finally, we carried out a regression analysis only on children who were early talkers at 13 months, predicting whether children would stay precocious or drop back toward the mean. The total variance accounted for was a large and reliable 45.2% ($p < .002$). However, none of the seven variables made a unique contribution when it was entered on the last step.

Discriminant analysis and classification.   In these analyses, we used the same seven predictors adopted in the earlier regressions. The purpose of discriminant analysis was (once again) to see how many individual cases were correctly classified using these predictors.

In the analysis of late-talker status at 20 months, 77.9% of the cases were classified correctly, and the overall prediction was highly reliable by a chi-square statistic, $\chi^2(3, N = 217) = 34.86$, $p < .00001$. Of the children who really qualified as late talkers at 20 months, 90.0% were correctly classified, but 10.0% were misassigned to the normal range (see Table 9). Of those children who were in the normal range at Time 2, 75.9% were assigned correctly, but 24.1% were misclassified as late talkers.

In the corresponding analysis of early-talker status at 20 months, 91.7% of the cases were classified correctly, a highly reliable prediction, $\chi^2(3, N = 217) = 107.20$, $p < .00001$. However, among those children who qualified for early-talker status at

TABLE 9
Prediction of Late-Talker Status Using Seven Predictor Variables

		Predicted Group Membership	
Actual Group	Number of Cases	Late Talker Time 2	Average Time 2
Late talker Time 2	30	27 (90.0%)	3 (10.0%)
Average Time 2	187	45 (24.1%)	142 (75.9%)

20 months, only 69.6% were classified correctly, whereas 30.4% were misassigned to the normal range (see Table 10). Among those children who fell below the 90th percentile at 20 months, 94.3% were correctly classified, but 5.7% were misassigned to the early-talker group.

Finally, we conducted a discriminant analysis using these seven variables to predict which children stayed precocious and which ones fell behind. The total prediction was reliable, in line with the previous regression analyses, $\chi^2(3, N = 44) = 23.18$, $p < .002$. Overall, 81.8% of the cases were correctly assigned. Of those early talkers who maintained their precocity from 13 to 20 months, 68.8% were classified correctly, but 31.3% were misassigned (see Table 11). Among those children who moved out of early-talker status into the normal range, 89.3% were correctly classified, whereas 10.7% were misassigned to the early-talker group.

Once again, we had clear evidence for continuity at the group level for late- and early-talker status, but the ability to predict the outcome for individual children was not very good. In most of these analyses, approximately two thirds of the target cases were correctly identified, but many children were misclassified. Whether these predictions were valuable or not depends on one's point of view: How much is at stake if even one case is missed? What harm is done if none are detected? We return to this point in the final discussion (labeled the The Pediatrician's Dilemma).

TABLE 10
Prediction of Early-Talker Status Using Seven Predictor Variables

		Predicted Group Membership	
Actual Group	Number of Cases	Early Talker Time 2	Average Time 2
Early talker Time 2	23	16 (69.6%)	7 (30.4%)
Average Time 2	194	11 (5.7%)	183 (94.3%)

TABLE 11
Prediction of Continuity of Early-Talker Status Using Seven Predictor
Variables

		Predicted Group Membership	
Actual Group	Number of Cases	Early Talker Times 1 and 2	Early Talker Time 1, Average Time 2
Early talker Time 1	16	11 (68.8%)	5 (3.3%)
Early talker Time 1, average Time 2	28	3 (10.7%)	25 (89.3%)

Meanwhile, we turn to fine-grained longitudinal data in Experiment 3 to get a clearer picture of the developmental trajectories observed in children who maintained late- or early-talker status across this period of development, compared with some cases in which children made dramatic changes in rate of language development, and in their rank relative to other children in the study.

EXPERIMENT 3

Method

Participants

Twenty-eight children (17 boys and 11 girls) were included in Experiment 3. The majority of the children (64%) were either firstborn or had no siblings in the same household. Thirty percent of the group were secondborn and 6% were third- or fourthborn.

The ethnic and racial distribution of the group was representative of the U.S. population as a whole. Nine percent of the children were African American, 27% were of various racial and ethnic combinations, and 64% were White. A range of educational and SES levels also was represented, including 12% of the sample who were from single-parent households.

Children were recruited through a participant pool, which contained names of parents who had responded to newspaper advertisements asking if they wished to participate in developmental studies, and through personal referrals. Children were not enrolled in the study if they were exposed to a second language on a regular basis. However, during the course of the study some of the children were exposed to a second language because of child-care arrangements.

Procedure

Experiment 3 used both of the MacArthur CDIs. CDIs were mailed to parents and were returned to the experimenter by mail each month. After the first form was filled out, the items checked on the form returned each month were filled in on the next form before it was sent. Thus, the data were cumulative. However, parents were permitted to remove checks from the CDIs if they had changed their minds about the status of that item since the last CDI was returned, and many did so. Children were analyzed descriptively with respect to their percentile on the national norms at each monthly datapoint. Percentiles for each child were calculated from the CDI Infant form when the children were between 8 and 16 months old, and from the CDI Toddler form when they were between 17 and 30 months old. Our goal was to examine continuity of status for individual children in a manner that would allow us to compare these children to the existing literature on late talkers (Paul, 1991; Rescorla & Schwartz, 1990; Thal, & Tobias, 1994; Thal, Tobias, & Morrison, 1991; Whitehurst, Fischell, Arnold, & Lonigan, 1992) and to the two experiments reported earlier. To do that, we identified the children in the sample who fell below the 10th percentile or above the 90th percentile between 18 and 24 months of age. Not only is this the age range typically used in studies of children at the lower extreme of language development, Experiment 2 also showed it is difficult to classify a child as delayed in language at 13 months because so few children have sufficiently large expressive vocabularies. By using 18 to 24 months as the age of identification of expressive delay in Experiment 3, we were able to gather additional evidence for stability over time (i.e., are late talkers still late when they are older) and also to look back to see if any variables were predictive of subsequent delay. To do this, we looked at language production at 30 months of age to examine whether status at 18 to 24 months was related to status at 30 months. We also looked back at word comprehension and gesture production for all children, and also at word production for early talkers, to see if there was continuity from the earlier months to the period from 18 to 24 months.

Results

Of the 28 children who participated in this experiment, 5 had word production scores below the 10th percentile at some point between 18 and 24 months of age, and 6 had word production scores above the 90th percentile for their age at some point within that period. Seventeen scored consistently between the 10th and 90th percentiles across the period from 18 to 24 months. Four of the late talkers were boys, and one was a girl; four of the early talkers were boys, and two were girls (see Table 12).

TABLE 12
Production Vocabulary Status at 30 Months of Age for 24 Participants Identified as Late,
Early, or Average Between 18 and 24 Months

| Participant | Sex | 18–24 Month Status | Percentile | |
			29 Month	30 Month
1	M	Late	Missing	12
2	M	Late	55	73
12	M	Late	8	8
28	F	Late	23	24
31	M	Late	17	26
7	F	Early	100	100
16	M	Early	100	100
19	M	Early	94	95
22	M	Early	98	99
27	F	Early	92	Missing
38	M	Early	96	98
4	F	Average	Missing	98
6	M	Average	60	54
10	F	Average	54	57
11	F	Average	87	88
13	M	Average	74	76
14	M	Average	70	Missing
15	F	Average	93	92
17	M	Average	Missing	64
24	F	Average	Missing	54
26	M	Average	95	96
30	F	Average	98	Missing
32	M	Average	Missing	12
34	M	Average	16	Missing
35	F	Average	92	Missing
36	F	Average	Missing	57
37	M	Average	17	13
41	M	Average	38	33

Note. Status is determined by percentile scores on the MacArthur Comunicative Development Inventory. M = male; F = Female.

Of the five late talkers, only one scored below the 10th percentile at 30 months of age; the remaining children were at the 12th, 24th, 26th, and 73rd percentile. Even if we regard the 12th percentile as close enough to qualify as a late talker, only 40% of the sample retained late-talker status in this longitudinal study—a result that is even poorer than the discriminant analysis results of Experiment 1.

By contrast, all six of the early talkers scored above the 90th percentile at 30 months of age (note that the 30-month datapoint was missing for one of the early talkers, so the assessment was based on the 29-month datapoint for that child). This is a much greater percentage than was seen in the discriminant analysis from Experiment 1 (see Table 12). Hence, early-talker status at 18 to 24 months predicted early-talker status at 30 months of age in this longitudinal sample.

Of the 17 children who fell within the average range from 18 to 24 months, 0 moved into the late-talker category by the end of the study (note that the 30-month datapoint was missing for 4 of these children, so this assessment was based on the 29-month datapoint for these cases; see Table 12). However, 5 of these 17 children moved into the early-talker category, according to cross-sectional norms on the MacArthur CDI. This finding reflects an upward drift for the longitudinal sample as a whole. The reason for this upward drift is unclear and may reflect the kind of fine-grained longitudinal method adopted in this study (cf. Goodman & Bauman, 1995; Goodman, Jahn-Samilo, & Bates, 1995).

Prediction of Outcome Using Word Production

Figure 1 illustrates progress in word production from 8 to 30 months for children who qualified as late, early, and average talkers at some point within the period from 18 to 24 months. A series of one-tailed t tests was conducted to determine when the early and late groups each differed significantly from the sample as a whole ($p < .05$). Results suggest that the six early talkers were not significantly different from the rest of the group prior to 18 months, although they retained a large and reliable advantage for the rest of the study. By contrast, late talkers were significantly below the other children in the study from 10 months of age (from 15 months of age using the Bonferroni correction), and their disadvantage as a group was maintained for the remainder of the study. Hence, we conclude there was some stability in expressive vocabulary for late talkers across the period from 15 (perhaps 10) to 30 months, even if the majority of individual late talkers moved above the 10th percentile (i.e., they lost their official late-talker status); stability of early-talker status was not evident until 18 months, but remained high after that point. Apparent differences between Experiment 2 and Experiment 3 in the onset and maintenance of late and early status may be related to the frequency of sampling (i.e., there were only 2 datapoints in Experiment 2, compared with up to 23 datapoints for each child in Experiment 3).

Prediction of Outcome Using Word Comprehension, Gesture Production, or Both

Can we predict who will become a late or early talker from progress in comprehension, gesture, or both before 18 months of age? Table 13 summarizes

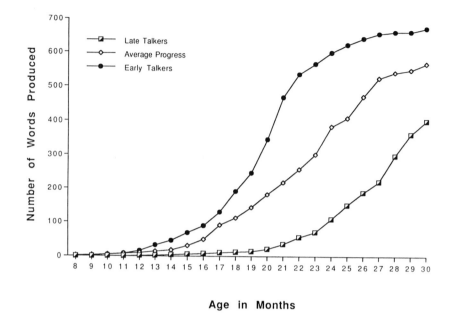

FIGURE 1   Mean number of words produced at each month from 8 to 30 months of age by children who were classified as late, early, or progressing at an average rate at some point between 18 and 24 months of age.

the percentile scores for each child in the experiment at 16 months of age, in word production, word comprehension, and gesture production.

As can be seen in the table, the five children who qualified as late talkers during the period from 18 to 24 months were all within the bottom 10% in comprehension at 16 months (i.e., the final datapoint on the Infant form). Four of these five children were also in the bottom 10% for gesture production at 16 months, and three were within the bottom 10% on word production. The fact that production was the weakest predictor undoubtedly was due to floor effects for production within this age range (i.e., there was far less variance in word production for the sample as a whole, which necessarily meant that production percentiles were less reliable).

Figure 2 illustrates progress in comprehension for the respective late, early, and average groups; and Figure 3 illustrates progress in gesture production. A series of one-tailed t tests were conducted to determine when the late talkers diverged from the average group in comprehension and gesture production (t tests for word production were reported previously). These tests showed (with the Bonferroni correction) that the late talkers were significantly below the other children at every

TABLE 13
Comprehension Vocabulary and Gesture Production Status at 16 Months of Age for 24
Participants Identified as Late, Early, or Average Between 18 and 24 Months

Participant	Sex	18–24 Month Status	16-Month Production Percentile	16-Month Comprehension Percentile	16-Month Gesture Production Percentile
1	M	Late	1	1	10
2	M	Late	41	9	25
12	M	Late	26	1	9
28	F	Late	2	1	3
31	M	Late	1	1	9
7	F	Early	18	97	45
16	M	Early	30	13	11
19	M	Early	25	5	17
22	M	Early	100	100	99
27	F	Early	57	31	85
38	M	Early	98	97	95
4	F	Average	50	24	60
6	M	Average	82	26	17
10	F	Average	78	33	60
11	F	Average	52	58	23
13	M	Average	33	33	13
14	M	Average	94	100	97
15	F	Average	23	34	99
17	M	Average	83	76	99
24	F	Average	87	52	5
26	M	Average	92	71	63
30	F	Average	21	22	24
32	M	Average	74	15	75
34	M	Average	28	27	16
35	F	Average	24	89	65
36	F	Average	53	64	95
37	M	Average	15	7	50
41	M	Average	23	77	90

Note. Status is determined by percentile scores on the MacArthur Communicative Development Inventory. M = male; F = female.

age from 8 through 16 months, in both comprehension and gesture production (see Figures 2 and 3). Hence, this particular sample of late talkers appears to be slow across the board, in all modalities.

Among the six children who qualified as early talkers between 18 and 24 months of age, Table 13 shows that only two were in the top 10% for vocabulary production at 16 months, three were in the top 10% for comprehension, and two were in the top 10% for gesture production. At the same time, several of the early-talkers-to-be had rather low scores for comprehension, gesture production, or both during this

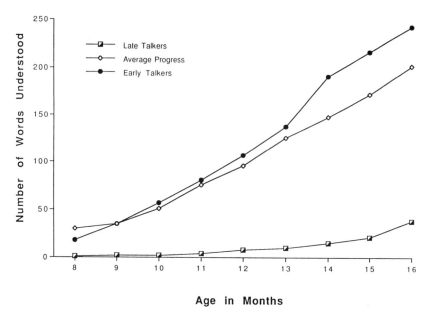

FIGURE 2   Mean number of words understood at each month from 8 to 30 months of age by children who were classified as late, early, or progressing at an average rate at some point between 18 and 24 months of age.

early phase of development. For example, Participant 19 had a 16-month percentile score of 5 for comprehension, 17 for gesture production, and 25 for word production; Participant 16 had a 16-month percentile score of 13 for comprehension, 11 for gesture production, and 30 for word production; Participant 7 had a high score of the 97th percentile for comprehension, but scored only at the 45th percentile for gesture production and at the 18th percentile for word production. In fact, only two of the early-talkers-to-be started off high across the board: Participant 22 had 16-month percentiles of 100 in comprehension, 99 in gesture production, and 100 in word production; and Participant 38 had 16-month percentiles of 97 in comprehension, 95 in gesture production, and 98 in word production. Once again, we conducted a series of one-tailed t tests, this time to determine when the early talkers diverged from the average group on either comprehension or gesture production (results of t tests for word production were reported earlier). Results of these t tests were very clear, and they were compatible with the wide variation documented in Table 13. That is, early talkers were not significantly different from the rest of the sample (collapsing across late and average talkers) on any measure, at any point from 8 to 16 months. This finding is illustrated in Figures 2 and 3, which show that late talkers were late from the beginning on both comprehension and gesture

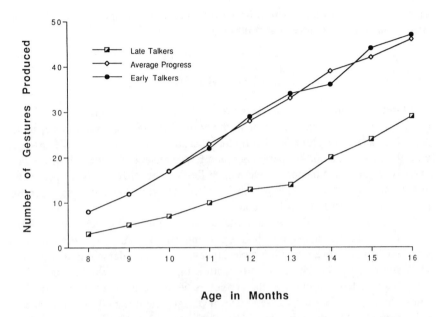

FIGURE 3   Mean number of gestures produced at each month from 8 to 30 months of age by children who were classified as late, early, or progressing at an average rate at some point between 18 and 24 months of age.

production, but early talkers were indistinguishable from children who later made average progress in word production.

Finally, we looked at the 8- to 16-month data for the children who made average progress in expressive vocabulary within the period from 18 to 24 months (see Table 13 and Figures 2 and 3). In comprehension at 16 months of age, one of the average-to-be children scored in the top 10%, and one was in the bottom 10%. In gesture production at 16 months of age, a total of five children scored within the top 10%, and one was in the bottom 10%. In word production, two children started out in the top 10%, and none were in the bottom 10%. We conclude there is a certain amount of regression toward the mean in this group, with some children moving out of the extremes and into the normal range. There also appears to be some asymmetry in the direction of movement. For example, high gesture scores were not a good index of eventual precocity in language, but low gesture scores were common in children who qualified as late talkers. In the same vein, low comprehension scores occurred even in children who ended up as early talkers, but very low comprehension scores characterized all the late talkers in this particular subsample.

Results of Experiment 3 differed in detail from those of Experiments 1 and 2, but one conclusion emerged clearly from all three: There was some continuity in language status across the period from 10 to 30 months of age, but our ability to predict outcomes for individual children was limited.

CONCLUSIONS

The three experiments provide clear support for the stability of individual differences for children at either extreme of the normal distribution from as early as 13 months of age at the group level, a finding that supports earlier work by Fenson et al. (1993, 1994). In both Experiment 1 and Experiment 2, children who were late or early at one of the datapoints were more likely to be late or early, respectively, at the other datapoint. However, the predictions were somewhat stronger for precocious toddlers than for late talkers.

In Experiments 1 and 2, we also attempted to identify variables that predicted stability of language status in both groups using demographic and communication factors. For the 20- to 26-month sample, however, few of the demographic variables were significant. For the 13- to 20-month sample, only early-talker status was reliably predicted, but many of the predictors were not in the expected direction. These findings reflect the current state of disagreement regarding predictors of outcome in the literature on late talkers (Paul, 1991; Rescorla & Schwartz, 1990; Thal, Tobias, & Morrison, 1991; Weismer, Murray-Branch, & Miller, 1994; Whitehurst et al., 1992). Because of these conflicting findings, we conclude that within the full range of middle-class toddlers sampled in Experiments 1 and 2, demographic factors had more effect on the likelihood that children would remain precocious rather than delayed, but, in either case, the effects were relatively small within the SES range that we sampled here.

Communication factors provided reliable predictors for both studies. For children examined at 20 and 26 months of age, total number of words produced, presence of word combinations, sentence complexity, and the mean of the three longest utterances were significantly related to remaining late or early. As a group, children who were late on these variables at 20 months were more likely to be late at 26 months, and vice versa. However, regression analyses in which each of these factors was entered into the equation last demonstrated that only the size of the expressive vocabulary contributed independent variance. The patterns of prediction were quite different for late and early talkers from 13 to 20 months. Again, all the communication measures (production vocabulary, comprehension vocabulary, gesture production, and the percentage of comprehension vocabulary produced) contributed to predicting outcome for both groups. However, regression analyses indicated that only production and comprehension vocabulary contributed unique variance for early talkers. For the late talkers, on the other hand, only gesture production and the percentage of comprehension vocabulary produced made unique contributions to continued delay. This is particularly interesting in light of findings by Bates et al. (this issue) regarding children with focal brain injury. In that study gesture production was significantly worse in children with right-hemisphere lesions, and the percentage of comprehension vocabulary produced was the only measure that was sensitive to left-hemisphere damage. In addition, left- and right-hemisphere damage was associated with different profiles of early language delay in the children with focal brain injury. These findings suggest that the nature of the delay in late talkers (and, potentially, in children with specific language impairment) may be due to central nervous system phenomena that are bilateral and diffuse. These speculations suggest interesting directions for future cross-population research.

Although the experiments reported here provide solid evidence for continuity at the group level, they do not provide evidence of the ability to predict outcome for individual children, a finding that supports Weismer et al. (1994). Discriminant analyses in Experiment 1 and Experiment 2 indicate poor prediction of Time 2 language status from variables measured 6 months earlier, and the descriptive analyses of individual children in the monthly longitudinal study (Experiment 3) show equally poor predictability for all late talkers and for early talkers below 18 to 24 months of age. This is demonstrated dramatically by Participants 7 and 19, for example, who scored at the 10th percentile for vocabulary production at 16 months and above the 90th percentile at 30 months of age.

Although predictive ability for individuals is not good, it is the case that the two late talkers who remained low at 30 months (one at the 10th percentile, the other at the 12th percentile) were delayed in both vocabulary comprehension and gesture production at 16 months of age. Thus, although delay in these variables does not indicate that a child will be delayed in language production at 30 months, the reverse is possible. That is, delays in these factors at an earlier time may be necessary for there to be a language delay at 30 months. This is yet another research direction that appears worth pursuing.

Professionals who have the responsibility of deciding whether children with early language delays should be referred for services want to be able to diagnose late talkers with some certainty. The limited value of any of the variables described previously for predicting future language status of individual children puts them in a difficult position. We label this phenomenon the Pediatrician's Dilemma. Briefly, because only 10% of all children meet late-talker criteria, one can be right 90% of the time by claiming that late talkers do not exist. In addition, because a limited percentage of late talkers retain that status, chances of being right are even higher. The critical question concerns whether this matters: Does it really make a difference if exceptional children are not identified before they are 3 or 4 years old? For linguistically precocious children the answer is probably *no*. However, for children who truly are language delayed and who are destined for learning difficulties in school, the long-term consequences of later identification could be serious. Clearly, carefully designed long-term studies are necessary to determine whether this is the case. However, because we know that the age and language variables identified in this set of studies, along with other factors such as family history, are predictive at a group level, it behooves us to treat them as we treat risk factors for afflictions such as cancer and heart disease. That is, given one or two of the risk factors, children should be carefully evaluated for the presence of others and should be monitored more frequently throughout the preschool years for the development of additional risk factors or a clear language disorder.

ACKNOWLEDGMENTS

This work was supported in part by grants P50 DC01289, DC00089, and DC00482, from the National Institutes of Health, and the John D. and Catherine T. MacArthur Foundation.

REFERENCES

Bates, E., Benigni, L., Bretherton, I., Camaioni, L., & Volterra, V. (1979). *The emergence of symbols: Cognition and communication in infancy.* New York: Academic.

Bates, E., Bretherton, I., & Snyder, L. (1988). *From first words to grammar: Individual differences and dissociable mechanisms.* New York: Cambridge University Press.

Bates, E., Dale, P. S., & Thal, D. (1995). Individual differences and their implications for theories of language development. In P. Fletcher & B. MacWhinney (Eds.), *Handbook of child language* (pp. 96–151). Oxford, England: Basil Blackwell.

Bates, E., Marchman, V., Thal, D., Fenson, L., Dale, P., Reznick, J. S., Reilly, J., & Hartung, J. (1994). Developmental and stylistic variation in the composition of early vocabulary. *Journal of Child Language, 21,* 85–124.

Bureau of the Census. (1991). *General population characteristics* (Vol. 1). Washington, DC: U.S. Government Printing Office.

Education of Handicapped Act Amendment, 100 Fed. Reg. 1145 (1986).

Fenson, L., Dale, P., Reznick, J. S., Bates, E., Thal, D., & Pethick, S. (1994). Variability in early communicative development. *Monographs of the Society for Research in Child Development, Serial, 59*(5, Serial No. 242).

Fenson, L., Dale, P., Reznick, J. S., Thal, D., Bates, E., Hartung, J., Pethick, S., & Reilly, J. (1993). *MacArthur Communicative Development Inventories: User's guide and manual.* San Diego, CA: Singular Publishing Group.

Gesell, A. (1925). *The mental growth of the preschool child: A psychological outline of normal development from birth to the sixth year, including a system of developing diagnosis.* New York: Macmillan.

Goldfield, B. (1987). The contributions of child and caregiver to referential and expressive language. *Applied Psycholinguistics, 8,* 267–280.

Goodman, J. C., & Bauman, A. (1995). Group uniformity and individual differences in the rate and shape of language development. *Society for Research in Child Development Abstracts, 10,* 112.

Goodman, J. C., Jahn-Samilo, J., & Bates, E. (1995). *Patterns of vocabulary acquisition: Evidence from a longitudinal study.* Manuscript in preparation.

Hampson, J., & Nelson, K. (1993). Relation of maternal language to variation in rate and style of language acquisition. *Journal of Child Language, 20,* 313–342.

Hardy-Brown, K. (1983). Universals and individual differences: Disentangling two approaches to the study of language acquisition. *Developmental Psychology, 19,* 610–624.

Hollingshead, A. (1965). *Two-factor index of social position.* New Haven, CT: Yale University Press.

Huttenlocher, J., Haight, W., Bryk, A., Seltzer, M., & Lyons, T. (1991). Early vocabulary growth: Relation to language input and gender. *Developmental Psychology, 27,* 236–248.

McCarthy, M (1954). Language development in children. In L. Carmichael (Ed.), *Manual of child psychology* (pp. 492–630). New York: Wiley.

Munro, B., & Page, E. (1993). *Statistical methods for health care research* (2nd ed.). Philadelphia: Lippincott

Paul, R. (1991). Profiles of toddlers with slow expressive language development. *Topics in Language Disorders, 11,* 1–13.

Plomin, R. (1989). Environment and genes: Determinants of behavior. *American Psychologist, 44,* 105–111.

Plunkett, K. (1993). Lexical segmentation and vocabulary growth in early language acquisition. *Journal of Child Language, 20,* 43–60.

Rescorla, L., & Schwartz, E. (1990). Outcome of toddlers with specific expressive language delay. *Applied Psycholinguistics, 11,* 393–408.

Robinson, N. M., Dale, P. S., & Landesman, S. (1990). Validity of Stanford–Binet IV with linguistically precocious toddlers. *Intelligence, 14,* 173–186.

Shore, C. (1995). *Individual differences in language development.* Thousand Oaks, CA: Sage.

Thal, D., & Bates, E. (1988). Language and gesture in late talkers. *Journal of Speech and Hearing Research, 31,* 115–123.

Thal, D., & Tobias, S. (1994). Relationships between language and gesture in normally developing and late-talking toddlers. *Journal of Speech and Hearing Research, 37,* 157–170.

Thal, D., Tobias, S., & Morrison, D. (1991). Language and gesture in late talkers: A one-year follow-up. *Journal of Speech and Hearing Research, 34,* 604–612.

Tuchman, R., Rapin, I., & Shinnar, S. (1991). Autistic and dysphasic children I: Clinical characteristics. *Pediatrics, 88,* 1211–1218.

Vihman, M., & Miller R. (1988). Words and babble at the threshold of language acquisition. In M. D. Smith & J. L. Locke (Eds.), *The emergent lexicon: The child's development of a linguistic vocabulary* (pp. 151–183). New York: Academic.

Weismer, S. E., Murray-Branch, J., & Miller, J. F. (1994). A prospective longitudinal study of language development in late talkers. *Journal of Speech and Hearing Research, 37,* 852–867.

Whitehurst, G., Fischell, J., Arnold, D., & Lonigan, C. (1992). Evaluating outcomes with children with expressive language delay. In S. Warren & J. Reichle (Eds.), *Causes and effects in communication and language intervention* (pp. 277–324). Baltimore: Paul Brookes.

DEVELOPMENTAL NEUROPSYCHOLOGY, *13*(3), 275–343

From First Words to Grammar in Children With Focal Brain Injury

Elizabeth Bates
University of California, San Diego

Donna Thal
San Diego State University
University of California, San Diego

Doris Trauner
University of California, San Diego

Judi Fenson
University of California, San Diego

Dorothy Aram
Emerson College

Julie Eisele
Skidmore College

Ruth Nass
New York University Medical Center

The effects of focal brain injury were investigated in the first stages of language development, during the passage from first words to grammar. Parent report, free-speech data, or both are reported for 53 infants and preschool children between 10 and 44 months of age. All children had suffered a single, unilateral brain injury to the left or right hemisphere, incurred before 6 months of age (usually in the pre- or perinatal period). This is the period in which one would expect to see maximal plasticity, but it is also the period in which the initial specializations of particular

---

Requests for reprints should be sent to Elizabeth Bates, Department of Psychology, University of California, San Diego, San Diego, CA 92093.

cortical regions ought to be most evident. In direct contradiction of hypotheses based on the adult aphasia literature, results from 10 to 17 months suggest that children with right-hemisphere injuries are at greater risk for delays in word comprehension and in the gestures that normally precede and accompany language onset. Although there were no differences between left- and right-hemisphere injury per se on expressive language, children whose lesions included the left-temporal lobe showed significantly greater delays in expressive vocabulary and grammar throughout the period from 10 to 44 months. No specific deficits were associated with left-frontal damage, but there was a significant effect of frontal lobe injury to either hemisphere in the period from 16 to 31 months, when normal children usually show a burst in vocabulary and grammar. This bilateral effect of frontal damage is independent of motor impairment. Hence, there are specific effects of lesion site in early language development, but they are consistent neither with the lesion-syndrome correlations observed in adults with homologous injuries nor with the literature on acquired lesions in older children. Results are used to argue against innate localization of linguistic representations, and in favor of an alternative view in which innate regional biases in style of information processing lead to familiar patterns of brain organization for language under normal conditions and permit alternative patterns to emerge in children with focal brain injury.

In 1861, Paul Broca described a case of nonfluent aphasia with preserved comprehension, associated with damage to a region of left-frontal cortex that now bears Broca's name. By 1874, Carl Wernicke had described a very different form of aphasia, a severe comprehension deficit with preserved fluency and melodic line (albeit with clear impairment of word retrieval). This syndrome was associated with damage to the posterior portion of the left-temporal lobe, a region now referred to as *Wernicke's area*. The reliability and significance of these two complementary lesion-syndrome mappings have been called into question many times (Freud 1891/1953; Goldstein, 1948; Head, 1963; Marie, 1906; Mohr et al., 1978), including recent studies using in vivo brain imaging that showed the classic lesion-syndrome correlations are violated at least 20% of the time (Basso, Capitani, Laiacona, & Luzzatti, 1980; Bates, Appelbaum, & Allard, 1991; Dronkers, Shapiro, Redfern, & Knight, 1992; Willmes & Poeck, 1993). Nevertheless, there is still broad consensus on four points.

1. The left hemisphere is specialized for language in over 95% of normal adults (Bryden, 1982; Damasio & Damasio, 1992; Galaburda, 1994; Gazzaniga, 1994; Hellige, 1993).
2. The perisylvian regions of the left hemisphere are particularly important for language (Damasio, 1989; Damasio & Damasio, 1992; Geschwind, 1972; Rasmussen & Milner, 1977), although they are not the only relevant areas (Ojemann, 1991).
3. The contrasting syndromes described by Broca and Wernicke are robust findings across natural languages (Bates & Wulfeck, 1989; Menn & Obler, 1990).

4. These syndromes are reliably, albeit imperfectly, correlated with anterior versus posterior lesion sites along the Sylvian fissure (Damasio, 1992; Goodglass, 1993; Naeser, Helm-Estabrooks, Haas, Auerbach, & Levine, 1984).

Given these findings in adults, it is not unreasonable to assume that the left hemisphere must be innately specialized for language, with privileged roles for the perisylvian areas that are implicated in the major forms of aphasia. On these grounds, one would expect to find forms of language impairment in small children with unilateral brain injury that are grossly analogous to the major categories of aphasia in adults, an expectation that can be framed in terms of three hypotheses.

1. The left-specialization hypothesis predicts the most severe language impairments overall in children with injuries to the left hemisphere.
2. The Broca hypothesis predicts severe deficits in language production among children with damage to the anterior regions of the left hemisphere (in particular, the perisylvian area of the left-frontal lobe).
3. The Wernicke hypothesis predicts severe deficits in language comprehension in children with damage to the posterior regions of the left hemisphere (in particular, the posterior portion of the left temporal lobe).

Although these adult-based hypotheses form a reasonable starting point for developmental research, they are largely unsupported by the literature on language development in children with focal brain injury (Alajouanine & Lhermitte, 1965; Almli & Finger, 1984; Annett, 1973; Aram, 1988, 1992; Aram, Ekelman, Rose, & Whitaker, 1985; Aram, Ekelman, & Whitaker, 1986; Aram, Meyers, & Ekelman, 1990; Bishop, 1981, 1983, 1992; Day & Ulatowska, 1979; Fletcher, 1993; Hammill & Irwin, 1966; Hecaen, 1976, 1983; Hecaen, Perenin, & Jeannerod, 1984; Isaacson, 1975; Janowsky & Finlay, 1986; Kohn, 1980; Kohn & Dennis, 1974; Marchman, Miller, & Bates, 1991; Reed & Reitan, 1969; Reilly, Bates, & Marchman, in press; Riva & Cazzaniga, 1986; Riva, Cazzaniga, Pantaleoni, Milani, & Fedrizzi, 1986; Smith, 1984; Stiles & Thal, 1993; Thal et al., 1991; Trauner, Chase, Walker, & Wulfeck, 1993; Vargha-Khadem, Isaacs, Papaleloudi, Polkey, & Wilson, 1991; Vargha-Khadem, Isaacs, van der Werf, Robb, & Wilson, 1992; Vargha-Khadem, O'Gorman, & Watters, 1985; Vargha-Khadem & Polkey, 1992; Woods, 1980; Woods & Carey, 1979; Woods & Teuber, 1978; Wulfeck, Trauner, & Tallal, 1991; for another view, see St. James-Roberts, 1979).

The first and most important challenge lies in the fact that most children with early unilateral brain injury go on to achieve levels of language performance that are within the normal range. This does not mean that early brain damage has no effect on language outcomes. However, the impairments observed in children with this neurological history are more subtle and less persistent than are the outcomes observed in adults with homologous injuries (for reviews, see Eisele & Aram, 1995; Fletcher, 1993; Riva, Milani, Pantaleoni, Devoti, & Zorzi, 1992; Satz, Strauss, & Whitaker, 1990; Stiles, 1995; Stiles & Thal, 1993; Vargha-Khadem & Polkey, 1992), and many children show no impairments at all (Dall'Oglio, Bates, Volterra, DiCapua, & Pezzini, 1994; Feldman, Holland, Kemp, & Janosky, 1992; Vargha-Khadem et al., 1991). Results vary from one study to another, depending on the measures used, the age range of interest, and the inclusionary and exclusionary criteria adopted in the study (e.g., age of lesion onset, etiology, presence or absence of children with seizures or seizure medication). In some studies, there are no significant differences of any kind between the focal-lesion population and normal controls. In other studies, children with focal brain injury score significantly lower as a group on a number of different language and cognitive measures, compared with controls matched for age, sex, and social class (i.e., brain damage often does exact a cost). However, one conclusion is clear across all these studies: Children with a history of early focal brain injury rarely meet the criteria required for a diagnosis of aphasia.

The second finding is the absence of a clear-cut difference between children with left- versus right-hemisphere injury. To be sure, some studies do report differences in the predicted direction, especially for expressive language, for tasks that involve subtle morphosyntactic contrasts, or both (e.g., Aram, Ekelman, Rose, & Whitaker, 1985; Aram et al., 1986, 1990; Aram, Ekelman, & Whitaker, 1987; Dennis, 1980, 1988; Dennis & Kohn, 1975; Dennis, Lovett, & Wiegel-Crump, 1981; Dennis & Whitaker, 1976, 1977; but see Bishop, 1983). However, these left-hemisphere findings often are complicated by other factors. For example, Eisele and Aram (1995) suggested that damage to anterior subcortical structures may be the strongest predictor of residual language and cognitive deficits in both left-hemisphere- and right-hemisphere-lesioned children. However, a small group of left-hemisphere children with anterior subcortical damage do present with more language-specific deficits than do right-hemisphere children with comparable damage (Aram & Eisele, 1994a, 1994b; Aram, Rose, Rekate, & Whitaker, 1983; Eisele & Aram, 1995; Eisele, Alexander, & Aram, 1997). Reilly, Marchman, and Bates (in press) reported a small but reliable left-hemisphere disadvantage in the production of complex syntax for children under 5 years of age, but they reported no effects of lesion site whatsoever in children after age 5—even though all the children in their study had the same etiology (i.e., lesion onset prior to 6 months of age). The issue is complicated even further by occasional findings in the opposite direction, that is, a significant disadvantage for children with right-hemisphere damage on some receptive language tasks (Eisele & Aram, 1993, 1994; Thal et al., 1991; Trauner et al., 1993; Wulfeck, Trauner, & Tallal, 1991).

The next finding is perhaps less surprising once one has digested the ambiguous results obtained for left-hemisphere versus right-hemisphere damage. That is, even in those cases in which a left–right difference was reported, there was little evidence in favor of site-specific effects within the left hemisphere (Eisele & Aram, 1995; Riva & Cazzaniga, 1986). Indeed, Thal et al. (1991) reported effects that run directly counter to the Broca hypothesis, with more severe and protracted delays in early word production in children with left-posterior damage. Putting this result together with the finding that comprehension deficits appear to be more likely in children with right-hemisphere damage (a disconfirmation of the Wernicke hypothesis), Thal et al. concluded it may be a mistake to expect the developing brain to yield brain–behavior correlations similar to those observed in the adult because the processes involved in language acquisition are quite different from processes required for fluent and efficient language use in a mature adult native speaker: "The regions that mediate language learning are not necessarily the same regions that mediate maintenance and use of language in the adult" (p. 499). A similar proposal was offered by Petersen, Fiez, and Corbetta (1992), who suggested that localization of function in adults may reflect the developmental status of a behavior (i.e., novice vs. expert, or controlled vs. automatic) instead of domain-specific content (see also Raichle, 1994).

Earlier reports on the recovery of language in children with focal brain injury led some investigators to conclude that the two hemispheres are initially equipotential for language (Lashley, 1950, 1951; Lenneberg, 1967; for some related comments, see Caplan & Hildebrandt, 1988; Kennard, 1936). On this view, the familiar pattern of left-hemisphere specialization does not emerge until some point after language has been acquired. Indeed, Lenneberg went so far as to suggest that the acquisition of language may be the cause rather than the effect of lateralization. Most modern investigators dispute this claim because there is at least some evidence for early differences in lateralization, and for early left-hemisphere specialization for speech stimuli. Such evidence includes those studies that show a disadvantage for children with left-hemisphere damage (cited previously), but it also includes neuroanatomical studies demonstrating structural differences between the left and right hemisphere at birth or in the first years of language learning, with special reference to perisylvian cortex (Geschwind & Levitsky, 1968; Witelson & Kigar, 1988), together with electrophysiological studies suggesting differential response of the left hemisphere to speech sounds in normal infants (Molfese, 1989, 1990; Molfese & Segalowitz, 1988).

In our view, the best argument for early left-hemisphere specialization is a logical one, based on findings from adults. Simply put, there has to be something special about left-perisylvian tissue that makes it particularly well suited for language learning and language use. If this were not the case, there would be no explanation for the huge bias toward left-hemisphere mediation observed in 95% of normal adults. But what is that "something"? How direct is the relation between the initial predispositions of the left hemisphere and the classic form of brain organization for language that is observed so often in adults?

In a book titled *Rethinking Innateness: Development in a Connectionist Perspective* (Elman et al., 1996) the authors proposed three levels at which it would be fair to say that a given function is "innate," or at least, "innately predisposed." Let us consider each of these three options in turn, with reference to the role of the left hemisphere in early language learning.

Innate representations.   Although strong proponents of nativism within linguistics and psycholinguistics were rarely explicit about the level at which innate ideas are implemented in the brain, the usual argument was that children are born with innate knowledge about basic principles of language, in general, and grammar, in particular (Crain, 1992; Lightfoot, 1991; Pinker, 1991, 1994a, 1994b). To be sure, this knowledge will be shaped by experience to some extent, perhaps in the form of "triggering" or "selecting" among predetermined options (Piatelli-Palmarini, 1989), and some maturation may have to take place before the innate knowledge can be used (Borer & Wexler, 1987; Spelke, Breinlinger, Macomber, & Jacobson, 1992). However, most of these investigators were clear in their belief that children are born with domain-specific representations laid out somewhere in the brain.

The most likely neural implementation for such innate knowledge would have to be in the form of fine-grained patterns of synaptic connectivity at the cortical level (i.e., cortical microcircuitry). To the best of our knowledge, this is how the brain stores its representations, whether they are innate or acquired. In this regard, Pinker (1994a) suggested that the "language instinct" is indeed based on detailed microcircuitry, and that the same is probably true for many other cognitive processes:

> It is a certain wiring of the microcircuitry that is essential.... If language, the quintessential higher cognitive process, is an instinct, maybe the rest of cognition is a bunch of instincts too—complex circuits designed by natural selection, each dedicated to solving a particular family of computational problems posed by the ways of life we adopted millions of years ago. (pp. 93, 97)

If this is the claim with regard to left-hemisphere specialization for language, it means that the left hemisphere starts with representations that are not present in the right hemisphere. To explain the fact that children who have lost these areas go on to achieve language abilities in the normal range, one would have to conclude that (a) partial representations also were available in the right hemisphere sufficient to support compensatory language learning; or (b) no representations are innately present in the right hemisphere, but that hemisphere can acquire representations "from scratch" that are adequate for language even though they are not optimal. In either case, it seems that these innate left-hemisphere representations are not necessary for normal language development to take place, which raises interesting questions concerning how they might have evolved in the first place.

In fact, evidence has been mounting against the notion of innate microcircuitry as a viable account of cortical development (i.e., against representational nativism). In a number of recent studies with vertebrate animals, investigators changed the nature of the input received by a specific area of the cortex, either by transplanting plugs of fetal cortex from one area to another (e.g., somatosensory to visual, or vice versa; O'Leary, 1993; O'Leary & Stanfield, 1989), by radically altering the nature of the input by deforming the sensory surface (Friedlander, Martin, & Wassenhove-McCarthy, 1991; Killackey, Chiaia, Bennett-Clarke, Eck, & Rhoades, 1994), or by redirecting inputs from their intended target to an unexpected area (e.g., redirecting visual inputs to auditory cortex; Frost, 1982, 1990; Pallas & Sur, 1993; Roe, Pallas, Hahm, & Sur, 1990; Sur, Garraghty, & Roe, 1988; Sur, Pallas, & Roe, 1990; see also Molnar & Blakemore, 1991). Surprisingly, under these aberrant conditions it is clear that fetal cortex takes on neuroanatomical and physiological properties that are appropriate for the information it receives ("When in Rome, do as the Romans do") and quite different from the properties that would have emerged if the default inputs had occurred. This suggests that cortex has far more representational plasticity than was believed previously. Indeed, recent studies have shown that cortex retains representational plasticity into adulthood (e.g., radical "remapping" of the somatosensory cortex after amputation, in humans and in infrahuman primates; Merzenich, Recanzone, Jenkins, Allard, & Nudo, 1988; Pons et al., 1991; Ramachandran, 1993; see also Greenough, Black, & Wallace, 1993; Greenough, McDonald, Parnisari, & Camel, 1986). Although one cannot entirely rule out the possibility that neurons are born "knowing" what kinds of representations they are destined to take on, the case for innate representations does not look very good right now. As Elman et al. (1996) noted, this means we have to search for other ways that genes might operate to insure species-specific forms of brain organization.

Innate architectures.   Although it now seems unlikely that regions of cortex contain detailed, innate representations, this does not mean that "all cortex is created equal." Regions can vary along a number of structural and functional parameters that have important implications for the kinds of computations they are able to carry out, and (by extension) for the kinds of representations they are likely to take on. Elman et al. (1996) described constraints at this level under the term "architectural constraints" (p. 27). To operationalize architectural constraints in real brains and in neural nets, they broke things down into three sublevels:

1. Basic computing units. In real brains, this sublevel refers to neuronal types, their firing thresholds, neurotransmitters, excitatory and inhibitory properties, and so forth. In neural networks, it refers to computing elements with their activation

function, learning algorithm, temperature, momentum and learning rate, and so forth.

2. Local architecture. In real brains, this sublevel refers to regional factors such as the number and thickness of layers, density of different cell types within layers, and type of neural circuitry (e.g., with or without recurrence). In neural networks, it refers to factors such as the number of layers, density of units within layers, presence or absence of recurrent feedback units, and so forth.

3. Global architecture. In real brains, this sublevel includes gross architectural facts such as the characteristic sources of input (afferent pathways) and patterns of output (efferent pathways) that connect brain regions to the outside world and to one another. In many neural network models, the size of the system is so small that the distinction between local and global architecture is not useful. However, in so-called modular networks or expert networks it often is useful to talk about distinct subnets and their interconnectivity.

If we assume the brain is an enormous and highly differentiated neural network, with many parts of the system activated in parallel, it is reasonable to assume that development is based in part on a process of competition among regions with somewhat different architectures (Changeux, Courrège, & Danchin, 1973; Changeux & Danchin, 1976; Churchland & Sejnowski, 1992; Edelman, 1987; Killackey, 1990). Through this competitive process, regions of the brain attract those inputs that they handle particularly well, and they are recruited for those tasks that require a particular form of computation (not unlike the process by which tall and agile children are recruited to play basketball). In a bidirectional cycle of cause and effect, each region goes on to form representations that are particularly well suited for the tasks they do best (through additive processes of synaptic growth and strengthening of existing connections, and through subtractive processes of synaptic pruning and cell loss; for a review, see Bates, Thal, & Janowsky, 1992). As a result, the suitability of specific regions for specific tasks will increase over time, above and beyond the predispositions that permitted them to "win" in the first place. In this way, an initial architectural bias can result in regional specialization at the representational level.

There are now several simulations of brain development in artificial neural networks that provide support for the idea that representational specializations emerge through experience in systems that differ only in their initial computational properties. One example (Jacobs, Jordan, Nowlan, & Hinton, 1991; Jacobs & Kosslyn, 1994) involved the development of two distinct visual systems, one for object recognition and another for motion detection, out of two subnetworks that initially differed only in their mode of processing. In other words, one of the best known examples of modularity in brain organization for higher cognitive functions (in this case, object recognition and spatial analysis) can be demonstrated in systems with relatively minimal innate predispositions (see also Hazeltine & Ivry, 1994).

As Freud (1891/1953) and Wernicke (1874) argued many years ago, innate constraints on input and output can also play a major role in brain organization for language. Specifically, perisylvian cortex may be destined to play a special role in language because of its proximity to the basic input and output systems of speech (i.e., primary auditory cortex; cortical and subcortical speech–motor output systems). If this is the case, we might expect to find a different pattern of intrahemispheric specialization in visuomanual languages such as American Sign Language—an idea that has some support (Bellugi & Hickok, 1995; Klima, Kritchevsky, & Hickok, 1993; Poizner, Klima, & Bellugi, 1987). Under this argument, it should also be possible for regions farther away from the privileged perisylvian zones to take over after localized brain injury if (and only if) they have access to the relevant information. The fact that so many children with perisylvian injuries eventually develop normal or near-normal language provides prima facie support for a process of this kind (for clear evidence of "long distance" reorganization in infant monkeys with lesions to specific areas of visual cortex, see Webster, Bachevalier, & Ungerleider, 1995).

Although the input–output argument can help to explain intrahemispheric organization for language, it does little to explain why the perisylvian areas of the left hemisphere play a more important role than do the perisylvian areas of the right hemisphere. Presumably, these two areas receive the same kind of information from the speech signal and from the world to which that signal refers. To explain the asymmetry of human language processing, we need to invoke some combination of input–output constraints and innate differences between the left and right hemispheres in local architecture. Together, these initial biases may set in motion a gradual "modularization" process, built on innate predispositions that are related only indirectly to the full form of brain organization for language observed in the adult (see also Karmiloff-Smith, 1992). An approach of this kind could explain why it is that the left hemisphere wins a primary role in mediation of language in 95% of normal adults. At the same time, it is compatible with the fact that children with focal brain injury can develop alternative forms of brain organization for language at surprisingly little cost if the default systems are damaged in some way. However, this leaves a number of unanswered questions about timing and temporal constraints on cortical plasticity, which brings us to the final point.

Innate scheduling. Elman et al. (1996) underscored the role of timing in all aspects of development (cf. Gould, 1977), with particular reference to the role that genes play in turning systems on and off at different points in the life span. In addition to the computational biases previously described, variations in timing can also play a role in the specialization of cortical regions for particular cognitive functions—what Elman et al. referred to as "chronotopic constraints" (see also Molnar & Blakemore, 1991). For example, regions of cortex may be recruited into a particular task (and may develop subsequent specializations for that task) simply because they are ready at the right time. Conversely, other areas of the brain may lose their ability to perform that task because they developed too late (i.e., after the job is filled). Differential rates of maturation have been invoked to explain the left-hemisphere bias for language under default conditions (Annett, 1973, 1985; Corballis & Morgan, 1978; Courchesne, Townsend, & Chase, 1994; Kinsbourne & Hiscock, 1983; Parmelee & Sigman, 1983; Simonds & Scheibel, 1989). For example, it has been suggested that the left hemisphere matures more slowly than the right in the 1st year of life, which could help explain why the right hemisphere plays a more important role in visuospatial functions that begin to develop at birth, whereas the left hemisphere takes a greater role in linguistic functions that start to develop many weeks or months after birth. The chronotopic argument also may be related to the subcortical findings reported by Aram et al. (1983; see also Eisele et al., 1997). That is, damage to certain subcortical structures may be more devastating in the early stages of language development (before cortical organization is established), compared with homologous subcortical injuries in the adult (after cortical organization for language is complete).

Genetic timing also has been invoked to explain critical-period effects in language learning (Johnson & Newport, 1989; Krashen, 1973; Lenneberg, 1967; Locke, 1993). However, there are at least two versions of the critical-period hypothesis that must be considered here, one that requires an extrinsic genetic signal and another that does not (Marchman, 1993; see also Oyama, 1993). On the "hard" maturational account, plasticity comes to an end because of some explicit and genetically determined change in learning capacity (e.g., a reduction in neurotrophic factors). In this case, the genetically timed stop signal is independent of the state of the system when the critical period comes to an end. On the "soft" maturational account, no extrinsic stop signal is required. Instead, reductions in plasticity are an end-product of learning itself, due to the process of progressive cortical specialization described earlier. In essence, the system uses up its learning capacity by dedicating circuits to particular kinds of tasks, until it reaches a point at which there are serious limitations on the degree to which the system can respond to insult.

An example of soft maturation comes from Marchman (1993), who simulated aspects of grammatical development in neural networks that were subjected to "lesions" (i.e., random elimination of 2% to 44% of all connections) at different points across the course of learning. Although there were always decrements in performance immediately following the lesion, networks with small lesions, early lesions, or both small and early lesions were able to recover to normal levels. However, late lesions (if they were large enough) resulted in a permanent impairment of language learning. Furthermore, this impairment was more severe for some aspects of the task than it was for others (e.g., regular verb inflections were more impaired than were irregular verbs). Notice that these findings mimic classical critical-period effects described for human language learning (e.g., Johnson & Newport, 1989), but without any extrinsic (hard) changes in the state of the system.

Instead, the network responds to the demands of learning through specialization, changing its structure until it reaches a point of no return, that is, a point at which the system can no longer start all over again to relearn the task without prejudice.

As Marchman (1993) pointed out, the respective hard and soft accounts of critical-period effects are not mutually exclusive. Both could contribute to the reductions in plasticity that are responsible for differences between children and adults in recovery from unilateral brain injury (see also Oyama, 1993). However, if the soft account is at least partially correct, it would help explain why the end of the critical period for language in humans has proven so difficult to find, with estimates ranging from 1 year of age to adolescence (e.g., Johnson & Newport, 1989; Krashen, 1973).

In this study, we examined the first stages of language development in children with early-onset focal brain injury, using the framework provided by Elman et al. (1996) to resolve apparent contradictions between plasticity and early specialization for language. We focused on children with unilateral lesions to the left or right hemisphere, incurred prenatally or before 6 months of life. We present results on early communication and language from 10 to 44 months of age, the period in which normally developing children make the transition from first words to grammar. This is the group that should (on the arguments provided previously) yield the strongest evidence for plasticity because these children acquire their lesions before language development has gotten underway (cf. Marchman, 1993). At the same time, this is also the period of development in which inherent regional specializations should be most apparent because the child has not yet had the time or occasion to develop alternative forms of brain organization. That is, we looked at children with focal brain injury during their first encounters with the language problem and watched them seek the best solution to that problem that they could find with limited neural resources.

This study was similar to an earlier study from our laboratories (Thal et al., 1991) on children with the same etiology, with a number of critical differences. First, we combined data for 18 of the 27 children studied by Thal et al. with 35 new participants added since 1991, yielding a total of 53 children with focal brain injury who participated in at least one of the three substudies described here. Hence, we had a sample that was approximately twice the size of that used by Thal et al. Second, the Thal et al. study focused on two periods of development, which we refer to as the infant phase (10–17 months) and the toddler phase (18–31 months). We looked again at these two periods, with a similar methodology, but in addition, we looked at free-speech data between 20 and 44 months. This means that the window of development under study extended all the way from first words to the point where the fundamentals of grammar are normally in place. Third, Thal et al. looked exclusively at early vocabulary, in comprehension and production. We looked at early vocabulary in this study as well, but we also examined the development of gestures (from 10–17 months) and the emergence of grammar (from 18–44 months). Fourth, and most important for our purposes here, Thal et al. analyzed the relation between language development and lesion site by looking at the presence or absence of damage to one of the four quadrants of the brain (i.e., left anterior, left posterior, right anterior, and right posterior). In this study, we took a more detailed look at lesion site within each hemisphere, examining the effects of the presence or absence of damage to each of the four cortical lobes (frontal, temporal, parietal, and occipital), with particular emphasis on frontal and temporal lesions, where the classical language zones are located. For many of the participants, we also had ancillary information on seizure history and on motor and visual symptoms (i.e., hemiparesis; visual field cuts).

Summarizing briefly, Thal et al. (1991) reported few differences in early language as a result of left- versus right-hemisphere injury, although there were some interesting and surprising trends. In their analyses of the infant phase, none of the right–left comparisons reached significance. In both lesion groups, there were more children at or below the 10th percentile for expressive vocabulary than would be expected by chance (the 10th percentile was used because this was the definition of "late talkers" in previous studies within this age range). In other words, it is difficult to get language production off the ground following damage to either hemisphere (see Marchman et al., 1991, for related results on babbling). Results for comprehension were somewhat different: In the right-hemisphere group there were significantly more children at risk for comprehension impairment than would be expected by chance (i.e., 4 of 6, or 67%, fell below the 10th percentile mark); this was not true in the left-hemisphere group, where 3 of 10, or 30%, of the sample were in the risk range ($p < .10$). This right-hemisphere disadvantage in comprehension is surprising in light of the adult aphasia literature (i.e., against the Wernicke hypothesis), but it is compatible with other reports for young children (Eisele & Aram, 1993, 1994; Trauner et al., 1993; Wulfeck et al., 1991).

In Thal et al.'s (1991) analyses of the toddler phase, the predicted left–right difference in word production was finally evident. However, there were no differences between children with and without left anterior damage (against the Broca hypothesis). Instead, significant delays in word production were found in children with injuries to left-posterior cortex, compared to right-hemisphere children and to left-hemisphere children without posterior involvement. In addition, Thal et al. reported that children with right-hemisphere injury, isolated left-anterior lesions, or both tended to produce a remarkably high number of "closed-class words" for their vocabulary size (e.g., prepositions, pronouns, articles, auxiliary and copular verbs, question words). This suggests that the ability to produce these "little words" may be greater if the posterior quadrant of the left hemisphere is intact.

Based on the theoretical framework described previously, and on earlier findings by Thal et al. (1991), our expectations in this study included the following.

Site-specific effects. We argued that there must be something special about the initial status of left-perisylvian tissue to explain the patterns of brain organization for language that are observed reliably in the adult. However, results to date have not revealed clear effects of lesion site in children with focal brain injury. Many studies found no effects at all, whereas others reported effects that do not map onto the adult literature (i.e., the left-specialization hypothesis, the Broca hypothesis, and the Wernicke hypothesis). In this study, we asked the same questions again with a more finely grained coding for lesion site. We framed our questions in a series of planned comparisons based on the adult literature (i.e., left–right comparisons, and presence or absence of left-frontal, left-temporal, or both left-frontal and left-temporal injuries) and then went back to search for patterns that do not follow the adult model.

Phase-specific effects. We were alerted to the possibility that effects of lesion site may change across the course of development for at least three reasons. First, the processes required for successful language learning are not necessarily the same processes required for efficient language use after learning is complete. Hence, regions that are important in one phase of development may be less important in another (see also Petersen et al., 1992; Raichle, 1994). Second, learning to gesture, learning to comprehend, and learning to produce speech may each call on different learning mechanisms, which (in turn) are different from the mechanisms required for gesture, comprehension, and production in the adult. Third, regional biases that are evident at the beginning of language learning may disappear over time, not only because the challenges of learning have changed, but also because alternative forms of brain organization have emerged to solve each learning problem. In other words, brain–behavior mapping is a moving target across the first years of life.

By putting together site-specific and phase-specific findings for infants with focal brain injury, we hoped to learn more about innate regional variations in style of computation that lead to brain organization for language in adults under normal conditions.

GENERAL METHOD

Participants

A total of 53 infants and toddlers with unilateral focal brain injury participated in the study, 36 with lesions to the left hemisphere and 17 with lesions to the right hemisphere.[1] For 27 of these children, data were available at only one time point; another 20 contributed data at two time points, and 6 children were represented in all three studies.[2] Total sample sizes across studies were 26 for Study 1 (language and gesture from 10–17 months), 29 for Study 2 (vocabulary and grammar from 17–31 months), and 30 for Study 3 (mean length of utterance [MLU] between 20 and 44 months). A breakdown of individual participants is provided in Table 1, indicating the substudies in which each child participated and whether that child contributed data to the previous report by Thal et al. (1991).

Children were selected from ongoing studies of language, cognition, and focal brain injury, at three different research sites (Language Research Center at University of California at San Diego and Children's Hospital in San Diego, Cornell University Medical Center in New York City, and the Rainbow Babies and Children's Hospital in Cleveland). In all cases, lesion onset occurred prenatally or within the first 6 months of life. In most cases, neurological data were consistent with pre- or perinatal stroke, although it often was difficult to diagnose the etiology or the age of lesion onset with precision. The presenting symptoms that led to such a diagnosis included motor weakness on one side, evidence of neonatal seizures, or both. Identification of lesion site was based on CT scan, magnetic resonance imaging, or both. Because participants were obtained from different sites, those measures could not be expected to be identical. However, in all cases there was sufficient information in the scan to derive information on the presence or absence of damage to each of the four lobes in the involved hemisphere. For a subset of these cases, the original scans on which a diagnosis of unilateral brain injury was based were not available for inspection. In those cases, codings of side and site were based on explicit notations in the radiological report (cases in which lobe information was absent were excluded from the study). All remaining scans were read by a pediatric neurologist who was blind to the language status of each participant.

Table 1 presents information on sex; lesion side (left hemisphere vs. right hemisphere); intrahemispheric lesion site (frontal, temporal, parietal, or occipital);

---

[1]This marked imbalance between left-hemisphere and right-hemisphere cases was noted in many other studies of pre- and perinatal brain injury, and it may reflect asymmetries in blood flow that are particularly marked during fetal development (Altman & Volpe, 1987).

[2]Because we had a mix of longitudinal and cross-sectional participants in the three studies reported here, it was important to determine whether the lesion-symptom correlations that we observed at each stage were produced by the same children or by different children with the same neurological characteristics. In particular, our results could be skewed artificially if a few very slow children happened to be among the longitudinal participants who contribute to more than one study. To determine whether this was the case, we divided the sample into longitudinal and nonlongitudinal participants (with *longitudinal* defined as participation in more than one of the three studies), and ran a series of preliminary one-way analyses of variance comparing these two groups on all our primary dependent variables, at each age level. There were no significant differences between longitudinal and cross-sectional participants in these comparisons, justifying our conclusion to group these cases together within each study.

and (where available) the presence or absence of subcortical involvement, seizure history, hemiparesis, and visual field cuts. In 44 cases there was evidence of subcortical involvement (including subcortical structures, deep white matter, or both), whereas for 7 cases the scan suggested subcortical sparing; for the remaining 2 cases, evidence for subcortical involvement was unavailable or inconclusive. Of the 53 children, 26 were known to have some form of hemiparesis, 11 children had no motor involvement, and information on motor involvement was not available for 16 cases. There was evidence of a hemianopia (i.e., visual field cut) in 5 cases, and 19 children had no evidence of visual involvement; field cut information was not available for the remaining 29 cases. Preliminary analyses showed the major neurological variables were not confounded with age or sex, and the lesion site variables were (with one exception) independent of seizure history, hemiparesis, or visual field cuts (see Table 1 for details). The single exception was a significant relation between the presence or absence of frontal injury and evidence for a visual field cut, with fewer children in the frontal category showing visual problems ($p <$ .04 by a chi-square likelihood ratio). This is not surprising because one would expect injuries with a more anterior distribution to spare visual functions. It is interesting to note, however, that there was no significant relation between visual symptoms and the presence or absence of occipital damage. There was also no relation between evidence for hemiparesis and the presence or absence of frontal damage.

Among the 30 cases known to have temporal involvement (in the left or the right hemisphere), there were 15 cases in which it was possible to judge whether the lesion compromised Wernicke's area (defined to include the posterior perisylvian region of the temporal lobe, near the parietal–occipital juncture). Of these 15 cases, 10 were judged to involve damage to Wernicke's area, whereas the same area appeared to be spared in another 5 cases. Among the 23 cases known to have frontal involvement (in the left or right hemisphere), there were 15 cases in which it was possible to determine whether Broca's area was involved (defined as the third convolution of the frontal lobe, near the Sylvian fissure). Of these 15 cases, 9 lesions were judged to involve Broca's area, whereas 6 lesions appeared to spare this region. In all the analyses described in the following sections, the effects of temporal or frontal damage (especially left-temporal damage) became numerically stronger when recalculated to reflect the presence or absence of damage to Broca's area or the presence or absence of damage to Wernicke's area. However, the effects also were weaker statistically because of reductions in sample size. Because these numbers were relatively small, and because there was not sufficient information to support a clear decision in many cases, tests of the Broca hypothesis and the Wernicke hypothesis were based on the presence or absence of damage to the frontal or temporal lobes, respectively.

Children were excluded from the study if there was any evidence of multiple lesions, trauma, or tumor, or if lesions were a product of disorders that might

TABLE 1
Neurological Information for Individual Participants

| | | | | Neurological Variables | | | | |
Participant Number	Sex	Side	Lobes Involved	Subcortical	Hemiparesis	Hemivisual	Seizure History	Studies[a]
1	M	R	T,P,O	Y	na	na	na	0,2
2	M	L	F	Y	N	N	N	0,3
3	F	R	T,P,O	Y	Y	na	N	2
4	M	L	P	Y	na	na	N	1,2,3
5	M	R	P	Y	N	N	N	1,2,3
6	M	L	F,T,P,O	Y	Y	N	N	2,3
7	M	L	P	Y	Y	N	N	0,3
8	M	L	P	na	na	na	na	0,1,3
9	M	R	F,T,P,O	Y	Y	N	Y	0,1,2,3
10	M	R	F	Y	Y	N	N	0,3
11	M	R	F,T,P	Y	na	na	na	2
12	M	L	—	Y	Y	N	N	3
13	F	L	F,T,P,O	Y	Y	N	N	1
14	M	L	P,O	Y	N	N	N	1,2,3
15	M	L	F,T	Y	N	N	N	3,4
16	M	L	F,T,P,O	Y	N	Y	N	2,3
17	M	L	T,P	Y	N	Y	N	1,2,3
18	M	L	T,O	Y	N	N	N	1
19	M	L	T,P	Y	na	na	na	0,2
20	M	L	F	Y	Y	N	N	3
21	M	R	F,T,P,O	Y	Y	N	N	1,2
22	M	L	T,P,O	Y	na	na	na	1,2
23	M	L	T	Y	Y	Y	N	3
24	F	L	P	N	na	na	na	0,1,2

25	M	R	P,O	Y	Y	na	Y	1
26	M	L	T,P,O	na	Y	na	Y	0,1,3
27	M	R	F,T	Y	na	na	Y	2,3
28	F	L	T,P,O	Y	na	na	na	0,2
29	M	R	F,T,P,O	N	Y	N	N	1
30	M	L	F,T,P	Y	Y	N	N	0,3
31	M	L	F,T,P	N	Y	Y	N	0,3
32	F	L	F,T,P,O	Y	N	na	N	2,3
33	M	L	F,T,P	Y	Y	N	N	0,3
34	F	R	F,T,P	Y	Y	N	N	2,3
35	F	L	—	Y	Y	na	N	1
36	F	L	—	Y	Y	Y	N	2,3
37	F	L	P	Y	Y	na	N	0,1,2
38	M	L	F,T,P	Y	Y	na	N	1,3
39	M	L	F	Y	Y	na	N	3
40	M	R	—	Y	Y	na	na	1
41	M	L	T,P	Y	na	na	na	0,1,2
42	F	R	P	N	na	na	N	0,1,2
43	M	L	P	Y	na	na	na	1,2
44	F	L	F,T,P,O	N	Y	Y	N	0,3
45	M	R	P	Y	na	na	na	1
46	F	L	F	Y	N	na	na	0,3
47	M	R	P	Y	N	na	na	1,2,3
48	F	L	F,T,P,O	Y	Y	na	na	3
49	F	L	—	Y	na	na	na	1
50	F	R	F,T,P	N	na	na	na	2
51	M	L	T	N	na	na	na	1,2
52	F	L	F	Y	Y	na	Y	2,3
53	F	R	F,T,P,O	Y	Y	Y	Y	1,2

Note. M = male; F = female; L = left; R = right; F = frontal; T = temporal; P = parietal; O = occipital; Y = yes; N = no; na = not applicable.

[a]Study 0 = Thal et al., 1991.

produce more diffuse brain damage. The latter included congenital viral infection, consistent problems during pregnancy, maternal drug or alcohol ingestion during pregnancy, bacterial meningitis, encephalitis, severe anoxia, and chronic lesions such as tumor or arteriovenous malformation. Children also were screened for visual and auditory sensory impairment. Children with severe or uncontrollable seizures were not included in this sample, although 9 of the 53 children did have a positive history of seizure activity (30 cases had no documented seizures; information on past seizure history was not available for 14 cases). In all cases, vision was 20/50 or better with correction, and hearing was present at 25 decibels at two or more pure tone frequencies. The resulting sample represented a range of social class and educational levels, although the sample mean was skewed toward middle-class families with at least 12 years of formal education.

In previous studies, we used a 5-point rating scale originally developed by Vargha-Khadem to assess lesion size. In the study by Thal et al. (1991) there was no linear effect of lesion size using this measure. We also applied the Vargha-Khadem measure in this study, but found no significant effects of lesion size in any of the analyses that follow. In the interests of brevity, these null results are not discussed further.

Although our sample size was small by the standards of traditional epidemiological studies, it represented the combined efforts of three different research laboratories, across an 8-year period, using the same stringent inclusionary and exclusionary criteria. As a result, we believe this is the largest and most homogeneous group of children with early focal brain injury ever described in this critical age range.

Materials and Procedure

Studies 1 and 2 were based on parental report data from the MacArthur Communicative Development Inventory (CDI; for details, see Fenson, Dale, Reznick, Bates, & Thal, 1994; Fenson et al. 1993). This instrument was developed over a 20-year period in laboratories across the United States, and it provides normative information (including separate percentile scores for girls and boys) based on a cross-sectional study of 1,803 English-speaking children between 8 and 30 months of age (excluding children with evidence of mental retardation or significant medical problems, ascertained by a family history questionnaire, and any child with significant exposure to a language other than English). The norming sample represents a broad range of social class and educational groups, although it (as was our focal-lesion sample) is skewed toward middle-class families with 12 or more years of formal education.

A variety of studies have demonstrated the reliability and validity of this instrument (Dale, 1991; Dale, Bates, Reznick, & Morisset 1989; for reviews, see

Fenson et al., 1994), enough to give us considerable confidence in the generality of these results. For example, the vocabulary checklists correlate positively and significantly with laboratory observations of vocabulary (from standard tests and free speech), with coefficients ranging from +.40 to +.80, depending on the study. The grammar measures obtained in Part 2 of the Toddler scale (see Method section) also are correlated strongly with laboratory measures of grammar. For example, Dale (1991) showed that the grammatical complexity scale correlates with a laboratory measure of MLU of +.88 at 20 months of age, and +.76 at 24 months of age. Details for the Infant and Toddler scales are presented later.

Study 3 was restricted to a report of MLU in morphemes, based on free-speech samples that were videotaped in the laboratory, across three standardized situations (book reading, having a snack, and free play on the floor). A minimum of 50 utterances were required for transcription and analysis; for children who were still producing little or no speech in the free-speech sample, a default score of 1.00 was assigned (indicating a MLU of only one morpheme). This was done to avoid biasing the sample by including only those children with productive language (which might give a spuriously high estimate of language abilities in children with focal brain injury). Transcriptions were made according to the Codes for the Human Analysis of Transcripts (CHAT) coding system of the Child Language Data Exchange System (MacWhinney, 1991). MLU in morphemes was calculated according to criteria recommended by Miller and Chapman (1981), which are based on the criteria recommended by Brown (1973). MLU scores were then transformed into age-based percentile scores, based on norms provided by Miller and Chapman for healthy, middle-class children across the age span covered in this study.

Data Analysis

Ideally, one would want to test for the effects of specific lesion sites by looking at children whose damage is restricted entirely to that site. Unfortunately, this ideal strategy is not realistic when one is dealing with rare accidents of nature. The injuries suffered by these children usually involve more than one lobe within the damaged hemisphere, and more than one neurological risk factor (see Table 1). For example, there were 19 cases of lesions restricted to a single lobe, 29 cases with injuries involving two or more lobes, and 5 cases of purely subcortical damage. Furthermore, some lesion sites are more common than others (due to the nature of the middle cerebral artery strokes that are responsible for many cases of early focal brain injury). The incidence of specific lesion sites in this sample breaks down as follows (from most to least frequent): 69.7% of all cases have parietal involvement, 56.5% have lesions involving the temporal lobe, 43.4% have frontal involvement,

34% have injuries that include the occipital lobe, and 9.4% have deep subcortical injuries that spare all four lobes (including their associated white matter). Chi-square tests showed that there was no significant relation between side of injury and probability of damage to any of these sites. In the results that follow, we treat specific neurological variables as risk factors, partitioning the same data in various ways, for example, presence or absence of a positive seizure history, presence or absence of evidence for hemiparesis, and presence or absence of damage to a particular lobe (e.g., presence or absence of left-temporal damage; presence or absence of left-frontal damage).

Because the same children contributed to each of these analyses (grouped in different ways), these cannot be viewed as independent tests. Protection against spurious effects can only come from the strength of the hypotheses being tested, and from the order in which tests are conducted. In each of the three substudies reported here the relations between neurological predictors and behavioral outcomes were assessed in a specified order, starting with planned comparisons based on the adult literature. In each of these analyses, the focal-lesion sample was grouped by the presence or absence of a risk factor (e.g., presence or absence of left-hemisphere damage, of left-temporal damage, etc.), so that subgroup served as the hypothetical "risk group," and the remaining cases in the sample served as controls.

First, differences between children with left-hemisphere versus right-hemisphere lesions were assessed with a one-tailed t test (assuming that left-hemisphere children should perform significantly worse on each variable, i.e., the left-specialization hypothesis). Second, comparisons were conducted with children regrouped to reflect the presence or absence of left-temporal damage, and (where sample size permitted) the presence or absence of left-frontal damage. Group comparisons that reached significance in these planned comparisons were regarded as "strong evidence." The same data also were examined from a nonparametric perspective, looking at the number of children within each subgroup who fell at or below the 10th percentile (defined as the "risk range"). It may be the case, for example, that more children with left-hemisphere damage fall in the risk range on a particular measure than would be expected by chance on a binomial test, whereas the same is not true for children with right-hemisphere damage. Conceptually, this is similar to the approach taken in several previous studies of early unilateral brain injury (e.g., Aram et al., 1985; Dennis & Kohn, 1975; Riva & Cazzaniga, 1986) in which children in each neurological group were compared with a separate set of normal controls. In the absence of a significant between-group comparison (e.g., a significant difference between left hemisphere and right hemisphere), significant findings using this binomial approach were regarded as "weak evidence."

After these planned comparisons, the data for each study were explored in a number of ways, including (a) control analyses comparing children with and without left-parietal injury (to determine whether any findings based on the "classical language lobes" were artifacts of lesion site or middle cerebral artery etiology), (b) regroupings based on the presence or absence of damage to the frontal lobes or the temporal lobes (independent of side), and (c) regroupings looking at the "mirror image" of our left-hemisphere tests (i.e., presence or absence of right-temporal and right-frontal damage). In addition, differences associated with seizure history, hemiparesis, visual field cuts, and subcortical involvement were assessed where there were enough cases to warrant statistical analysis.

Our interpretation of results for each of these studies depends crucially on background information about the mean age at which early language milestones are attained in normal children, and on the range of variation that can be observed in children without focal brain injury. Therefore, we begin our discussion of each study with a brief synopsis of normal development for each of the variables in question, as background for the focal-lesion findings that follow.

STUDY 1: FIRST WORDS AND GESTURE

Background

For children who are developing on a normal schedule, systematic evidence for word comprehension usually appears between 8 and 10 months of age, although there is enormous variation. For example, Fenson et al. (1994) reported that 10-month-olds in their norming sample already had a mean receptive vocabulary of 36 words, but the range extended from 0 to more than 150 items. Vocabulary production develops much more slowly, with the first words appearing between 10 and 12 months, and there is much less variation at the beginning. For example, the mean at 12 months in the Fenson et al. sample was 10 words, with a range from 0 to just over 50. However, many children moved sharply ahead of their age mates after this point, so the mean at 16 months was 64 words, with a range from 0 to more than 200.

There is also ample evidence for a marked dissociation between comprehension and production in this age range (Bates, Dale, & Thal, 1995; Benedict, 1979). Indeed, some normally developing children are reported to have receptive vocabularies of 200 words or more, even though they still produce little or no meaningful speech. One of the questions that we ask in this study (following Thal et al., 1991) concerns whether such dissociations are correlated with lesions to particular areas of the left or right hemisphere. In this study, the relation between comprehension and production was operationalized with a ratio of expressive to receptive vocabulary (i.e., the proportion of words reported in language comprehension that also are produced by the child).[3]

This is also the age range in which children begin to produce communicative gestures, including universal gestures such as giving, showing, and pointing, as well as cultural conventions like waving good-bye. At the same time, they also start to produce conventional gestures associated with familiar objects, inside and outside a communicative situation (e.g., putting telephone receiver to the ear, stirring with spoons, and putting a teddy bear to bed). Studies with normally developing children and with several clinical populations suggest these gestural categories are correlated with the onset of first words (Acredolo & Goodwyn, 1988, 1990; Bates, Benigni, Bretherton, Camaioni, & Volterra, 1979; Bates, O'Connell, & Shore, 1987; Bates & Thal, 1991; Brownell, 1988; Shore, O'Connell, Beeghly, Bretherton, & Bates, 1990), although the correlation between gesture and comprehension tends to be higher in this age range than does the correlation between gesture and production (Bates, Thal, Whitesell, Fenson, & Oakes, 1989; Fenson et al., 1994). In adults with focal brain injury, impairments in the ability to imitate familiar gestures, produce them on command, or both (sometimes called *ideomotor apraxia*) are associated with damage to the left hemisphere (Duffy & Duffy, 1981; Goodglass, 1993; see also Bates, Bretherton, Shore, & McNew, 1983; Milner, 1994). To date, little is known about the relation between early gesture and lesion type in children with focal brain injury (but see Aram & Eisele, 1985; Marchman et al., 1991, for preliminary evidence that early gestural development may be at risk in this population).

Participants

A total of 26 infants with focal brain injury participated in this study, 16 with left-hemisphere damage and 10 with right-hemisphere damage, with a mean age of 13.8 months (*SD* = 1.9, range = 10 to 17). The sample included 7 children whose

---

[3]On the MacArthur CDI's Infant scale there is a single-word checklist with separate columns for *understands* and *understands and says*. The list does not allow for a category representing *says but does not understand*. According to Fenson et al. (1993), parents of normally developing children who participated in earlier studies with predecessors of this inventory were unable to distinguish between *saying with understanding* and *saying without understanding;* most parents assume that a child who says a word has some understanding of its meaning. Therefore, to avoid ambiguity, the third option was eliminated in the final form of the scale. This means, of course, that there is no direct mechanism for detecting rote, or parrot-like, production in the absence of understanding. Indirect estimates of comprehension-free production have been made in regression designs, partialing out comprehension totals from analyses looking at the correlates of production (see Fenson et al., 1994, for some examples). For our purposes, the main point is that a simple ratio of words produced to words comprehended can be interpreted as the percentage of those words that children understand that they can also produce.

infant data were included in Thal et al. (1991). Of the children with left-hemisphere damage, 8 had lesions that included the left-temporal cortex, and 2 of these also had damage to the left-frontal cortex. Of the children with right-hemisphere involvement, 4 had lesions that included the right-temporal cortex, and the same 4 had lesions involving the right-frontal lobe. There were no frontal cases without accompanying temporal damage in this sample, in either the left-hemisphere or the right-hemisphere group (for details, see Table 1).

Method

Data for this study were based on the CDI: Words and Gestures scale (formerly called the CDI: Infants). This instrument comes in two parts. Part 1 is a checklist of 396 words that are among the first to appear in the vocabularies of young English-speaking children. Next to each word, the parent is asked to indicate if the child (a) understands that word, and (b) understands and produces that word. The checklist is divided into 19 semantic categories: sound effects (e.g., *moo* and *vroom*), animal names, vehicle names, toys, food items, articles of clothing, body parts, furniture, household objects, outside things and places to go, people (including proper nouns), routines and games (e.g., *peekaboo*), verbs, words for time, adjectives, pronouns, question words, prepositions, and quantifiers. All forms are presented in their "citation form" (e.g., verbs are listed as stems). Part 2 is a checklist of 63 communicative or symbolic gestures that also develop in this age range. Data from Part 2 were not available for 6 of the children, leaving a total sample size of 20 for all gestural analyses.

We provide information concerning mean raw scores for comprehension, production, and gesture. However, because the children vary in age, all neurological analyses were based on percentile scores (separately normed by age and sex). In addition, we analyze results for the percentage of comprehension vocabulary that was realized in production, a proportion score that takes age-based variance in vocabulary totals into account.

Results

Correlations among measures. Pearson product–moment correlations were calculated among the four key measures in this study (comprehension, production, and gesture percentile scores; percentage of word comprehension that also is produced), across all 26 children in the focal-lesion sample. Results are consistent in direction (although not always in magnitude) with several correlational studies of normal controls (Bates et al. 1989; Bates, Bretherton, & Snyder, 1988; Fenson et al., 1994; Thal, Bates, Goodman & Jahn-Samilo, this issue). The relation between comprehension and production fails to reach significance with a sample of 26 (+.18, *ns*). This means that the focal-lesion sample displays the same dissociation between lexical comprehension and production that is so often observed for normally developing infants in this age range. Gesture is strongly related to comprehension (+.71, *p* < .001), but its relation to production falls below significance (+.35, *p* < .10), another finding that often is reported for normally developing infants. The production–comprehension ratios are positively and significantly correlated with total production (+.73, *p* < .001), but they are uncorrelated with total comprehension (−.25, *ns*) and gesture (−.01, *ns*). Despite the high correlation between the ratio scores and total production, a longitudinal study with normal controls showed that this ratio is a significant predictor of language ability 6 months later even after variance from raw production and comprehension scores is removed (Thal et al., this issue). So it appears that this proportion score can yield unique information of relevance for the neurological analyses that follow. We turn now to separate results for each of the four measures.

Word comprehension.   Children in this sample were reported to understand an average of 93 words (*SD* = 67.6, range = 20 to 232). The mean percentile score for the sample as a whole was 32.7 (*SD* = 29.3), with a range from 4 to 94. In other words, our focal-lesion sample spans the full range of variation observed in the CDI norming sample of 659 infants. However, of the 26 children in our study, 8 children, or 31% of the sample, scored at or below the 10th percentile in word comprehension for their age. A binomial test indicated that this is more than would be expected by chance (*p* < .002).

A planned one-tailed *t* test comparing percentile scores for children with left- versus right-hemisphere damage did not reach significance. In fact, results were not even in the direction one would predict based on the adult literature. Children in the left-hemisphere group actually scored higher in word comprehension (*M* = 36) than did children in the right-hemisphere group (*M* = 28), against the Wernicke hypothesis but in the same direction reported in some developmental studies (Eisele & Aram, 1994; Thal et al., 1991; Trauner et al., 1993). These results are displayed in Figure 1.

This tendency emerges more clearly when we take a nonparametric look at the same data. Within the left-hemisphere group, 3 of 16 children, or 19% of the sample, fell at or below the 10th percentile on word comprehension. A binomial test revealed that this was no more than would be expected by chance if the left-hemisphere sample had been drawn randomly from the normal population. However, within the right-hemisphere group, 5 of 10 children, or 50% of the sample, were at or below the 10th percentile, far more than would be expected by chance (*p* < .004). These differences are illustrated in Figure 2. This is the same result reported by Thal et al. (1991) for a smaller sample of children with focal brain injury (including 7 of

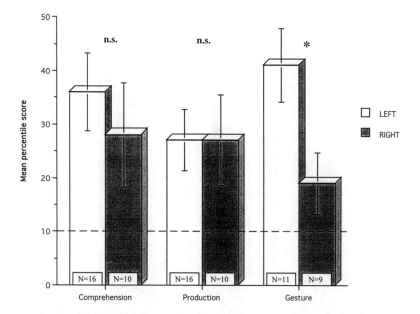

FIGURE 1   Mean percentile scores for word comprehension, word production, and gesture as a function of left- versus right-hemisphere damage. * = group difference is p < .05. ns = group difference not significant.

the 26 children in our study). However, a likelihood ratio comparing the number of left-hemisphere versus right-hemisphere children who did or did not fall below the 10th percentile failed to reach significance ($p < .10$). So this is only weak evidence for a right-hemisphere disadvantage in comprehension.

As planned, we also conducted a one-tailed t test comparing comprehension percentile scores for children with and without left temporal damage—a direct test of the Wernicke hypothesis. There was no significant difference ($p < .18$), and, in any case, results were in the opposite direction from what would be expected based on the adult literature: a mean comprehension score of 27 for children without left-temporal damage, compared with a mean of 46 for children whose lesions extended into the left-temporal cortex (see Figure 3). A nonparametric look at the same data (see Figure 4) indicates that 8 of the 18 children without left-temporal damage (i.e., 44%) fell at or below the 10th percentile, significant by a binomial test ($p < .001$), but 0 of the 8 children with left-temporal damage fell within this range (i.e., 0%), a finding that directly contradicts the Wernicke hypothesis. A likelihood ratio comparing children with and without left-temporal damage who fell above or below the 10th percentile was significant ($p < .007$), which means that children with damage to the left-temporal lobe are actually less likely to suffer from comprehension delays than are children whose lesions spare this area!

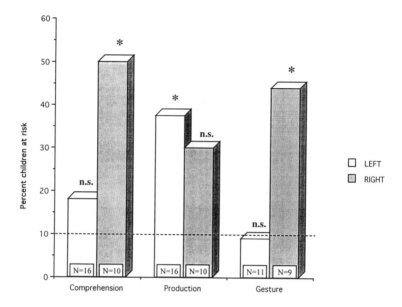

FIGURE 2 Percentage of children at or below the 10th percentile (i.e., in the "risk range") as a function of left- versus right-hemisphere damage. * = group difference is $p < .05$. ns = group difference not significant.

There were only 2 children with lesions involving the left-frontal lobe, too few to justify a separate statistical analysis. However, it is interesting to note that the mean comprehension percentile score for the 2 children with left-frontal involvement was 65.5, compared with a mean of 30.0 for children without this kind of lesion. If we put this finding together with the left-temporal analysis presented earlier, it seems that damage to the classical language zones within the left hemisphere has little impact on the early development of word comprehension. If anything, right-hemisphere damage is a greater risk factor in early comprehension, whereas children with left-frontal lesions, temporal lesions, or both are well within the normal range.

To explore the possibility that particular sites within the right hemisphere may be involved in this effect, we looked separately at data for the 10 right-hemisphere children, comparing those with and without damage involving the right-temporal lobe. For the 6 right-hemisphere children with sparing of the temporal lobe, the mean comprehension score was 30; for the 4 right-hemisphere children with temporal lobe involvement, the mean score was 25. Although this is in the direction one might predict (based on the idea that the homologue of Wernicke's area is important in early comprehension), the difference was not reliable by a one-tailed t test. The same children with right-temporal involvement also had right-frontal

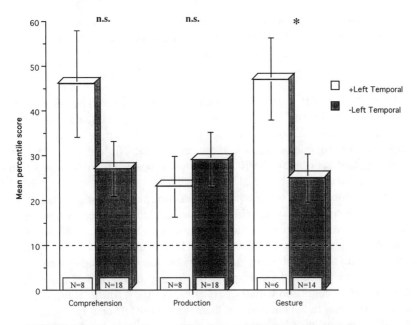

FIGURE 3   Mean percentile scores for word comprehension, word production, and gesture as a function of the presence or absence of left-temporal lobe damage. * = group difference is $p < .05$. *ns* = group difference not significant.

involvement, and there were no isolated right-frontal cases, so we could not ask about separate contributions of right-temporal versus frontal areas in this sample. Because 9 of 10 right-hemisphere cases had some parietal involvement, it was not possible to conduct a control analysis separating out the effects of parietal damage from other sites. An analysis comparing children with and without right-occipital damage failed to reach significance.

Finally, we used two-tailed *t* tests to look separately at the effects of the presence or absence of a seizure history, hemiparesis, and subcortical involvement (sample sizes for each comparison varied depending on the availability of information; see Table 1). None of these effects reached significance. There were too few children in this sample with documented visual field cuts to support a separate analysis of this neurological variable.

To summarize, we found an apparent disconfirmation of the Wernicke hypothesis: Children with left-hemisphere damage were not at significant risk for comprehension deficits. Even more important, none of the children with damage to the left-temporal lobe (the presumed site of Wernicke's area) were significantly delayed in word comprehension. In fact, there was weak support in these data for the idea that the right hemisphere is more important for early word comprehension (in line with three other development studies; viz. Eisele & Aram, 1994; Thal et al., 1991; Trauner et al., 1993). However, we found no evidence implicating particular sites within the right hemisphere.

Word production.   The mean number of words produced by children in this sample was 9.3 (SD = 13.7, range = 0 to 61). This corresponds to a mean percentile score of 27.2 (SD = 23.9), with a range from 4 to 90 —just as impressive as the range observed for comprehension. However, 9 of the 26 children, or 35% of the sample, scored at or below the 10th percentile, significantly more than would be expected by chance on a binomial test ($p < .0001$).

A planned one-tailed t test comparing production percentile scores for left-hemisphere versus right-hemisphere children failed to reach significance—not surprising because the mean scores for the two groups were identical (left-hemisphere mean = 27; right-hemisphere mean = 27). These data are graphed in Figure 1, to facilitate comparison with word comprehension and with the other measures that follow. In the left-hemisphere sample, 6 of 16 cases, or 37.5%, fell at or below the 10th percentile, compared with 3 of 10 cases, or 30.0%, of the right-hemisphere sample. Binomial tests indicated that there were more left-hemisphere children in the risk range than would be expected by chance ($p < .006$), but the corresponding statistic failed to reach significance in the right-hemisphere group. This was a difference in the predicted direction, but it was confounded by the fact that the right-hemisphere group was smaller. A likelihood ratio comparing left-hemisphere and right-hemisphere children who do or do not fall at or below the 10th percentile failed to reach significance. Although these left–right differences were not significant, they are included in Figure 2 to facilitate comparison across measures.

We also conducted a planned comparison of children with and without left-temporal damage (without left-temporal damage M = 29; with left-temporal damage M = 23) and found no significant difference by a one-tailed t test (see Figure 3). Within the group without left-temporal damage, 6 of 18, or 33.3% of the sample, fell at or below the 10th percentile, significantly more than would be expected by chance ($p < .02$). Within the group with left-temporal damage, 3 of 8 cases, or 37.5% of the sample, fell in the same risk range, missing significance by a binomial test ($p < .08$). A likelihood ratio comparing the presence or absence of left-temporal damage in children under and over the 10th percentile failed to reach significance. In other words, we had little evidence for a specific left-temporal effect on the production of first words (see Figure 4).

Because there were only 2 children in this sample with left-frontal involvement, we could not justify statistical analyses looking at the presence or absence of this risk factor. Examination of mean percentile scores suggested that children with lesions extending into the left-frontal lobe may be somewhat worse off (without left-frontal lobe lesion M = 28; with left-frontal lobe lesion M = 17). However, these

2 children also had left-temporal involvement, so there was no evidence to support the idea of a special role for the left-anterior cortex in this stage of word production (i.e., no support for the Broca hypothesis).

We also took an exploratory look at sites within the right hemisphere. Children with lesions involving the right-temporal zone were somewhat worse off in word production ($M = 20.5$), compared with those whose right-temporal lobe was spared ($M = 31.0$), but a two-tailed t test showed that the difference was not reliable. Because temporal and frontal damage always coincided in this right-hemisphere sample, the results provided no information supporting the idea that right-hemisphere homologues to the classical language zones play an important role in the production of first words. And because all but 1 of the 10 right-hemisphere cases had parietal involvement, we could not determine whether right-parietal injuries play any special role. A comparison of children with and without right-occipital damage failed to reach significance.

Similar to our findings for word comprehension, a series of separate t tests was conducted to look for possible effects of seizure history, hemiparesis, or subcortical involvement. None of these effects was significant. There were (as noted) too few cases with visual field cuts to permit analysis.

To summarize, children with focal brain injury, as a group, were markedly delayed in the onset of word production (left hemisphere and right hemisphere), although some children performed very well despite their injuries. In direct contradiction of hypotheses based on the adult literature (the left-specialization hypothesis and the Broca hypothesis), we found little evidence to suggest that left-hemisphere sites are particularly important for the production of first words. However, as indicated later in this article, site-specific evidence emerges when production is viewed in a different way, that is, as that percentage of comprehension vocabulary that children are able to produce.

Gesture.   Children in this sample produced an average of 28 gestures out of the 63 total on the CDI scale ($SD = 10.5$, range = 5 to 45). The corresponding mean percentile score was 31.4 ($SD = 22.8$), with a range from 4 to 88. Once again, this is a very wide range for a sample this small. Of the 20 children for whom gesture data were available, 5 children (i.e., 25% of the sample) fell at or below the 10th percentile. This was *not* significantly more than would be expected by chance, although it was in the expected direction ($p < .09$).

Based on the adult literature, one would expect more left-hemisphere involvement in the production of communicative and symbolic gestures (Duffy & Duffy, 1981; Goodglass, 1993; Milner, 1994). We therefore conducted a planned comparison of gesture percentile scores for left hemisphere versus right hemisphere, predicting a disadvantage in the left-hemisphere sample. T tests results were robust and reliable—but in precisely the opposite direction ($t = 2.38$, $p < .03$, two-tailed)! For the 11 left-hemisphere children for whom gesture data were available, the mean score was 41; 1 of the 11 children (9% of the sample) fell at or below the 10th percentile, no more than would be expected by chance on a binomial test. For the 9 right-hemisphere children for whom we had gesture scores, the mean was 19; 4 of 9, or 44% of the sample, were at or below the 10th percentile, which was (despite the small sample size) more than would be expected by chance ($p < .02$). However, a likelihood ratio comparing left–right damage with performance above or below the 10th percentile failed to reach significance ($p < .07$). Parametric data for individual children are presented in Figure 1, together with the group means for the respective left-hemisphere versus right-hemisphere groups. Nonparametric data are illustrated in Figure 2.

Following the plan of analysis outlined earlier, we also compared gesture scores for children with and without left-temporal damage. Results missed significance by a two-tailed test ($t = -2.09, p < .067$), and we were not entitled to use a one-tailed test because these results were not in the predicted direction (without left-temporal damage $M = 25$; with left-temporal damage $M = 47$). This analysis was simply a weak reconfirmation of the surprising finding reported earlier, that is, an association of gestural delays with right-hemisphere damage. Results are graphed in Figure 3, to facilitate comparison across measures.

Taking a nonparametric look at the same contrasts (Figure 4), we found that 5 of the 14 children whose lesions spared the left-temporal cortex (including all the

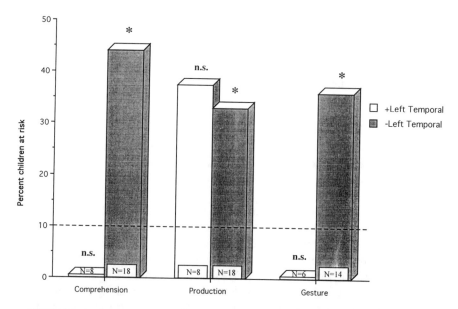

FIGURE 4   Percentage of children at or below the 10th percentile (i.e., in the "risk range") as a function of the presence or absence of left-temporal lobe damage. * = group difference is $p < .05$. ns = group difference not significant.

right-hemisphere children) fell at or below the 10th percentile. This corresponded to 36% of the sample and was significantly more than would be expected by chance on a binomial test ($p < .02$). Of the 6 children whose lesions involved the left-temporal cortex, 0 fell at or below the 10th percentile for gesture, which definitely suggests that the left-temporal cortex is not crucial for symbolic or communicative gesture in this age range. A chi-square likelihood ratio comparing children with and without left-temporal damage who fell above or below the 10th percentile was reliable ($p < .04$).

Mean scores for children with and without lesions involving the left-frontal cortex also suggested a relative sparing of gesture, although the numbers were too small for a statistical comparison. The 2 children with left-frontal involvement had a gestural mean of 59, compared with a mean of 28 for the rest of the sample. At the very least, it appears that left-frontal damage does not make things worse in the gestural domain.

To explore the possibility that sites within the right hemisphere may be particularly important for gesture, we looked at the data in several ways. First, we compared results for children with and without right-temporal damage. Results confirmed that performance was indeed significantly worse for the group with right-temporal damage ($M = 12.5$, $n = 4$) compared to the group without right-temporal damage ($M = 36.1$, $n = 16$), a difference that reached significance by a two-tailed test ($t = 3.62$, $p < .002$). Because the right temporal cases all had frontal damage as well, this result did not discriminate between right-temporal and right-frontal damage. When the data were re-grouped to reflect the presence or absence of right-parietal damage, results were slightly weaker (with right-parietal damage = 21.3, $n = 9$; without right-parietal damage = 38.1, n = 11) and failed to reach significance by a two-tailed test ($p < .086$). Finally, because gesture involves the visual modality, it seemed appropriate to compare children with and without right-occipital damage (with right-occipital damage = 11.2, $n = 5$; without right-occipital damage = 38.13, $n = 15$). This difference was reliable by a two-tailed test ($t = 4.22$, $p < .001$). It is worth noting that there was no trace of an occipital effect in the left-hemisphere sample; in fact, there was a trend in the opposite direction from what one would predict if injuries to visual cortex in either hemisphere caused delays in gestural development (with left-occipital damage = 55.5, $n = 4$; without left-occipital damage = 25, $n = 16$; $t = -2.44$, $p < .07$, two-tailed). Similar to our findings for comprehension, we must conclude that right-hemisphere children have a significant disadvantage in early gestural development (indeed, a stronger disadvantage than we found for word comprehension). There is little evidence for site-specific effects within the right hemisphere, although right-occipital damage may be a risk factor.

Finally, we looked at the presence or absence of seizure history, hemiparesis, or subcortical involvement on gesture percentile scores and obtained no significant effects. There were too few children with visual field cuts to permit statistical analysis.

To summarize, we found an apparent disadvantage for gesture in children with right-hemisphere damage, in direct contradiction of expectations based on the adult literature. However, one aspect of this finding is compatible with studies of early gesture in normally developing children. As we noted earlier, the correlation between gesture and word comprehension was invariably higher in this age range than was the correlation between gesture and word production in normal children (Fenson et al., 1994). We already have seen that comprehension deficits are somewhat more likely in children with right-hemisphere damage, and now we have seen that gestural deficits are also more likely with injuries to the right hemisphere. This raises the intriguing possibility that early gesture and word comprehension may have a common neurological base, with the right hemisphere playing a role that is not evident later in life. We return to this idea in the final discussion.

Proportion of receptive vocabulary that is produced.   It is usually the case in this age range that children comprehend far more words than they are able to say. In the CDI norming sample (based on 659 children), the average percentage of receptive vocabulary that children can also produce is 15% ($SD = 17\%$), although the range goes all the way from 0% to 100%. This ratio is moderately correlated with age across the large norming sample ($r = +.40, p < .001$). In the focal-lesion sample, the mean was 11% ($SD = 12\%$, range = 0% to 45%), and these ratios were not significantly related to age, although there was a trend in that direction ($r = +.26, p < .10$).

A planned comparison of left-hemisphere and right-hemisphere children on these percentage scores was not significant, although there was a tendency for left-hemisphere children to produce a smaller proportion of their receptive vocabulary (9%) compared with right-hemisphere children (14%). Results are graphed in Figure 5.

In contrast, the planned comparison of children with left-temporal involvement and children with left-temporal sparing did reach significance ($t = 2.12, p < .022$, one-tailed). This reflects a mean score of 6% for children with left-temporal involvement versus 13% for children whose lesions spared that area. Results are graphed in Figure 4, to facilitate comparison of this significant left-temporal contrast with the nonsignificant left–right contrast described earlier. The 2 children who also had left-frontal involvement were at an even greater disadvantage, producing only 3% of their receptive vocabularies (vs. 12% for the rest of the sample). Recall, however, that these children had large left-hemisphere lesions involving both the temporal and the frontal zones, so this does not give us clear information about the role of the left-anterior cortex.

This finding appears to offer some support for the idea that the left-temporal cortex plays a special role in the development of expressive language. However,

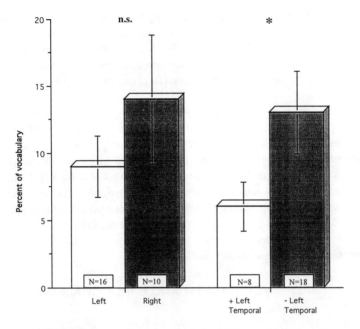

FIGURE 5 Percent of receptive vocabulary that is expressed in speech as a function of left- versus right-hemisphere damage and presence/absence of left temporal lobe damage. * = group difference is $p < .05$. *ns* = group difference not significant.

such temporal injuries are usually caused by middle cerebral artery strokes that involve other brain regions. For example, 6 of the 8 children in this sample with left-temporal damage also had damage to the left-parietal lobe; conversely, 6 of the 12 children with left-parietal damage had injuries that included the left-temporal cortex (see Table 1). Although we did not find a gross association between lesion size and delays in language, the possibility remains that risks associated with left-temporal damage may be an epiphenomenon of damage to adjacent areas. To control for this possibility, we repeated the same paired comparison using the presence or absence of left-parietal damage as a grouping factor. A *t* test revealed no evidence for specific effects of left-parietal injury ($t = 0.59$, $p < .56$). This control analysis bolsters our confidence that the process of turning comprehension into speech is delayed in children with damage involving the left-temporal lobe.

Following these comparisons, we took an exploratory look at children with damage to specific sites within the right hemisphere. Scores were slightly higher for the 8 right-hemisphere children without frontal or temporal involvement (16%) than they were for 4 right-hemisphere children with damage to both these regions

(12%), but the difference was not reliable. Regroupings based on the presence or absence of right-parietal or right-occipital damage also yielded null results.

Finally, we found no evidence of a difference in performance as a function of seizure history, hemiparesis, or subcortical involvement. We could not conduct analyses on the presence or absence of visual field cuts due to limitations on sample size.

To summarize, even though there were no site-specific effects on percentile scores for total word production, we found a difference when production was analyzed as a proportion of receptive vocabulary. Specifically, children with left-temporal damage produced a smaller percentage of the words they knew, a tendency that was even greater when lesions included both the temporal and frontal zones. This is the only strong evidence we obtained in Study 1 for some version of the left-specialization hypothesis. However, the left-temporal finding runs against the Wernicke hypothesis in its original form (i.e., the prediction that left-temporal injuries affect comprehension, whereas left-frontal injuries affect production). We return to this point in the summary and conclusion.

STUDY 2: VOCABULARY AND EARLY GRAMMAR

Background

In normally developing children, language development undergoes a dramatic change from 16 to 30 months of age. Most children display a marked acceleration in vocabulary development during this period, a nonlinear increase that sometimes is referred to as the *vocabulary burst*. This acceleration usually begins by 18 months of age (e.g., Dromi, 1987), although there are enormous individual differences in onset and rate of growth (Bates et al., 1988; Nelson, 1973). For example, Fenson et al. (1994) reported a mean vocabulary of 312 words at 24 months, with a range from fewer than 50 words to more than 500. It is during this period of development that Thal et al. (1991) observed particularly marked delays in word production among children with left-posterior injuries.

This is also the period in which most normal children make the transition from first words to grammar. First word combinations typically appear between 18 and 20 months, with a marked increase in the use of grammatical inflections and function words between 24 and 30 months of age. Recent studies suggest the onset of grammar is linked tightly to vocabulary growth in the normal population (Bates et al., 1994; Fenson et al., 1994). For example, the transition from single words to word combinations is predicted better by vocabulary size than by age (i.e., most children start to produce sentences when their vocabularies exceed 50 words). The tight relation between vocabulary growth and grammar continues after this point, with studies reporting correlations ranging from +.76 to +.88 for grammatical complexity and vocabulary size between 20 and 28 months of age (see also Bates et al., 1988). This strong association contrasts markedly with the dissociations between comprehension and production that so often are observed in early language development. At this point, very little is known about the emergence of grammar or its relation to vocabulary size in children with focal brain injury, although in preliminary observations Eisele and Aram (1995) suggested that both domains are at risk in the focal-lesion population (cf. Feldman et al., 1992).

Another measure examined in this study is the proportion of total vocabulary comprising grammatical function words (also known as closed-class words). This is a particularly interesting and controversial measure in the literature on early child language. At first glance, one might expect the early appearance of function words to index early emergence of productive control over grammar. However, studies show that this is not the case for English-speaking children in the first stages of language acquisition (Bloom et al., 1991; Bloom, Lightbown, & Hood, 1975; Peters, 1983). For example, in a longitudinal study by Bates et al. (1988), percentage use of closed-class words at 20 months was correlated significantly and negatively with the very same measure at 28 months. Bates et al. (1994) showed that this age-related change in the meaning of "closed-class style" actually reflects a transition in vocabulary size. For children with vocabularies of fewer than 400 words, closed-class style is completely unrelated to current or later grammar. For children with vocabularies of more than 400 words, the very same measure is an excellent index of current and later grammatical abilities. To explain these peculiar findings, Bates et al. (1994) suggested that the early use of function words actually reflects a tendency for some children to produce rote and formulaic structures that have not yet been broken down into their constituent elements; for this reason, children who start with telegraphic speech actually have conducted a more detailed analysis of their input (i.e., they have decided which elements they can afford to leave out).

Early use of closed-class words may be related to a continuum of individual differences that have been described for normally developing children in the period from 18 to 24 months (Bloom, 1970, 1973; Nelson, 1973, 1981), with children at one extreme who avoid grammatical function words, restricting themselves to "telegraphic speech" (e.g., "Mommy sock"; Bloom, 1970), whereas children at the other extreme tend to specialize in well-practiced routines, the reproduction of acoustic details they do not fully understand (a tendency that has been called "rote," "expressive" or "pronominal style"; Bloom et al., 1975), or both. Bates et al. (1995) speculated that individual differences in auditory memory may be responsible for this pattern of variation. In this regard, it is interesting to note that Thal et al. (1991) found that children with right-hemisphere damage had higher ratios of closed-class elements in their speech, suggesting that this style is associated with greater reliance on left-hemisphere processes.

Participants

Data on vocabulary and grammar were analyzed for 29 toddlers with focal brain injury, with a mean age of 26.5 months (*SD* = 3.2, range = 19 to 31). Vocabulary data for 8 of these children were reported in the study by Thal et al. (1991); 15 children also contributed data to Study 1. A total of 17 children had left-hemisphere damage, and 12 children had right-hemisphere damage. Of the 17 left-hemisphere cases, 10 had damage involving the left-temporal lobe, and 5 had injuries involving the frontal lobe. Of these 5 left-frontal cases, 4 also had left temporal damage, which made it impossible to disentangle the effects of left-frontal injury from the effects of left-temporal lobe injury (similar to the problem faced in Study 1). Of the 10 right-hemisphere cases, 9 had lesions involving the right-temporal lobe, and 6 of these also had damage to the frontal lobe (for details, see Table 1).

Materials

Parents of all the children in the study completed the CDI: Words and Sentences scale (previously known as the CDI: Toddlers). This scale also is composed of two sections. Part 1 is a checklist of 680 words (including the 396 words from the Infant list). In contrast with the Infant form, the Toddler form only asks about word production (previous research in our laboratories showed that most parents of normally developing children are unable to track word comprehension after 16 months of age). The Toddler list is divided into 22 semantic categories. In addition to the 19 categories from the Infant checklist, the Toddler list also contains separate sections for helping verbs (auxiliaries and modals) and conjunctions, and the Infant category *outside things and places to go* is divided into two separate sections, *outside things* and *places.*

Part 2 of the Toddler scale looks at early grammar from several different points of view (for a detailed discussion, see Dale 1991; Fenson et al., 1994; Marchman & Bates, 1994). It begins with a single question regarding the onset of word combinations: Parents are asked to check *not yet, sometimes,* or *often.* If the child reportedly is producing any word combinations at all, parents are asked to continue to a series of questions about the nature of word combinations and grammatical forms. These include a checklist of verbs and nouns in regular and irregular inflected forms, a section in which parents are asked to provide the three longest utterances their child produced in the last few weeks, and a separate section on grammatical complexity. The complexity section is made up of 37 sentence pairs, each reflecting a minimal contrast in grammatical complexity (e.g., "Kitty sleeping" vs. "Kitty is sleeping"). Parents are asked to indicate which alternative within each pair "sounds most like the way that your child is talking right now." The minimal contrasts tapped by this subscale include the presence or absence of copulae, auxiliaries, modals, possessives, plurals, tense markers, prepositions, and articles in obligatory contexts. It also includes a few items in which both items are grammatically correct but vary in complexity (e.g., "Lookit me!" vs. "Lookit me dancing!"). Scores can vary from 0 (parents always check the simpler alternative) to 37 (parents always check the more complex alternative). As noted earlier, this scale is highly correlated with laboratory measures of MLU. Finally, parents are asked to provide examples of the three longest utterances they have heard their child produce in the past 2 weeks. These were scored manually, according to procedures of the Child Language Data Exchange System (MacWhinney, 1991) for calculation of MLU in morphemes. We refer to this measure as *M3L*. Preliminary analyses have shown that M3L and the complexity scale are highly correlated. To avoid redundant analyses that would capitalize on chance, we restricted ourselves to an analysis of M3L because that measure bears a more transparent relation to the MLU scores used in Study 3. Both vocabulary and M3L scores are expressed as percentiles, based on the MacArthur CDI norms. Finally, percentile scores also were assigned for the ratio of function words to total vocabulary, based on data from the same large norming study.

Results

Correlations among measures.   Pearson product–moment correlations were calculated among three key measures (vocabulary percentiles, M3L percentiles, and percentiles for closed-class proportion scores), across all 30 children in this study. In line with findings for normal controls (Fenson et al., 1994), there was a very strong correlation between M3L and vocabulary ($+.77$, $p < .0001$), providing very little evidence for a dissociation between grammatical and lexical development in this age range. However, the closed-class proportion scores were unrelated to the other two measures ($+.07$ for vocabulary and closed-class scores, *ns*; $+.27$ for M3L and closed-class scores, *ns*).

Word production.   Mean vocabulary size in the focal-lesion sample was 251 words ($SD = 217$, range = 2 to 670). This corresponds to a mean percentile score (based on age and sex) of 27.5 ($SD = 28$, range = 4 to 96). Once again, it is interesting that our sample of 29 covers the same large range in vocabulary development observed in normal controls. However, 11 of the 29 children, or 38% of the sample, obtained scores at or below the 10th percentile, significantly more than would be expected by chance on a binomial test ($p < .00001$).

The mean vocabulary percentile score for left-hemisphere children was 25, compared with a mean score of 31 for right-hemisphere children (see Figure 6). This difference was not reliable by a planned one-tailed *t* test. Within the left-hemisphere group, 7 of 17 cases, or 41% of the sample, fell at or below the 10th percentile, more than would be expected by chance if these children were drawn from the normal population ($p < .002$). However, 4 of 12 children with right-hemi-

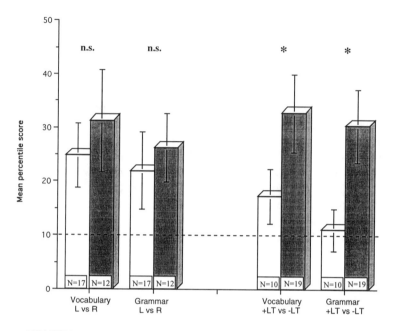

FIGURE 6 Mean percentile scores for vocabulary and grammar as a function of left- versus right-hemisphere damage and the presence or absence of left-temporal lobe damage. * = group difference is $p < .05$. ns = group difference not significant.

sphere damage (or 33% of that sample) were also at or below the 10th percentile, which approaches significance in a binomial test ($p < .06$). A likelihood ratio comparing left hemisphere versus right hemisphere on performance above or below the 10th percentile failed to reach significance. The nonparametric data are illustrated in Figure 7.

A second planned comparison involved children with left-temporal lesions ($N = 10$, mean percentile = 17) versus children whose lesions spared the left-temporal cortex ($N = 19$, mean percentile = 33). This difference was significant by a one-tailed t test ($t = 1.75, p < .05$, one-tailed), which means that children with left-temporal lesions are at greater risk for delays in vocabulary development during the crucial period from 19 to 31 months, when normally developing children pass through the vocabulary burst. Results for this left-temporal analysis are plotted in Figure 6 to facilitate comparison with the nonsignificant left–right comparison.

A nonparametric look at the same data showed that 6 of 19 cases (32%) of children without left-temporal involvement were at or below the 10th percentile, significant in a binomial test ($p < .02$). Among the children whose lesions involved the left-temporal zone, 5 of 10 (50%) were in the bottom 10th, highly reliable in a binomial test ($p < .0033$). A likelihood ratio comparing children with or without

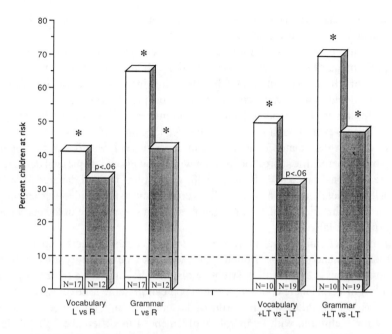

FIGURE 7   Percentage of children at or below the 10th percentile (i.e., in the "risk range") for vocabulary and grammar as a function of left- versus right-hemisphere damage and the presence or absence of left-temporal lobe damage. * = group difference is $p < .05$. ns = group difference not significant.

left-temporal involvement who were or were not in the bottom 10th failed to reach significance. The nonparametric data are presented in Figure 7 to facilitate comparison with the left–right analysis.

In this sample we had only 1 case of isolated left-frontal damage. However, we had four cases in which the lesion involved both left temporal and left-frontal zones, so we could at least look at whether left frontal and left-temporal damage had an additive effect. Among the 5 children with left-frontal involvement, the mean vocabulary percentile score was 11, compared with a mean of 31 for the rest of the sample (i.e., all right-hemisphere children and all left-hemisphere children with frontal sparing). This difference was significant by a one-tailed t test ($t = 2.36, p < .032$, one-tailed). When we restricted ourselves only to children with a left-hemisphere lesion, the difference between those with and without frontal involvement also was significant ($t = 2.00, p < .035$, one-tailed; without left-frontal involvement $M = 30$, with left-frontal involvement $M = 11$). However, when we looked only at those children who had left-temporal involvement ($n = 10$), the 4 with frontal extension were not significantly worse than the 6 without ($t = 0.67, p < .53$; without frontal extension $M = 20$, with frontal extension $M = 13.2$). Hence, this is best viewed as weak evidence for the Broca hypothesis due to the confound between frontal and temporal involvement.

To control for the possibility that our left-temporal and frontal effects were epiphenomena of lesion size, we regrouped the children to reflect the presence or absence of left-parietal damage. Of the 10 children in this sample with left-temporal damage, 8 had injuries that also involved the left-parietal zone; conversely, of the 13 children with left-parietal damage, 8 had injuries extending into the temporal lobe. Hence, even though the overlap between lesion sites was substantial, there were enough dissociated cases to permit separate analyses. A t test comparing vocabulary percentile scores for children with and without left-parietal damage did not reach significance ($t = -0.16$, $p < .88$; without left-parietal damage $M = 28.2$, with left-parietal damage $M = 26.5$). This control analysis provided further support for the idea that the classical language lobes play a specific role in the early stages of expressive language.

Having determined that there were weak but reliable effects implicating the left-temporal and (perhaps) frontal zones, we took an exploratory look at the role of homologous areas within the right hemisphere. Results were rather surprising. Of 12 right-hemisphere children, the mean percentile score for expressive vocabulary was 39 for 3 children with sparing of the temporal zone, compared with a mean of 29 for 9 children with temporal involvement. This difference failed to reach significance by a two-tailed t test ($p < .75$). Of the same 12 right-hemisphere children, the mean score was 49.5 for 6 without frontal involvement, compared with a low of 13.0 for 6 whose lesions involved the right-frontal cortex. This difference approached significance by a two-tailed test ($t = 2.23$, $p < .07$). Although these were only trends, it appeared that right-frontal injuries were associated with delays in expressive vocabulary that were just as severe as those that we saw with left-frontal damage.

This pattern led to the hypothesis that any form of frontal damage (left or right) may result in expressive language delays from 19 to 31 months. To explore this possibility further, we carried out a direct comparison of children with and without injuries involving the frontal lobe, without regard to side of lesion. Because this was not a planned comparison, we used a two-tailed test, but we still found a robust and reliable difference ($t = 3.03$, $p < .006$, two-tailed), reflecting a mean percentile score of 37 in 18 children with frontal sparing versus a mean of 12 in 11 children with frontal involvement. This finding is illustrated in Figure 8. Figure 9 illustrates the same information broken down by side of lesion. By contrast, when we conducted a similar analysis comparing 10 children without temporal involvement ($M = 36$) and 19 children with temporal injuries ($M = 23$), the difference was not reliable ($t = 1.15$, $p < .27$, ns). In other words, frontal involvement is a significant risk factor for expressive vocabulary, for both left- and right-hemisphere cases. Temporal involvement does not show the same degree of bilateral risk. To facilitate

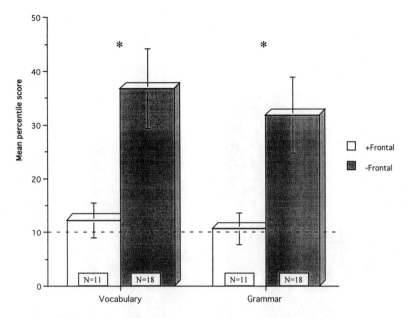

FIGURE 8   Mean percentile scores for vocabulary and grammar as a function of frontal lobe damage to either hemisphere. * = group difference is $p < .05$.

comparison with the significant bilateral effects for frontal involvement, the Side × Temporal breakdown is illustrated in Figure 10.

Finally, we also looked for differences associated with subcortical involvement, seizure history, hemiparesis, or visual field cuts. None of the comparisons were reliable.

To summarize, left-hemisphere injury per se did not appear to be a significant risk factor for expressive vocabulary. A significant number of children were at risk (i.e., at or below the 10th percentile) in both the left-hemisphere and right-hemisphere groups. There was, however, a small but reliable effect of injuries involving the left-temporal zone, a difference that was magnified if the lesion also involved the left-frontal cortex. Similar effects were not found when children were regrouped according to the presence or absence of left-parietal injury. All of these results were in the direction one would predict, based on the adult aphasia literature. However, there was also a surprising mirror image of these perisylvian findings in the right-hemisphere group. In particular, it seemed that injuries to either side of the frontal cortex could result in marked delays in expressive vocabulary, at least during this phase of development. Results were in the same direction for the temporal cortex (i.e., temporal injuries on the right also resulted in lower scores), but they were not reliable.

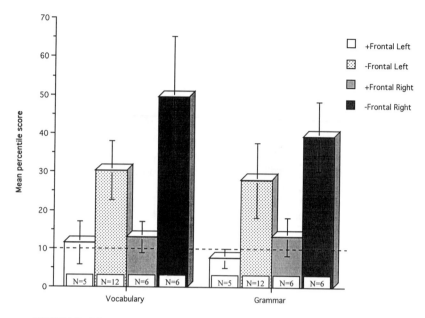

FIGURE 9 Mean percentile scores for vocabulary and grammar as a function of the presence or absence of frontal lobe damage to the left and right hemispheres. * = group difference is $p < .05$.

M3L.   For children in the focal-lesion sample, the three longest utterances in morphemes averaged 3.55 in length ($SD = 2.74$, range = 1.00 to 12.33). This corresponded to a mean percentile score of 23.7 ($SD = 26.4$, range = 4 to 88). The range was just as impressive as we had seen for lexical development and grammar. However, 16 of the 29 children, or 55% of the sample, fell at or below the 10th percentile, far more than would be expected by chance ($p < .00001$).

A planned comparison of left-hemisphere versus right-hemisphere children on the M3L measure failed to reach significance ($t = -0.45$, *ns*; left-hemisphere $M = 22$; right-hemisphere $M = 26$). This difference (or absence of a difference) is presented in Figure 6 (alongside the effects and noneffects of lesion site on vocabulary). Within the left-hemisphere group, 11 of 17 cases, or 65% of the sample, fell at or below the 10th percentile, highly reliable by a binomial test ($p < .00001$). However, it was also true that 5 of 12 cases, or 42% of the right-hemisphere sample, fell at or below the 10th percentile, another reliable finding by a binomial test ($p < .009$). A likelihood ratio comparing left-hemisphere damage versus right-hemisphere damage on the number of children above or below the 10th percentile failed to reach significance. The nonparametric data are presented in Figure 7 to facilitate comparison of results for vocabulary and grammar.

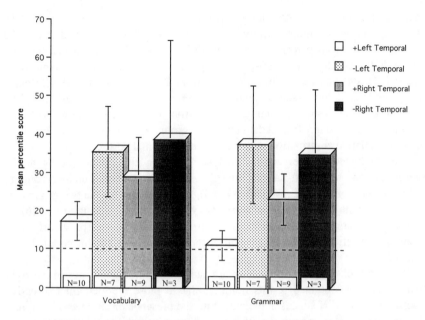

FIGURE 10   Mean percentile scores for vocabulary and grammar as a function of the presence or absence of temporal lobe damage to the right and left hemispheres. * = group difference is $p < .05$. *ns* = group difference not significant.

We then conducted a planned comparison of children with and without left-temporal involvement and obtained a reliable difference ($t = 2.47$, $p < .02$, one-tailed). This reflected a mean M3L percentile score of 30 for children with sparing of the left-temporal zone, compared with a mean of 11 for children with left-temporal involvement. Data are illustrated in Figure 8, where grammar and vocabulary can be compared.

A nonparametric look at the same data showed that 7 of the 10 children with left-temporal involvement (or 70%) were at or below the 10th percentile for this measure of grammar, a reliable result by a binomial test ($p < .00001$). However, 6 of the 19 children without left-temporal involvement (or 32%) were in the same risk range, a smaller proportion but still a reliable finding ($p < .02$). So there were children at risk in both groups, even though the numbers were greater with left-temporal injury. A likelihood ratio comparing the two groups on numbers above and below the 10th percentile mark failed to reach significance. The nonparametric data are presented in Figure 9, where vocabulary and grammar are compared.

The data were regrouped to see whether left-frontal involvement increased the magnitude of effects. Among the 24 children without left-frontal injuries, the mean percentile score was 27; for the 5 children who had left-frontal involvement, the mean grammar score was 7.5. This group difference was reliable ($t = 3.18, p < .004$). If we restrict our attention entirely to children with left-hemisphere damage, the corresponding mean percentile scores were 28 without left-frontal involvement versus 8 for children with left-frontal injury, an effect that was reliable by a one-tailed test (based on the Broca hypothesis; $t = 2.05, p < .04$, one-tailed). Hence, it appeared that delays associated with left-temporal injury were exacerbated if the children also had lesions extending into the frontal cortex. Because we had only one case of isolated left-frontal damage in this group, we cannot say anything more about the relative contribution of temporal versus frontal cortex.

We conducted another control analysis grouping children according to the presence or absence of left-parietal injury. Results of a t test based on this grouping did not reach significance ($t = 0.49, p < .63$), and the means for the two groups are very close (with left-parietal injury = 21; without left-parietal injury = 26). It therefore appears that the left-temporal and frontal effects reported previously were relatively specific and were not by-products of lesion size within the left hemisphere.

We also took an exploratory look at results for homologous sites in the right hemisphere and obtained results quite similar to those reported for expressive vocabulary. The differences associated with the presence or absence of temporal damage were not large: a mean of 35 in right-hemisphere children without temporal involvement versus 23 in children with temporal lesions, a nonsignificant difference ($t = 0.64$, ns). By contrast, mean scores were 39 for 6 right-hemisphere children without frontal involvement, compared with a mean of only 13 in 6 right-hemisphere children with frontal damage, a reliable difference ($t = 2.52, p < .04$, two-tailed).

Once again, this pattern led us to hypothesize that frontal injuries may create delays in expressive language regardless of side. A t test comparing children with and without frontal lesions was reliable by a two-tailed test ($t = 2.76, p < .011$). This reflects a without-frontal-lesion mean of 32 and a with-frontal-lesion mean of 11, illustrated in Figure 8 (see also Figure 9 where the left-frontal and right-frontal effects are plotted separately). By contrast, a comparison based on the presence or absence of temporal lesions (regardless of side) failed to reach significance by a two-tailed test ($t = 1.66, p < .12$), although the difference was in the same direction and was similar in magnitude (without temporal lesion $M = 37$; with temporal lesion $M = 17$). Although this Side × Temporal breakdown was not reliable, it is presented in Figure 10 to facilitate comparison with the bilateral frontal effect.

Finally, there were no significant differences on the M3L measure as a function of seizure history, hemiparesis, visual field cuts, or the presence or absence of subcortical damage. It is also worth noting that the mean for children without evidence of motor involvement was 16.75, compared with a mean of 32.00 for children with some kind of hemiparesis. Although this difference was not reliable, it can be used to argue that gross motor involvement per se is not a significant risk factor for early grammar and cannot be responsible for the left-temporal effect or the bilateral frontal effects described previously.

To summarize, these findings for early grammar paralleled the findings reported for vocabulary development from 19 to 31 months. Although there were no significant differences associated with left- versus right-hemisphere injury, children with damage to the left-temporal lobe were at a significant disadvantage. No such disadvantage was seen when children were regrouped to reflect the presence or absence of left-parietal damage. The left-temporal disadvantage was even greater if left-temporal lesions were accompanied by left-frontal involvement. However, these frontal effects appeared to be bilateral. That is, significant delays in the emergence of grammar were observed with damage to the frontal region, with equivalent delays for left-frontal and right-frontal cases.

Proportion of vocabulary comprising grammatical function words. As noted earlier, this measure is not related to productive control over grammar during the first stages of combinatorial speech. Instead, it has been argued that a (proportionally) high ratio of grammatical function words indicates a tendency for children to produce rote formulae and unanalyzed acoustic details they still do not understand.

In this study, the average ratio of function words to total vocabulary was 12.7% (*SD* = 20.6%, range = 1.8% to 100%). This enormous range reflects nothing more than the volatility of percentile scores when denominators are very small. For example, a child with only two words ("No!" and "Up!") would obtain a function word percentage score of 100%. For this reason, Bates et al. (1994) recommended the use of percentile scoring based on total vocabulary size instead of raw percentages, and they noted these percentile scores should only be assigned to children whose vocabularies are greater than 70 words. Before that point, percentile scoring is subject to floor effects. Following these recommendations, percentile scores for function words as a percentage of total vocabulary were available for only 16 of the 29 children in the sample. For these children, the average percentile score was 56.4 (*SD* = 33.6, range = 4 to 96). Three of these 16 children (19% of the sample) had percentile scores at or below the 10th percentile, and another 2 (13%) had percentile scores at or above the 90th percentile. Neither of these figures was greater than would be expected by chance, which means that we did not have an abnormal number of children at either extreme of the hypothesized continuum from telegraphic speech to formulaic style.

Although we did not have an abnormal number of cases at the extreme ends of the distribution on these closed-class percentile scores, we did have effects of lesion side. Based on the adult literature, one might expect less use of grammatical function words in children with left-hemisphere damage. In fact, the mean percentile score (controlling for total vocabulary size) was 33 for the left-hemisphere group versus

75 for the right-hemisphere group, a significant difference by a one-tailed t test ($t = -3.21, p < .004$). Results are presented in Figure 11.

Although this is the direction one would predict if left-hemisphere children were at a significant disadvantage in the early use of function words, this particular result actually looked less like a left-hemisphere disadvantage and more like a right-hemisphere advantage (with a mean of 75). In fact, a likelihood ratio comparing left-hemisphere versus right-hemisphere children who were above or below the median was reliable (i.e., 2 above and 6 below in the left-hemisphere group, 7 above and 1 below in the right-hemisphere group, $p < .01$).

No further analyses of lesion type were conducted on this measure because the sample size within specific lesion sites was too small to warrant statistical analyses (recall that the overall sample for the closed-class style analysis was only 16). It is worth noting, however, that the 3 children with left-temporal involvement had relatively low closed-class scores ($M = 29$), compared with a mean of 60 for the rest of the sample. For the 3 children in this subsample who had left-frontal involvement, the mean closed-class score was 40, compared with 57 for the rest of the sample. Hence, there was a trend in the direction of less closed-class style with left-temporal (but not left-frontal) damage.

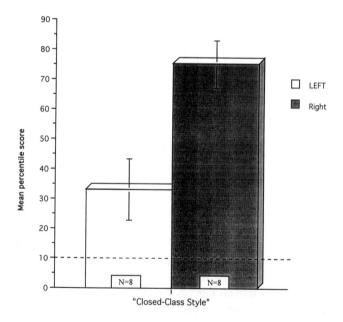

FIGURE 11   Mean percentile scores for closed-class style as a function of left- versus right-hemisphere damage. * = group difference is $p < .05$. ns = group difference not significant.

To summarize, we found a significant difference between left-hemisphere and right-hemisphere children on function words as a proportion of expressive vocabulary. In this period of development, a high score on this measure has been interpreted to reflect rote, unanalyzed reproduction of acoustic details the child does not yet understand. This interpretation was supported in this study by the fact that M3L was only weakly correlated with function word percentile scores. In fact, our results did not look like a selective disadvantage for left-hemisphere children (which one would expect if this were a form of developmental agrammatism). Rather, it appeared to reflect a selective advantage for right-hemisphere children, that is, a marked tendency for children in the right-hemisphere group to engage in rote or formulaic speech. We offer some possible explanations for this finding in the final discussion.

STUDY 3: GRAMMAR IN FREE SPEECH

Background

As already noted, there was a dramatic surge in the use of inflections and function words between 24 and 30 months. By 3 years of age, most normal children can engage in intelligible conversations with adults from outside the family, using a wide range of grammatical constructions. By 4 years of age, it is usually safe to conclude that all the basic principles of grammar have been mastered. This is true not only in English but in all the world's languages that have been studied to date (MacWhinney & Bates, 1989; Slobin, 1985). Hence, the period between 18 and 48 months represents a critical time in grammatical development, a period in which we are most likely to observe delays that might be associated with regional specializations for language learning.

There are hundreds of measures that can be, and have been, applied to free-speech development during this period (MacWhinney, 1991). However, MLU in morphemes is the most widely used measure, particularly in studies of children acquiring English. Although this measure has severe limitations after 4 years of age, it is an excellent index during the period in which most grammatical forms are mastered, correlating highly with more detailed and labor-intensive measures (e.g., indexes of morphological productivity, sentence complexity, and propositional complexity; for a discussion, see Bates et al., 1988, chap. 12). According to Miller and Chapman (1981), the MLU in morphemes at 20 months is less than 1.5 (referred to by Brown, 1973, as *Early Stage 1*), and there is usually little or no productive control over grammatical morphemes. By 44 months of age, the MLU in morphemes is 4.0 (referred to by Brown as *Stage 4*), and all the basic structures of English appear to be intact (including the complex system of modal verbs and difficult syntactic structures such as the passive). This is the period covered by our third and final study.

Participants

Free-speech data were available for 30 children, with a mean age of 30.5 months ($SD = 6.2$, range = 20 to 44 months). Eleven of these 30 children had participated in the study by Thal et al. (1991), 9 were included in Study 1, and 14 were included in Study 2 (see Table 1 for details). The total sample included 24 children with left-hemisphere damage and only 6 with right-hemisphere damage. Because the left–right imbalance was particularly large in this substudy, analyses based on side of lesion must be interpreted with caution. For additional details, see Table 1.

Procedure

For information concerning the procedure used in Study 3, please refer to the General Method section of this article.

Results

Children in the focal-lesion sample had a MLU of 1.98 ($SD = .94$, range = 1.00 to 4.38). Although the mean age of our sample was 30.5 months, these MLU scores correspond to a mean language age of 26.9 months ($SD = 7.6$, range = 19.0 to 45.6). In other words, the children with focal brain injury, as a group, were approximately 4 months behind their normal age mates. Expressed in terms of z scores, the mean for our sample was –0.88 (i.e., almost 1 SD below the mean for normally developing children), but the range was once again very broad ($SD = 1.48$, range = –3.17 to +2.15). A z score of –1.28 or less would correspond to a percentile score of 10 or less, which would be comparable to the risk range we adopted in the two previous studies. By this metric, 16 of the 30 children, or 53% of the sample, were at or below the 10th percentile, far more than would be expected by chance ($p < .00001$). By contrast, only 3 of 30 children fell at or above the 90th percentile—exactly what would be expected if children were drawn by chance from the normal population.

A planned comparison of children with left- versus right-hemisphere injury failed to reach significance ($t = -0.83$, ns), although the respective group means were in the predicted direction (left-hemisphere $M = -0.99$; right-hemisphere $M = -0.44$). These results are presented in Figure 12 with the results for individual children in each group. Within the left-hemisphere group, 15 of 24, or 62% of the sample scored, at or below the 10th percentile (with z scores less than –1.28). This

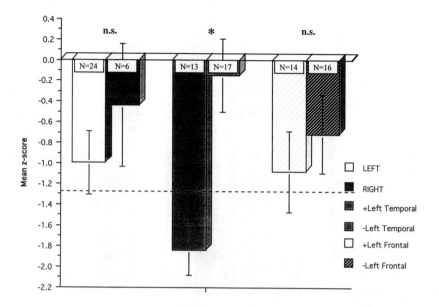

FIGURE 12 Mean z scores as a function of lesion side and lesion type. * = group difference is $p < .05$. ns = group difference not significant.

was far more than would be expected by chance if these children were drawn from the normal population ($p < .00001$). Within the right-hemisphere group, only 1 child out of 6 (or 17%) fell in the same risk range, a chance finding on a binomial test. A likelihood ratio comparing left-hemisphere and right-hemisphere children who were above or below the 10th percentile was significant ($p < .04$). Nonparametric results are presented in Figure 13.

Another planned comparison of children with and without left-temporal involvement reached significance ($t = 3.96$, $p < .0005$, one-tailed). This reflected a MLU z score of -0.15 for children without left-temporal involvement, compared with a mean of -1.84 for children with left-temporal injuries. These data are presented in Figure 12, where they can be compared with the nonsignificant results for left hemisphere versus right hemisphere.

From a nonparametric perspective, 5 of the 17 children without left-temporal injuries, or 29% of the sample, fell at or below the 10th percentile, reliable by a binomial test ($p < .05$). By comparison, 11 of the 13 children with left-temporal injuries, or 85% of the sample, fell in the same risk range, far more than would be expected by chance ($p < .00001$). A likelihood ratio comparing children with and without left-temporal injury who were above or below the 10th percentile was reliable ($p < .002$). The nonparametric data are presented in Figure 13, next to results for the left-hemisphere/right-hemisphere comparison.

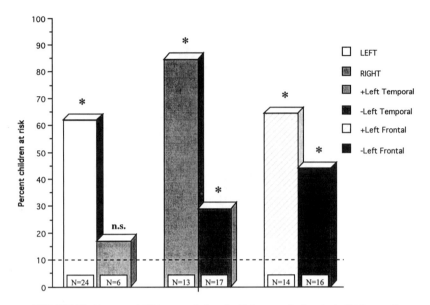

FIGURE 13   Percent of children at or below the 10th percentile (i.e., in the "risk range")
for mean length of utterance as a function of lesion size and type. * = group difference is
$p < .05$. ns = group difference not significant.

In this study (unlike the previous two), we had enough children with left-frontal
involvement but no involvement of the left-temporal lobe to warrant separate
analyses. A planned comparison of children with and without left-frontal injuries
did not reach significance ($t = 0.66$, ns), although mean scores were in the predicted
direction (without left-frontal involvement = -0.72; with left-frontal involvement
= -1.08). These data are graphed in Figure 12 to facilitate comparison with the
left-hemisphere/right-hemisphere and the without-left-temporal-involvement/with-
left-temporal-involvement findings discussed previously.

Taking a nonparametric look at the same data, we found that 7 of 16 children,
or 44% of those without left-frontal involvement, were at or below the 10th
percentile, substantially more than would be expected by chance ($p < .001$). This
compared with 9 of 14, or 64% of children with left-frontal injuries, also highly
reliable on a binomial test ($p < .00001$). In other words, a high proportion of these
children were at risk, whether or not they had injuries to the left-frontal cortex. A
likelihood ratio comparing children with and without left-frontal damage who were
above or below the 10th percentile failed to reach significance.

Based on our findings in Study 2, we carried out an exploratory comparison of
children with and without frontal damage, regardless of side, and found no significant effects by a two-tailed test ($t = 0.98$, $p < .34$; without frontal damage $M = -0.57$;
with frontal damage $M = -1.12$). We then conducted a complementary analysis

comparing children with and without temporal damage, again regardless of side. In this case, the finding was reliable by a two-tailed test ($t = 2.88$, $p < .008$; without temporal damage $M = -0.13$; with temporal damage $M = -1.54$).

To learn more about the specificity of our left-temporal effects, children were regrouped to reflect the presence or absence of left-parietal damage. Among the 13 children with left-temporal injuries, 9 also had damage to the parietal zone; conversely, among the 14 children with left-parietal damage, 9 had injuries extending into the left-temporal cortex. Hence, there was considerable overlap between these two lesion types, but enough separation to warrant separate analyses. In contrast with our findings in Studies 1 and 2, a t test comparing MLU z scores for children with and without left-parietal damage did reach significance (with left-parietal damage $M = -1.61$; without left-parietal damage $M = -.24$, $t = 2.89$, $p < .01$). Hence, the effects of left-temporal and left-parietal damage appeared to be confounded. To pull apart these confounds, we conducted two separate analyses of covariance. In the first analysis, we looked at the MLU z scores as a function of the presence or absence of left-temporal damage, controlling for the presence or absence of left-parietal injury. The effect of the left-parietal covariate was reliable, $F(1, 29) = 9.38$, $p < .01$, but so was the effect of left-temporal damage after left-parietal effects were controlled, $F(1, 29) = 6.29$, $p < .002$. In the converse analysis, the effect of the left-temporal covariate was reliable, $F(1, 29) = 14.07$, $p < .001$, but the effect of left-parietal injury was not reliable when left-temporal contributions were controlled, $F(1, 29) = 1.60$, ns. Hence, we concluded that left-temporal injuries represent a significant and unique risk factor for grammatical development in this age range.

Because there were only 6 children with right-hemisphere damage in this sample, a statistical search for specific sites of risk within the right hemisphere was not warranted. However, the raw data were largely compatible with our findings for grammar in Study 2. For the 3 right-hemisphere children with right-frontal sparing, the MLU z score was +.45, whereas the mean for right-hemisphere children with right-frontal involvement was –1.32. This was in the same direction that we reported in Study 2, suggesting that bilateral frontal effects may still have been operating, although they had begun to ebb. For the 3 right-hemisphere children with right-temporal sparing, the mean score was –.66, compared with a score of –.21 for the 3 right-hemisphere children with right-temporal involvement. This was in the opposite direction from what one might predict if there was a right-hemisphere mirror image of our left-temporal effects.

Finally, we looked for possible effects of the presence or absence of seizure history, hemiparesis, and visual field cuts and found no significant differences. Because there were only 2 children in this sample without some kind of subcortical involvement, no statistical analyses were conducted on this factor.

To summarize, these data provided only weak support for a left-hemisphere disadvantage in MLU during the period from 19 to 44 months (i.e., the effect was not significant on a parametric test, although a likelihood ratio showed that more left-hemisphere children fell at or below the 10th percentile). There was much stronger support for a site-specific disadvantage for children with injuries to the left-temporal lobe, in line with our findings for Studies 1 and 2. By contrast, there was no evidence for a specific left-frontal contribution (against the Broca hypothesis), and only a trend toward the kind of bilateral frontal effect that emerged in Study 2.

SUMMARY AND CONCLUSION

We began this article by pointing out a paradox: Most cases of adult aphasia are associated with injuries to the left hemisphere; however, infants who have suffered massive injuries to the same left-hemisphere sites usually go on to achieve language abilities within the normal range. Why are these left-hemisphere sites so important for adults if they are not necessary for normal language acquisition? The results presented here point toward a possible solution. In line with the taxonomy of innate constraints provided by Elman et al. (1996), and with a number of earlier proposals on the origins of lateralization (e.g., Annett, 1985; Bradshaw & Nettleton, 1981; Bryden, 1982), we propose that the human capacity for language is not localized at birth. Instead, it emerges indirectly out of innate variations in the way that information is processed in different regions of the brain, an example of what Elman et al. (1996) called "architectural constraints" (p. 27). New information about the existence and nature of these regional variations in architecture can be inferred from the site-specific and phase-specific effects of early focal brain injury that are observed during the passage from first words to grammar.

As a point of departure in the search for site-specific effects in children, we derived three straightforward predictions from the adult aphasia literature.

1. The left-specialization hypothesis predicts more severe language impairments overall in children with injuries to the left hemisphere.
2. The Broca hypothesis predicts more severe deficits in language production among children with damage to the anterior regions of the left hemisphere (in particular, the perisylvian area of the left-frontal lobe).
3. The Wernicke hypothesis predicts more severe deficits in language comprehension in children with damage to the posterior regions of the left hemisphere (in particular, the posterior portion of the left-temporal lobe).

The developmental literature to date provides surprisingly little support for any of these hypotheses, and the same is true for this study. In contrast with a number of previous studies, we found clear positive evidence for site-specific effects during particular periods in development. However, these effects do not map onto the adult aphasia literature in a straightforward fashion, and they vary depending on the kind of language problem the child is trying to solve at each point in time.

Table 2 provides a summary of neurological findings for each of the three studies presented here. Robust findings are indicated by a double arrow, which means a particular neurological risk factor is associated with a significant between-group difference (comparing children with that risk factor to the rest of the focal-lesion sample). Weak findings are indicated by a single arrow, indicating that children with that risk factor are more likely to fall in the risk range than would be expected by chance, even though between-group comparisons did not reach significance.

Starting with the emergence of first words and gesture from 10 to 17 months, we found only modest evidence in favor of an early left-hemisphere specialization for language (Hypothesis 1). In fact, some of our findings ran in the opposite direction, suggesting the right hemisphere may play a unique and important role in the first stages of language comprehension and gestural communication. Right-hemisphere lesions were associated with a robust disadvantage in gestural devel-opment—precisely the opposite of what would be expected based on the adult literature on communicative and pantomimic gesture (Duffy & Duffy, 1981; Goodglass, 1993). Right-hemisphere lesions also were associated with a weak disadvantage for word comprehension (i.e., more children with right-hemisphere damage fell at or below the 10th percentile than would be expected by chance, something that was not true for the left-hemisphere sample). Furthermore, none of

TABLE 2
Summary of Neurological Findings

	+ Left Lesion	+ Right Lesion	+Left-Temporal Lesion	+Left-Frontal Lesion	+Right-Frontal Lesion
Study 1: 10–17 months					
Gesture	—	↓↓	—	—	—
Word comprehension	—	↓	—	—	—
Word production	↓	—	—	—	—
% of comprehended words produced	—	—	↓↓	—	—
Study 2: 19–31 months					
Vocabulary	↓	—	↓↓	↓↓	↓↓
Grammar	↓	↓	↓↓	↓↓	↓↓
Closed-class style	—	↑↑	na	na	na
Study 3: 19–44 months					
Mean length of utterance in morphemes	↓	–	↓↓	—	—

Note: ↑ = weak advantage; ↑↑ = strong advantage; ↓ = weak disadvantage; ↓↓ = strong disadvantage; na = not applicable.

the children with left-temporal injuries were in the risk range for word comprehension, solid evidence against the Wernicke hypothesis (Hypothesis 3).

We found a weak disadvantage for word production in the left-hemisphere group (i.e., more of these children were at or below the 10th percentile than would be expected by chance), but the left–right comparison was not reliable (against Hypothesis 1). However, the Broca hypothesis (Hypothesis 2) did not fare very well. There was a robust disadvantage for the left-temporal group on a measure that reflects the proportion of comprehended words that the child is able to produce for him- or herself. In fact, as just noted, the left-temporal group did very well in word comprehension. Their problem seems to involve the process by which a normal receptive vocabulary is converted into speech, and it may be related to the sharp dissociations between comprehension and production that so often are reported in the normal population (e.g., Bates et al., 1988).

Study 2 focused on the passage from first words to grammar from 19 to 30 months, a particularly dramatic period of development in normal children. Here we found a number of additional surprises.

First, we found no evidence for a dissociation between grammar and vocabulary in this population. This finding is in line with reports for normal children (Fenson et al., 1994) and for several other clinical groups (e.g., Williams syndrome; Singer Harris et al. this issue). In fact, one might argue that the absence of a grammar–vocabulary dissociation is tautological, that is, that the correlations observed in the normal population mean that it would be impossible to find a dissociation in any clinical group. However, Singer Harris et al. report significant dissociations in the Down syndrome population, with grammar falling far behind the levels one would expect for normal children at the same vocabulary level. If grammar and vocabulary were governed by separate brain regions, we might have expected to find at least a few dissociated cases in our focal-lesion sample. Instead, we found no evidence for a dissociation between grammar and the lexicon in this period of development, and no evidence for differential effects of lesion side or site on these two domains.

Second, the results of Study 2 provide a further disconfirmation of Hypotheses 1 to 3. One of the biggest surprises in this dataset is an effect of frontal-lobe injury on progress in vocabulary and grammar that appears to be independent of lesion side (i.e., it was equally strong for left-hemisphere and right-hemisphere children). One might speculate that this bilateral frontal effect reflects nothing more than gross motor impairment, slowing children down in a period that normally is marked by the rapid acceleration of vocabulary and first word combinations. However, we found no relation between frontal damage and the presence or absence of hemiparesis in this sample of children (see General Method, and Table 1).

Assuming that the bilateral frontal effect is not a by-product of gross motor impairment, are there any other explanations? There are at least three possibilities, and they are not mutually exclusive. First, even though gross motor impairments apparently are not responsible for the bilateral frontal effect, there could be motor impairments specific to the motor speech system. A second and closely related possibility is that children with frontal damage are more likely to sustain damage to anterior subcortical systems (in particular, the basal ganglia), structures that may be particularly important in this phase of development. Unfortunately, we do not have detailed information on subcortical structures for this sample of children, but this remains a viable hypothesis for future research (Aram & Eisele, 1994b; Aram et al., 1983; Eisele et al., 1997). A third possibility is that children with frontal injuries are impaired in planning and sequencing (i.e., the so-called executive functions; Diamond, 1988; Milner, Petrides, & Smith, 1985; Shimamura, Janowsky, & Squire, 1990; Welsh & Pennington, 1988). Regardless of the explanation for this bilateral frontal effect, we underscore that the result is reliable only in this particular phase of language development, albeit a very important and dramatic phase for normally developing children. The result is important primarily because it suggests that Broca's area and associated regions in the left-frontal cortex have not yet assumed the special role they are known to play in adult language processing.

Study 2 provides limited evidence for left-hemisphere specialization in early expressive vocabulary and grammar (in favor of Hypothesis 1), but this unilateral finding is due almost entirely to lesions involving the left-temporal lobe (against Hypotheses 2 and 3). Children with lesions involving the left-temporal lobe were delayed significantly in both vocabulary and grammar, a continuation of the left-temporal delays observed from 10 to 17 months in the percentage of receptive vocabulary that children were able to realize in speech. Although there was a trend toward a mirror image effect on the right side, the right-hemisphere temporal effect was not reliable. Hence, the effect of temporal lobe damage appears to be asymmetrical, unlike the frontal lobe effects discussed earlier. Control analyses comparing children with and without left-parietal injury did not reach significance, bolstering our confidence that the left-temporal effects are real and quite specific.

Study 2 also replicated an interesting trend reported earlier by Thal et al. (1991): Children with right-hemisphere damage produce a higher proportion of grammatical function words than do children with left-hemisphere damage, controlling for total vocabulary size. As we noted earlier, this measure looks (at first glance) like an index of emerging grammar. However, studies of normally developing children confirmed that the early use of function words (closed-class style) is either unrelated or negatively related to progress in grammar several months later (Bates et al., 1988). The same measure also was unrelated to concurrent vocabulary and grammar in this study. So what does this peculiar measure mean? In a review of the literature on stylistic differences in early language, Bates et al. (1995) proposed that closed-class style (also called *pronominal style;* Bloom et al., 1975) may occur in children who can perceive, store, and reproduce passages of speech they still do not understand. They suggested that this propensity may reflect variations in auditory short-term memory, an acute capacity for perceptual detail, or both. If it is the case that children with right-hemisphere damage are forced to rely more on left-hemisphere processes, and if it is the case that the left hemisphere plays a critical role in the extraction and reproduction of perceptual detail, we may have an explanation for the prevalence of closed-class style in the right-hemisphere population—an explanation with interesting implications for the occurrence of this style in normal children.

The bilateral frontal effects observed in Study 2 did not reach significance in Study 3 (which looked at free speech, with an age range extending from 19 through 44 months of age), although results were in the same direction. However, the left-temporal effect on expressive language observed in Studies 1 and 2 was still operating in Study 3. If anything, the disadvantage associated with left-temporal involvement was even greater in this phase of development, with this particular measure of language ability (i.e., MLU in morphemes). The same finding could not be seen in a simple left–right comparison, and we also found no effects of left-parietal injury when left-temporal involvement was controlled. These results provide further evidence that the left-temporal lobe is central to the emergence of left-hemisphere specialization for language.

In a separate study of grammar and discourse in 30 children with early focal brain injury (including 10 children from this study), Reilly, Bates, and Marchman (in press) reported a left-hemisphere disadvantage in grammar between 3 and 6 years of age, a disadvantage that is due almost entirely to children with left-temporal involvement. It is interesting to note that they found no sign whatsoever of this left-temporal effect after age 6, on grammar or on any other measure of language in a storytelling task. When data were collapsed across the range from 3 to 12 years of age, no side or site of lesion effects of any kind were detectable in their data, for lexical, grammatical, or discourse measures. Children with focal brain injury scored (as a group) significantly lower on a host of language measures, compared with normal controls, although their performance was well within the normal range in all but a few cases. For this reason, Reilly et al. concluded that early focal brain injury does exact a price; the alternative forms of brain organization for language that these children have developed work very well in most cases, but they are not optimal. However, the Reilly et al. findings agree with many other studies of language in the focal-lesion population, with very limited evidence for site-specific effects after 5 to 7 years of age.

These are all cross-sectional findings (although a few children appeared in consecutive studies), and they must be replicated in a longitudinal design before we can draw strong conclusions about development and recovery over time. However, the picture that emerges when results from all these studies are combined is one in which site-specific effects come and go over time depending on the task at hand. Eventually all these children find a solution to the problems of language acquisition, a solution that is workable even if it is not optimal (see Webster et al., 1995, for similar findings in lesion studies with primate infants and adults). Putting our data together with those of Reilly et al. (in press), we propose that these solutions are relatively stable by 5 to 7 years of age, when the fundamental principles of oral language are well established in the normal population. Before this point, we find interesting site-specific effects, with particular emphasis on (a) right-hemisphere mediation of some processes that usually are handled in the left hemisphere among adults, (b) bilateral frontal effects during the most dramatic period of vocabulary expansion and early grammar, with (c) left-temporal effects on expressive (but not receptive) language that are visible across the period from 10 to 60 months of age. After age 6, these site-specific effects are difficult to detect in children with pre- or perinatal brain injury, suggesting that a substantial degree of interhemispheric reorganization, intrahemispheric reorganization, or both has taken place (Rasmussen & Milner, 1977; Webster et al., 1995).

We must stress that our conclusions pertain only to children with early (prelinguistic) lesion onset, the group for whom it is reasonable to assume maximal plasticity with minimal commitment. It is not clear when the capacity for reorganization disappears, although there are good reasons to believe that later lesions have a more severe and, perhaps, irreversible effect (Hecaen, 1976, 1983; Marchman, 1993). We also underscore the fact that brain damage does exact a price, even in cases of early lesion onset. Thus, for example, the children studied by Reilly et al. (in press) were significantly behind their age mates on a host of language measures, even though they were still well within the normal range. The capacity of the human brain to reorganize and redistribute language functions is not total. But it is certainly impressive, raising problems for any theory that presupposes innate localization of linguistic knowledge.

Although it will no doubt prove difficult to find a unifying account of all these findings, we propose that they reflect regional differences in architecture and, perhaps, in timing, biases that are related only indirectly to the functional and representational specializations that are evident in adult language processing (specializations that can be set up in other places if the child has no other choice). This framework could explain the apparent paradox between the adult aphasia literature and decades of research on language recovery in children with homologous injuries. Can we be more specific about the nature of these putative biases? A full account will require the collaborative efforts of behavioral scientists and developmental neurobiologists, delineating the computational properties of specific regions in the infant cortex and their functional consequences. However, we can offer a few speculations and a possible place to start.

Following a proposal by Stiles and Thal (1993), we suggest that the left- and right-temporal cortices differ at birth in their capacities to support perceptual detail (enhanced on the left) and perceptual integration (enhanced on the right). The site-specific effects that we see in early language development reflect the differential importance of detail and integration at various stages in the learning process. Although it was once believed that the right hemisphere is specialized innately for visuospatial analysis, most researchers now agree that the two hemispheres contribute equally to the analysis of visual displays—but they do so in markedly different ways. For example, a number of recent studies have shown that lesions to the right hemisphere lead to problems in the integration of elements in a perceptual array, whereas lesions to the left hemisphere create problems in the analysis of perceptual details in the same array (e.g., Robertson & Lamb, 1991). Asked to reproduce a triangle made up of many small squares, adult patients with left-hemisphere damage tend to reproduce the global figure (i.e., the triangle) but ignore information at the local level. Adult patients with right-hemisphere damage display the opposite profile, reproducing local detail (i.e., a host of small squares) but failing to integrate these features into a coherent whole. Stiles and Thal reported that children with focal brain injury behave very much like their adult counterparts on the local–global task, suggesting that the differential contribution of left- and right-hemisphere processes on this task may be a developmental constant. It is interesting to note that this double dissociation is most evident in patients with temporal involvement (on the left or on the right; J. Stiles, personal communication, September 1994).

We suggest that a relatively simple bias in style of computation may underlie the left-temporal effects observed in visual perception in adults by Robertson and Lamb (1991) and in children by Stiles and Thal (1993), and the left-temporal effects on language observed in this study. In the first stages of word comprehension and, perhaps, recognition and reproduction of familiar gestures, the ability to integrate information within and across modalities may be particularly helpful and important. After all, learning the meaning of the word *elephant* for the first time is quite different from the passive and automatic processes that underlie word recognition in the adult. Unlike the adult, the child can and must integrate information from many different sources and modalities to make sense of this new word (e.g., the sight of the elephant, accompanying sounds and smells, the context of the zoo and memories of being there before, and parental gestures and facial expressions as the word is spoken). Perhaps for this reason, integrative processes in the right hemisphere may predominate in word comprehension from 10 to 17 months, placing children with right-hemisphere injuries at a special (but temporary) disadvantage.

The learning process changes markedly when children have to convert the same sound patterns into motor output. At this point, perceptual detail may be of paramount importance (i.e., it is one thing to recognize the word *elephant,* but it is quite another thing to pull out each phonetic detail and construct a motor template). If it is the case that the left-temporal cortex plays a critical role in the extraction, storage, and reproduction of perceptual detail (visual, acoustic, or both), children with left-temporal injuries will be at a greater disadvantage in this phase of learning (see also Galaburda & Livingstone, 1993, Galaburda, Menard, & Rosen, 1994; Tallal, Sainburg, & Jernigan, 1991). However, once the requisite patterns finally are constructed and set into well-learned routines, the left-temporal disadvantage may be much less evident.

SOME CAVEATS

Although we believe these results raise some important questions for future research, we close by underscoring some limitations of this study.

First, the population of children with early unilateral brain injuries was quite small. Indeed, it took us 8 years in three large cities to accumulate the data reported here, which means (among other things) there was considerable variability in the quality of the CT scans and magnetic resonance imaging scans used to derive lesion information. All these findings must be replicated with separate samples of children, and with state-of-the-art techniques for three-dimensional lesion reconstruction.

Second, in contrast with adult aphasics, whose acquired lesions usually are diagnosed soon after the incident occurs, the onset time and etiology of the lesions in our children often were unknown. In addition, the distribution of left- versus right-hemisphere lesions was highly skewed, and within each group, there was considerable overlap in lesion location. Hence, some of our more interesting findings regarding the role of left-temporal structures must be qualified by the fact that the left-temporal lobe was also one of the most probable sites of injury, with obvious consequences for sample size and statistical power (although it is comforting that parallel analyses involving the presence or absence of left-parietal injury did not show the same pattern because parietal sites are even more common than temporal ones). To replicate the left-temporal effect, and to explore some of the unexpected findings uncovered here (e.g., the right-hemisphere effects in Study 1 and the bilateral frontal effects in Study 2), it would be useful to investigate a larger and more balanced population of children with focal brain injury, with special emphasis on the separate contributions of temporal and frontal damage.

Third, the results we report here are cross-sectional in nature. Before we can conclude with conviction that the site-specific effects observed in Studies 1 to 3 resolve by 5 to 7 years of age, we need to follow the same longitudinal sample of children across this hypothesized transition point.

Fourth, we must remember that development involves change at many levels, including changes in brain structure. For example, there are some cases in which a small lesion that is apparent on an early scan seems to have disappeared when the same child is studied many years later. Perhaps the early scan was wrong and the later scan was right, but it is also possible that tissue changes have taken place as a consequence of that early lesion. In fact, very little is known about the functional and structural changes that occur as a result of early focal brain injury. Possibilities include compensatory sprouting in other regions; retaining of exuberant neurons, axons, and synapses that might have been eliminated in the absence of early injury;

and "reprogramming" of areas that would have behaved quite differently if the lesion had never occurred. There also are occasional changes in a more negative direction, for example, children with early focal brain injury who go on to develop neurological problems (including seizures) that were not evident in the period of development we studied. For this reason, the null effects of lesion size, seizure history, and motor involvement that we report here for children in the age range from 10 to 44 months may underestimate the long-term contribution of these factors. These facts underscore the need for larger samples, and for long-term longitudinal studies.

What are the practical solutions to these problems? One possibility would be to redefine and expand our definition of focal brain injury. For example, we could obtain a larger sample of children with frontal injuries (unilateral or bilateral) if we were to include cases of tumor or trauma. However, that would also guarantee an increase in the heterogeneity of the sample, due to the introduction of complications that we did not face in this study (i.e., diffuse damage from closed-head injury, side effects of radiation or chemotherapy). In our view, the best solution to the problem of sample size lies in large-scale collaborations across clinical and research sites, permitting researchers to standardize their diagnostic criteria and pool data on robust and reliable neurological and behavioral measures. Some preliminary efforts in that direction are already underway.

At the very least, results of this study confirm that detailed neuroanatomical and neurophysiological studies of children with focal brain injury could yield extremely important information about the developmental processes that lead to brain organization for language in adults. If the correlations between lesion localization and behavioral outcome observed in children were identical to those observed in adults, developmental studies would have little to add (beyond a confirmation of strong claims about the innate bases of language). Conversely, if there were no correlations whatsoever between lesion type and behavioral outcome, further developmental studies would not take us very far (beyond a confirmation of strong claims about brain plasticity). Our results suggest that both these extreme views are wrong. We have a great deal to learn about the neural bases of language development, and research on children with early focal brain injury is one promising line of inquiry.

ACKNOWLEDGMENTS

This research was supported by National Institutes of Health/ National Institute on Deafness and Other Communication Disorders Program Project P50 DC01289–0351, Origins of Communicative Disorders, to Elizabeth Bates, and by a grant from the John D. and Catherine T. MacArthur Foundation. We are grateful to Larry Juarez and Meiti Opie for assistance in manuscript preparation.

REFERENCES

Acredolo, L. P., & Goodwyn, S. W. (1988). Symbolic gesturing in normal infants. *Child Development, 59,* 450–456.

Acredolo, L. P., & Goodwyn, S. W. (1990). Sign language among hearing infants: The spontaneous development of symbolic gestures. In V. Volterra & C. Erting (Eds.), *From gesture to language in hearing and deaf children* (pp. 68–78). Berlin: Springer-Verlag.

Alajouanine, T., & Lhermitte, F. (1965). Acquired aphasia in children. *Brain, 88,* 553–562.

Almli, C., & Finger, S. (1984). *Early brain damage.* New York: Academic.

Altman, D., & Volpe, J. (1987). Cerebral blood flow in the newborn infant: Measurement and role in the pathogenesis of periventricular and intraventricular hemorrhage. *Advances in Pediatrics, 34,* 111–138.

Annett, M. (1973). Laterality of childhood hemiplegia and the growth of speech and intelligence. *Cortex, 9,* 4–33.

Annett, M. (1985). *Left, right, hand and brain: The right shift theory.* Hillsdale, NJ: Lawrence Erlbaum Associates, Inc.

Aram, D. M. (1988). Language sequelae of unilateral brain lesions in children. In F. Plum (Ed.), *Language, communication, and the brain* (pp. 171–197). New York: Raven.

Aram, D. M. (1992). Brain injury and language impairment in childhood. In P. Fletcher & D. Hall (Eds.), *Specific speech and language disorders in children.* London: Whurr.

Aram, D. M., & Eisele, J. A. (1994a). Intellectual stability in children with unilateral brain lesions. *Neuropsychologia, 32,* 85–95.

Aram, D. M., & Eisele, J. A. (1994b). Limits to a left-hemisphere explanation for specific language impairment. *Journal of Speech and Hearing Research, 37,* 824–830.

Aram, D. M., Ekelman, B., Rose, D., & Whitaker, H. (1985). Verbal and cognitive sequelae following unilateral lesions acquired in early childhood. *Journal of Clinical and Experimental Neuropsychology, 7,* 55–78.

Aram, D. M., Ekelman, B., & Whitaker, H. (1986). Spoken syntax in children with acquired unilateral hemisphere lesions. *Brain and Language, 27,* 75–100.

Aram, D. M., Ekelman, B., & Whitaker, H. (1987). Lexical retrieval in left- and right-brain-lesioned children. *Brain and Language, 28,* 61–87.

Aram, D. M., Meyers, S. C., & Ekelman, B. L. (1990). Fluency of conversational speech in children with unilateral brain lesions. *Brain and Language, 38,* 105–121.

Aram, D. M., Rose, D. F., Rekate, H. L., & Whitaker, H. A. (1983). Acquired capsular/striatal aphasia in childhood. *Archives of Neurology, 40,* 614–617.

Basso, A., Capitani, E., Laiacona, M., & Luzzatti, C. (1980). Factors influencing type and severity of aphasia. *Cortex, 16,* 631–636.

Bates, E., Appelbaum, M., & Allard, L. (1991). Statistical constraints on the use of single cases in neuropsychological research. *Brain and Language, 40,* 295–329.

Bates, E., Benigni, L., Bretherton, I., Camaioni, L., & Volterra, V. (1979). *The emergence of symbols: Cognition and communication in infancy.* New York: Academic.

Bates, E., Bretherton, I., Shore, C., & McNew, S. (1983). Names, gestures and objects: Symbolization in infancy and aphasia. In K. Nelson (Ed.), *Children's language* (Vol. 4, pp. 59–123). Hillsdale, NJ: Lawrence Erlbaum Associates, Inc.

Bates, E., Bretherton, I., & Snyder, L. (1988). *From first words to grammar: Individual differences and dissociable mechanisms.* New York: Cambridge University Press.

Bates, E., Dale, P. S., & Thal, D. (1995). Individual differences and their implications for theories of language development. In P. Fletcher & B. MacWhinney (Eds.), *Handbook of child language* (pp. 96–151). Oxford, England: Basil Blackwell.

Bates, E., Marchman, V., Thal, D., Fenson, L., Dale, P., Reznick, J. S., Reilly, J., & Hartung, J. (1994). Developmental and stylistic variation in the composition of early vocabulary. *Journal of Child Language, 21,* 85–124.

Bates, E., O'Connell, B., & Shore, C. (1987). Language and communication in infancy. In J. Osofsky (Ed.), *Handbook of infant development* (2nd ed., pp. 149–203). New York: Wiley.

Bates, E., & Thal, D. (1991). Associations and dissociations in child language development. In J. Miller (Ed.), *Research on child language disorders: A decade of progress* (pp. 145–168). Austin, TX: Pro-Ed.

Bates, E., Thal, D., & Janowsky, J. (1992). Early language development and its neural correlates. In I. Rapin & S. Segalowitz (Eds.), *Handbook of neuropsychology: Vol. 7. Child neuropsychology* (pp. 69–110). Amsterdam: Elsevier.

Bates, E., Thal, D., Whitesell, K., Fenson, L., & Oakes, L. (1989). Integrating language and gesture in infancy. *Developmental Psychology, 25,* 1004–1019.

Bates, E., & Wulfeck, B. (1989). Comparative aphasiology: A cross-linguistic approach to language breakdown. *Aphasiology, 3,* 111–142, 161–168.

Bellugi, U., & Hickok, G. (1995). Clues to the neurobiology of language. In R. Broadwell (Vol. Ed.), *Decade of the brain series: Vol. 1. Neuroscience, memory and language* (pp. 87–107). Washington, DC: Library of Congress.

Benedict, H. (1979). Early lexical development: Comprehension and production. *Journal of Child Language, 6,* 183–200.

Bishop, D. V. M. (1981). Plasticity and specificity of language localization in the developing brain. *Developmental Medicine and Child Neurology, 23,* 251.

Bishop, D. V. M. (1983). Linguistic impairment after left hemidecortication for infantile hemiplegia? A reappraisal. *Quarterly Journal of Experimental Psychology, 35A,* 199–207.

Bishop, D. V. M. (1992). The biological basis of specific language impairment. In P. Fletcher & D. Hall (Eds.), *Specific speech and language disorders in children.* London: Whurr.

Bloom, L. (1970). *Language development: Form and function in emerging grammars.* Cambridge, MA: MIT Press.

Bloom, L. (1973). *One word at a time: The use of single-word utterances before syntax.* The Hague, Netherlands: Mouton.

Bloom, L., Capatides, J. B., Fiess, K., Gartner, B., Hafitz, J., Holzman, L., Lahey, M., Lifter, K., Lightbown, P., Merkin, S., Miller, P., Rispoli, M., Rocissano, L., Tackeff, J., & Wootten, J. (1991). *Language development from two to three.* Cambridge, England/New York: Cambridge University Press.

Bloom, L., Lightbown, L., & Hood, L. (1975). Structure and variation in child language. *Monographs of the Society for Research in Child Development, 40*(2, Serial No. 160).

Borer, H., & Wexler, K. (1987). The maturation of syntax. In T. Roeper & E. Williams (Eds.), *Parameter setting* (pp. 123–172). Dordrecht, The Netherlands: Reidel.

Bradshaw, J., & Nettleton, N. (1981). The nature of hemispheric specialization in man. *Behavioral and Brain Sciences, 4,* 51–91.

Brown, R. (1973). *A first language: The early stages.* Cambridge, MA: Harvard University Press.

Brownell, C. (1988). Combinatorial skills: Converging developments over the second year. *Child Development, 59,* 675–685.

Bryden, M. (1982). *Laterality: Functional asymmetry in the intact brain.* New York: Academic.

Caplan, D., & Hildebrandt, N. (1988). *Disorders of syntactic comprehension.* Cambridge, MA: MIT Press.

Changeux, J. P., Courrège, P., & Danchin, A. (1973). A theory of the epigenesis of neural networks by selective stabilization of synapses. *Proceedings of the National Academy of Sciences USA, 70,* 2974–2978.

Changeux, J. P., & Danchin, A. (1976). Selective stabilization of developing synapses as a mechanism for the specification of neuronal networks. *Nature, 264,* 705–712.

Churchland, P. S., & Sejnowski, T. J. (1992). *The computational brain.* Cambridge, MA: MIT Press.

Corballis, M., & Morgan, M. (1978). On the biological basis of human laterality: Evidence for a maturational left–right gradient. *Behavioral and Brain Sciences, 1,* 261–269.

Courchesne, A., Townsend J., & Chase, C. (1994). Neurodevelopmental principles guide research on developmental psychopathologies. In D. Cicchetti & D. Cohen (Eds.), *A manual of developmental psychology* (pp. 195–226). New York: Wiley.

Crain, S. (1992). Language acquisition in the absence of experience. *Behavioral and Brain Sciences, 14,* 597–611.

Dale, P. S. (1991). The validity of a parent report measure of vocabulary and syntax at 24 months. *Journal of Speech and Hearing Sciences, 34,* 565–571.

Dale, P. S., Bates, E., Reznick, S., & Morisset, C. (1989). The validity of a parent report instrument of child language at 20 months. *Journal of Child Language, 16,* 239–249.

Dall'Oglio, A., Bates, E., Volterra, V., DiCapua, M., & Pezzini, G. (1994). Early cognition, communication and language in children with focal brain injury. *Developmental Medicine and Child Neurology, 36,* 1076–1098.

Damasio, A. (1989). Time-locked multiregional retroactivation: A systems-level proposal for the neural substrates of recall and recognition. *Cognition, 33,* 25–62.

Damasio, A., & Damasio, H. (1992, September). Brain and language. *Scientific American, 267,* 88–95.

Day, P. S., & Ulatowska, H. K. (1979). Perceptual, cognitive, and linguistic development after early hemispherectomy: Two case studies. *Brain and Language, 7,* 17–33.

Dennis, M. (1980). Capacity and strategy for syntactic comprehension after left or right hemidecortication. *Brain and Language, 10,* 287–317.

Dennis, M. (1988). *Language and the young damaged brain.* Washington, DC: American Psychological Association.

Dennis, M., & Kohn, B. (1975). Comprehension of syntax in infantile hemiplegics after cerebral hemidecortication. *Brain and Language, 2,* 472–482.

Dennis, M., Lovett, M., & Wiegel-Crump, C. (1981). Written language acquisition after left or right hemidecortication in infancy. *Brain and Language, 12,* 54–91.

Dennis, M., & Whitaker, H. A. (1976). Language acquisition following hemidecortication: Linguistic superiority of the left over the right hemisphere. *Brain and Language, 3,* 404–433.

Dennis, M., & Whitaker, H. A. (1977). Hemispheric equipotentiality and language acquisition. In S. J. Segalowitz & F. A. Gruber (Eds.), *Language development and neurological theory* (pp. 93–106). New York: Academic.

Diamond, A. (1988). Abilities and neural mechanisms underlying AB performance. *Child Development, 59,* 523–527.

Dromi, E. (1987). *Early lexical development.* New York: Cambridge University Press.

Dronkers, N. F., Shapiro, J. K., Redfern, B., & Knight, R. T. (1992, February). *The third left frontal convolution and aphasia: On beyond Broca.* Paper presented at the 20th annual meeting of the International Neuropsychological Society, San Diego, CA.

Duffy, R., & Duffy, J. (1981). Three studies of deficits in pantomimic expression and pantomime recognition in aphasia. *Journal of Speech and Hearing Research, 46,* 70–86.

Edelman, G. (1987). *Neural Darwinism: The theory of neuronal group selection.* New York: Basic Books.

Eisele, J. A., Alexander, M. P., & Aram, D. M. (1997). *Anterior capsulostriatal lesions predict residual language and cognitive deficits in children.* Manuscript submitted for publication.

Eisele, J. A., & Aram, D. (1993). Differential effects of early hemisphere damage on lexical comprehension and production. *Aphasiology, 7,* 513–523.

Eisele, J. A., & Aram, D. (1994). Comprehension and imitation of syntax following early hemisphere damage. *Brain and Language, 46,* 212–231.

Eisele, J. A., & Aram, D. (1995). Lexical and grammatical development in children with early hemisphere damage: A cross-sectional view from birth to adolescence. In P. Fletcher & B. MacWhinney (Eds.), *Handbook of child language* (pp. 664–690). Oxford, England: Basil Blackwell.

Elman, J., Bates, E., Johnson, M., Karmiloff-Smith, A., Parisi, D., & Plunkett, K. (1996). *Rethinking innateness: Development in a connectionist perspective.* Cambridge, MA: MIT Press/Bradford Books.

Feldman, H., Holland, A., Kemp, S., & Janosky, J. (1992). Language development after unilateral brain injury. *Brain and Language, 42,* 89–102.

Fenson, L., Dale, P. A., Reznick, J. S., Bates, E., & Thal, D. (1994). Variability in early communicative development. *Monographs of the Society for Research in Child Development, 59*(5, Serial No. 242).

Fenson, L., Dale, P., Reznick, J. S., Thal, D., Bates, E., Hartung, J., Pethick, S., & Reilly, J. (1993). *The MacArthur Communicative Development Inventories: User's guide and technical manual.* San Diego. CA: Singular Publishing Group.

Fletcher, J. M. (1993). Afterword: Behavior–brain relationships in children. In S. H. Broman & J. Grafman (Eds.), *Atypical cognitive deficits in developmental disorders: Implications for brain function* (pp. 297–326). Hillsdale, NJ: Lawrence Erlbaum Associates, Inc.

Freud, A. (1953). *On aphasia: A critical study.* New York: International Universities Press. (Original work published 1891)

Friedlander, M. J., Martin, K. A. C., & Wassenhove-McCarthy, D. (1991). Effects of monocular visual deprivation on geniculocortical innervation of area 18 in cat. *The Journal of Neuroscience, 11,* 3268–3288.

Frost, D. O. (1982). Anomalous visual connections to somatosensory and auditory systems following brain lesions in early life. *Developmental Brain Research, 3,* 627–635.

Frost, D. O. (1990). Sensory processing by novel, experimentally induced cross-modal circuits. *Annals of the New York Academy of Sciences, 608,* 92–112.

Galaburda, A. M. (1994). Language areas, lateralization and the innateness of language. *Discussions in Neuroscience, 10*(1–2), 118–124.

Galaburda, A. M., & Livingstone, M. (1993). Evidence for a magnocellular defect in neurodevelopmental dyslexia. *Annals of the New York Academy of Sciences, 682,* 70–82.

Galaburda, A. M., Menard, M. T., & Rosen, G. D. (1994). Evidence for aberrant auditory anatomy in developmental dyslexia. *Proceedings of the National Academy of Sciences USA, 91,* 8010–8013.

Gazzaniga, M. (1994). Language and the cerebral hemispheres. *Discussions in Neuroscience, 10*(1–2), 136–149.

Geschwind, N. (1972, April). Language and the brain. *Scientific American, 226,* 76–83.

Geschwind, N., & Levitsky, W. (1968). Human brain: Left–right asymmetries in temporal speech region. *Science, 161,* 186–187.

Goldstein, K. (1948). *Language and language disturbances.* New York: Grune & Stratton.

Goodglass, H. (1993). *Understanding aphasia.* San Diego, CA: Academic.

Gould, S. J. (1977). *Ontogeny and phylogeny.* Cambridge, MA: Harvard University Press.

Greenough, W. T., Black, J. E., & Wallace, C. S. (1993). Experience and brain development. In M. Johnson (Ed.), *Brain development and cognition: A reader* (pp. 290–322). Oxford, England: Blackwell.

Greenough, W. T., McDonald, J. W., Parnisari, R. M., & Camel, J. E. (1986). Environmental conditions modulate degeneration and new dendrite growth in cerebellum of senescent rats. *Brain Research, 380,* 136–143.

Hammill, D., & Irwin, O. C. (1966). I.Q. differences of right and left spastic hemiplegic children. *Perceptual and Motor Skills, 22,* 193–194.

Hazeltine, E., & Ivry, R. (1994, March). *A connectionist model of sequential and laterality effects*. Paper presented at the first annual meeting of the Cognitive Neuroscience Society, San Francisco, CA.

Head, H. (1963). *Aphasia and kindred disorders of speech*. New York: Hafner.

Hecaen, H. (1976). Acquired aphasia in children and the ontogenesis of hemispheric functional specialization. *Brain and Language, 3,* 114–134.

Hecaen, H. (1983). Acquired aphasia in children: Revisited. *Neuropsychologia, 21,* 581–587.

Hecaen, H., Perenin, M., & Jeannerod, H. (1984). The effects of cortical lesions in children: Language and visual functions. In C. Almli & S. Finger (Eds.), *Behavioral biology of early damage* (Vol. 1). New York: Academic.

Hellige, J. (1993). *Hemispheric asymmetry*. Cambridge, MA: Harvard University Press.

Isaacson, R. L. (1975). The myth of recovery from early brain damage. In N. G. Ellis (Ed.), *Aberrant development in infancy* (pp. 1–26). New York: Wiley.

Jacobs, R., Jordan, M., Nowlan, S., & Hinton, G. (1991). Adaptive mixtures of local experts. *Neural Computation, 3,* 79–87.

Jacobs, R., & Kosslyn, S. (1994). Encoding shape and spatial relations: The role of receptive field size in coordinating complementary representations. *Cognitive Science, 18,* 361–386.

Janowsky, J., & Finlay, B. (1986). The outcome of perinatal brain damage: The role of normal neuron loss and axon retraction. *Developmental Medicine and Child Neurology, 28,* 375–389.

Johnson, J., & Newport, E. (1989). Critical-period effects in second language learning. *Cognitive Psychology, 21,* 60–99.

Karmiloff-Smith, A. (1992). *Beyond modularity: A developmental perspective on cognitive science*. Cambridge, MA: MIT Press.

Kennard, M. (1936). Age and other factors in motor recovery from precentral lesions in monkeys. *American Journal of Physiology, 115,* 138–146.

Killackey, H. P. (1990). Neocortical expansion: An attempt toward relating phylogeny and ontogeny. *Journal of Cognitive Neuroscience, 2,* 1–17.

Killackey, H. L., Chiaia, N. L., Bennett-Clarke, C. A., Eck, M., & Rhoades, R. (1994). Peripheral influences on the size and organization of somatotopic representations in the fetal rat cortex. *Journal of Neuroscience, 14,* 1496–1506.

Kinsbourne, M., & Hiscock, M. (1983). The normal and deviant development of functional lateralization of the brain. In M. Haith & J. Campos (Eds.), *Handbook of child psychology* (Vol. 2, 4th ed., pp. 157–280). New York: Wiley.

Klima, E. S., Kritchevsky, M., & Hickok, G. (1993, October). The neural substrate for sign language. In U. Bellugi (Chair), *Neural systems underlying spatial language and spatial cognition*. Symposium conducted at the 31st annual meeting of the Academy of Aphasia, Tucson, AZ.

Kohn, B. (1980). Right-hemisphere speech representation and comprehension of syntax after left cerebral injury. *Brain and Language, 9,* 350–361.

Kohn, B., & Dennis, M. (1974). Selective impairments of visuospatial abilities in infantile hemiplegics after right cerebral hemidecortication. *Neuropsychologia, 12,* 505–512.

Krashen, S. (1973). Lateralization, language learning, and the critical period: Some new evidence. *Language Learning, 23,* 63–74.

Lashley, K. S. (1950). In search of the engram. In *Symposia of the Society for Experimental Biology: No. 4. Physiological mechanisms and animal behaviour* (pp. 454–482). New York: Academic.

Lashley, K. S. (1951). *Central mechanisms in behavior*. New York: Wiley.

Lenneberg, E. H. (1967). *Biological foundations of language*. New York: Wiley.

Lightfoot, D. (1991). The child's trigger experience: Degree-0 learnability. *Behavioral and Brain Sciences, 14,* 364.

Locke, J. (1993). *The child's path to spoken language*. Cambridge, MA: Harvard University Press.

MacWhinney, B. (1991). *The CHILDES Project: Tools for analyzing talk*. Hillsdale, NJ: Lawrence Erlbaum Associates, Inc.

MacWhinney, B., & Bates, E. (Eds.). (1989). *The cross-linguistic study of sentence processing*. New York: Cambridge University Press.

Marchman, V. (1993). Constraints on plasticity in a connectionist model of the English past tense. *Journal of Cognitive Neuroscience, 5*, 215–234.

Marchman, V., & Bates, E. (1994). Continuity in lexical and morphological development: A test of the critical mass hypothesis. *Journal of Child Language, 21*, 339–366.

Marchman, V., Miller, R., & Bates, E. A. (1991). Babble and first words in children with focal brain injury. *Applied Psycholinguistics, 12*, 1–22.

Marie, P. (1906). Révision de la question de l'aphasie: La troisième circonvolution frontale gauche ne joue aucun rôle spécial dans la fonction du langage [The question of aphasia revised: The third left frontal convolution plays no special part in language function.] *Semaine Médicale, 26*, 241.

Menn, L., & Obler, L. K. (Eds.). (1990). *Agrammatic aphasia: Cross-language narrative sourcebook.* Amsterdam/Philadelphia: Benjamins.

Merzenich, M., Recanzone, G., Jenkins, W., Allard, T., & Nudo, R. (1988). Cortical representational plasticity. In P. Rakic & W. Singer (Eds.), *Neurobiology of neocortex* (pp. 41–67). New York: Wiley.

Miller, J. F., & Chapman, R. (1981). The relation between age and mean length of utterances in morphemes. *Journal of Speech and Hearing Research, 24*, 154–161.

Milner, B. (1994). Carotid-amytal studies of speech representation and gesture control. *Discussions in Neuroscience, 10*(1–2), 109–117.

Milner, B., Petrides, M., & Smith, M. (1985). Frontal lobes and the temporal organization of behavior. *Human Neurobiology, 4*, 137–142.

Mohr, J., Pesssin, M., Finkelstein, S., Funkenstein, H., Duncan, G., & Davis, K. (1978). Broca aphasia: Pathologic and clinical. *Neurology, 28*, 311–324.

Molfese, D. (1989). Electrophysiological correlates of word meanings in 14-month-old human infants. *Developmental Neuropsychology, 5*, 70–103.

Molfese, D. (1990). Auditory evoked responses recorded from 16-month-old human infants to words they did and did not know. *Brain and Language, 38*, 345–363.

Molfese, D., & Segalowitz, S. J. (1988). *Brain lateralization in children: Developmental implications.* New York: Guilford.

Molnar, Z., & Blakemore, C. (1991). Lack of regional specificity for connections formed between thalamus and cortex in coculture. *Nature, 351*, 475–477.

Naeser, M., Helm-Estabrooks, N., Haas, G., Auerbach, S., & Levine, H. (1984). Relationship between lesion extent in "Wernicke's area" on computed tomographic scan and predicting recovery of comprehension in Wernicke's aphasia. *Archives of Neurology, 44*, 73–82.

Nelson, K. (1973). Structure and strategy in learning to talk. *Monographs of the Society for Research in Child Development, 38*(1–2, Serial No. 149).

Nelson, K. (1981). Individual differences in language development: Implications for development and language. *Developmental Psychology, 17*, 170–187.

Ojemann, G. A. (1991). Cortical organization of language. *Journal of Neuroscience, 11*, 2281–2287.

O'Leary, D. D. (1993). Do cortical areas emerge from a protocortex? In M. Johnson (Ed.), *Brain development and cognition: A reader* (pp. 323–337). Oxford, England: Blackwell.

O'Leary, D. D., & Stanfield, B. B. (1989). Selective elimination of axons extended by developing cortical neurons is dependent on regional locale: Experiments utilizing fetal cortical transplants. *Journal of Neuroscience, 9*, 2230–2246.

Oyama, S. (1993). The problem of change. In M. Johnson (Ed.), *Brain development and cognition: A reader* (pp. 19–30). Oxford, England: Blackwell.

Pallas, S. L., & Sur, M. (1993). Visual projections induced into the auditory pathway of ferrets: 2. Corticocortical connections of primary auditory cortex. *Journal of Comparative Neurology, 337*, 317–333.

Parmelee, A., & Sigman, M. (1983). Perinatal brain development and behavior. In M. Haith & J. Campos (Eds.), *Handbook of child psychology* (Vol. 2, 4th ed., pp. 95–155). New York: Wiley.

Peters, A. (1983). *The units of language acquisition.* Cambridge, England: Cambridge University Press.

Petersen, S., Fiez, J., & Corbetta, M. (1992). Neuroimaging. *Current Opinion in Neurobiology, 2,* 217–222.

Piatelli-Palmarini, M. (1989). Evolution, selection and cognition: From "learning" to parameter setting in biology and the study of language. *Cognition, 31,* 1–44.

Pinker, S. (1991). Rules of language. *Science, 253,* 530–535.

Pinker, S. (1994a). *The language instinct: How the mind creates language.* New York: Morrow.

Pinker, S. (1994b). On language. *Journal of Cognitive Neuroscience, 6,* 84–91.

Poizner, H., Klima, E., & Bellugi, U. (1987). *What the hands reveal about the brain.* Cambridge, MA: MIT Press/Bradford Books.

Pons, T. P., Garraghty, P. E., Ommaya, A. K., Kaas, J. H. Taub, E., & Mishkin M. (1991). Massive cortical reorganization after sensory deafferentation in adult macaques. *Science, 252,* 1857–1860.

Raichle, M. (1994). Positron emission tomography studies of verbal response selection. *Discussions in Neuroscience, 10*(1–2), 130–135.

Ramachandran, V. S. (1993). Behavioral and magnetoencephalographic correlates of plasticity in the adult human brain. *Proceedings of the National Academy of Sciences USA, 90,* 10413–10420.

Rasmussen, T., & Milner, B. (1977). The role of early left brain injury in determining lateralization of cerebral speech functions. *Annals of the New York Academy of Sciences, 299,* 355–369.

Reed, J. C., & Reitan, R. M. (1969). Verbal and performance differences among brain-injured children with lateralized motor deficits. *Perceptual and Motor Skills, 29,* 747–752.

Reilly, J., Bates, E., & Marchman, V. (in press). Narrative discourse in children with early focal brain injury. *Brain and Language.*

Riva, D., & Cazzaniga, L. (1986). Late effects of unilateral brain lesions before and after the first year of life. *Neuropsychologia, 24,* 423–428.

Riva, D., Cazzaniga, L., Pantaleoni, C., Milani, N., & Fedrizzi, E. (1986). Acute hemiplegia in childhood: The neuropsychological prognosis. *Journal of Pediatric Neurosciences, 2,* 239–250.

Riva, D., Milani, N., Pantaleoni, C., Devoti, M., & Zorzi, C. (1992). Gli esiti a distanza delle lesioni cerebrali emisferiche congenite ed adquisite [Late effects of hemispheric cerebral congenital and acquired lesions]. In A. Benton, H. Levin, G. Moretti, & D. Riva (Eds.), *Neuropsicologia in età evolutiva* (pp. 185–197). Milan: FrancoAngeli.

Robertson, L. C., & Lamb, M. R. (1991). Neuropsychological contributions to theories of part/whole organization. *Cognitive Psychology, 23,* 299–330.

Roe, A. W., Pallas, S. L., Hahm, J. O., & Sur, M. (1990). A map of visual space induced in primary auditory cortex. *Science, 250,* 818–820.

Satz, P., Strauss, E., & Whitaker, H. (1990). The ontogeny of hemispheric specialization: Some old hypotheses revisited. *Brain and Language, 38,* 596–614.

Shimamura, A., Janowsky, J., & Squire, L. (1990). Memory for the temporal order of events in patients with frontal lobe lesions and amnesic patients. *Neuropsychologia, 28,* 803–813.

Shore, C., O'Connell, B., Beeghly, M., Bretherton, I., & Bates, E. (1990). Vocal and gestural symbols: Similarities and differences from 13 to 28 months. In V. Volterra & C. J. Erting (Eds.), *From gesture to language in hearing and deaf children* (pp. 79–91). New York: Springer-Verlag.

Simonds, R. J., & Scheibel, A. B. (1989). The postnatal development of the motor speech area: A preliminary study. *Brain and Language, 37,* 42–58.

Slobin, D. (Ed.). (1985). *The crosslinguistic study of language acquisition* (Vols. 1 & 2). Hillsdale, NJ: Lawrence Erlbaum Associates, Inc.

Smith, A. (1984). Early and long-term recovery from brain damage in children and adults: Evolution of concepts of localization, plasticity, and recovery. In C. R. Almli & S. Finger (Eds.), *Early brain damage* (pp. 299–324). New York: Academic.

Spelke, E., Breinlinger, K., Macomber, J., & Jacobson, K. (1992). Origins of knowledge. *Psychological Review, 99*, 605–632.

St. James-Roberts, I. (1979). Neurological plasticity, recovery from brain insult, and child development. In H. W. Reese (Ed.), *Advances in child development and behavior* (pp. 253–319). New York: Academic.

Stiles, J. (1995). Plasticity and development: Evidence from children with early focal brain injury. In B. Julesz & I. Kovacs (Eds.), *Maturational windows and cortical plasticity in human development: Is there reason for an optimistic view?* (pp. 217–237). Reading, MA: Addison-Wesley.

Stiles, J., & Thal, D. (1993). Linguistic and spatial cognitive development following early focal brain injury: Patterns of deficit and recovery. In M. Johnson (Ed.), *Brain development and cognition: A reader* (pp. 643–664). Oxford, England: Blackwell.

Sur, M., Garraghty, P. E., & Roe, A. W. (1988). Experimentally induced visual projections into auditory thalamus and cortex. *Science, 242*, 1437–1441.

Sur, M., Pallas, S. L., & Roe, A. W. (1990). Cross-modal plasticity in cortical development: Differentiation and specification of sensory neocortex. *Trends in Neuroscience, 13*, 227–233.

Tallal, P., Sainburg, R. L., & Jernigan, T. (1991). The neuropathology of developmental dysphasia: Behavioral, morphological, and physiological evidence for a pervasive temporal processing disorder. *Reading and Writing, 3*, 363–377.

Thal, D., Marchman, V. A., Stiles, J., Aram, D., Trauner, D., Nass, R., & Bates, E. (1991). Early lexical development in children with focal brain injury. *Brain and Language, 40*, 491–527.

Trauner D., Chase, C., Walker, P., & Wulfeck, B. (1993). Neurologic profiles of infants and children after perinatal stroke. *Pediatric Neurology, 9*, 383–386.

Vargha-Khadem, F, Isaacs, E. B., Papaleoudi, H., Polkey, C. E., & Wilson, J. (1991). Development of language in 6 hemispherectomized patients. *Brain, 114*, 473–495.

Vargha-Khadem, F., Isaacs, E., van der Werf, S., Robb, S., & Wilson, J. (1992). Development of intelligence and memory in children with hemiplegic cerebral palsy: The deleterious consequences of early seizures. *Brain, 115*, 315–329.

Vargha-Khadem, F., O'Gorman, A., & Watters, G. (1985). Aphasia and handedness in relation to hemispheric side, age at injury and severity of cerebral lesion during childhood. *Brain, 108*, 677–696.

Vargha-Khadem, F., & Polkey, C. E. (1992). A review of cognitive outcome after hemidecortication in humans. In F. D. Rose & D. A. Johnson (Eds.), *Recovery from brain damage: Advances in experimental medicine and biology: Vol. 325. Reflections and directions* (pp. 137–151). New York: Plenum.

Webster, M. J., Bachevalier, J., & Ungerleider, L. G. (1995). Development and plasticity of visual memory circuits. In B. Julesz & I. Kovacs (Eds.), *Proceedings of the Santa Fe Institute studies in the sciences of complexity* (Vol. 25, pp. 73–86). Reading, MA: Addison-Wesley.

Welsh, M. C., & Pennington, B. F. (1988). Assessing frontal lobe functioning in children: Views from developmental psychology. *Developmental Neuropsychology, 4*, 199–230.

Wernicke, C. (1966). The symptom complex of aphasia: A psychological study on an anatomic basis. In R. S. Cohen & M. W. Wartofsky (Eds.), *Boston studies in the philosophy of science, Proceedings of the Boston colloquium for the philosophy of science: 1966–68* (Vol. 4, pp. 34–97). New York: Humanities Press. (Original work published 1874)

Wernicke, C. (1977). The aphasia symptom complex: A psychological study on an anatomic basis. (N. Geschwind, Trans.) In G. H. Eggert (Ed.), *Wernicke's works on aphasia: A sourcebook and review*. The Hague, Netherlands: Mouton. (Original work published 1874)

Willmes, K., & Poeck, K. (1993). To what extent can aphasic syndromes be localized? *Brain, 116*, 1527–1540.

Witelson, S., & Kigar, D. (1988). Asymmetry in brain function follows asymmetry in anatomical form: Gross, microscopic, postmortem, and imaging studies. In F. Boller & J. Grafman (Eds.), *Handbook of neuropsychology* (Vol. 1, pp. 111–142). Amsterdam: Elsevier.

Woods, B. (1980). The restricted effects of right-hemisphere lesions after age one: Wechsler test data. *Neuropsychologia, 18,* 65–70.

Woods, B., & Carey, S. (1979). Language deficits after apparent clinical recovery from childhood aphasia. *Annals of Neurology, 6,* 405–409.

Woods, B., & Teuber, H. (1978). Changing patterns of childhood aphasia. *Annals of Neurology, 3,* 272–280.

Wulfeck, B., Trauner, D., & Tallal, P. (1991). Neurologic, cognitive and linguistic features of infants after focal brain injury. *Pediatric Neurology, 7,* 266–269.

DEVELOPMENTAL NEUROPSYCHOLOGY, *13*(3), 345–370

Contrasting Profiles of Language Development in Children With Williams and Down Syndromes

Naomi G. Singer Harris

San Diego State University
The Salk Institute for Biological Studies
Laboratory for Cognitive Neuroscience

Ursula Bellugi

The Salk Institute for Biological Studies
Laboratory for Cognitive Neuroscience

Elizabeth Bates

University of California, San Diego

Wendy Jones and Michael Rossen

The Salk Institute for Biological Studies
Laboratory for Cognitive Neuroscience

We describe language acquisition in two distinct genetically based syndromes. Parents of children with Williams syndrome (WMS) and Down syndrome (DNS) were given the MacArthur Communicative Development Inventory (CDI), a parental report measure of child language development. Although both groups of children were found to be equally delayed according to normative standards, differential patterns of language acquisition emerged. Early in language development, the groups were differentiated primarily by a proclivity for gesture production by the children with DNS. Later in language development, the groups were cleaved by grammatical development: Children with WMS displayed a significant advantage over children

---

Request for reprints should be sent to Ursula Bellugi, The Salk Institute for Biological Studies, Laboratory for Cognitive Neuroscience, 10010 North Torrey Pines Road, La Jolla, CA 92037.

with DNS. These findings are striking given the marked differences observed between adolescents and adults with WMS and DNS: Individuals with WMS exhibit linguistic skills superior to those of matched DNS controls despite significant but comparable cognitive deficits.

Williams syndrome (WMS), a genetically based neurodevelopmental disorder, is characterized by a unique neuropsychological profile in which language appears to "decouple" from other higher cognitive functions (Bellugi, Bihrle, Jernigan, Trauner, & Doherty, 1990; Bellugi, Bihrle, Neville, Jernigan, & Doherty, 1992; Bellugi, Wang, & Jernigan, 1994; Karmiloff-Smith, Klima, Bellugi, Grant, & Baron-Cohen, 1995; Mervis & Bertrand, in press; Wang & Bellugi, 1993). Despite average IQ scores ranging from 50 to 70, adolescents and adults with WMS display surprisingly good mastery of complex linguistic structures, as compared to Down syndrome (DNS) individuals matched for age and IQ. Furthermore, individuals with WMS have profound spatial cognitive deficits that exceed their levels of general cognitive impairment; a notable exception to this is their relatively unimpaired performance on tests of facial recognition (Bellugi et al., 1992, 1994; Jones, Singer, Rossen, & Bellugi, 1993). In addition, individuals with WMS tend to be quite sociable and affectively expressive (Reilly, Klima, & Bellugi, 1991; Udwin & Yule, 1990). These factors all contribute to a highly unusual neuropsychological profile exhibiting peaks and valleys in domains of higher cognitive functioning.

The contrast between WMS and DNS goes beyond different behavioral profiles. Both syndromes have a unique genetic basis: DNS generally involves an additional chromosome; WMS recently has been understood as deletion of one copy of the gene for elastin on Chromosome 7, plus surrounds (Ewart et al., 1993; Morris, 1995). The incidence of WMS (1 in 25,000) is considerably rarer than that of DNS, however (1 in 600). In addition, magnetic resonance imaging studies indicate that each syndrome appears to leave its own distinct morphological "stamp" on the brain, with WMS exhibiting relatively spared frontal, limbic, and cerebellar regions, and DNS exhibiting relatively preserved basal ganglia and diencephalic structures (Jernigan, Bellugi, Sowell, Doherty, & Hesselink, 1993; Wang, Hesselink, Jernigan, Doherty, & Bellugi, 1992). Thus, multiple levels of investigation point to behavioral, neuroanatomic, and genetic distinctions between these two neurodevelopmental disorders, providing clues to the relation between genes, brain, and behavior.

A missing piece thus far has been research on the early acquisition of language and other cognitive functions, and the developmental profiles of these two syndromes. As described previously, most of the research to date examined individuals with WMS and DNS in adolescence and adulthood. Studies of younger children with WMS and DNS are of particular importance because by examining differences between the two syndromes in the early stages of cognitive and language development, insights can be obtained into the factors responsible for the very different neuropsychological profiles evidenced in the steady state. Critical questions that drive such investigations of younger children with WMS and DNS are: What happens early in development that leads these two groups to such very different endpoints? How do their developmental trajectories differ? By examining differential aspects of language development in WMS and DNS, this study is one of the first and is the largest to begin to address these important questions.

A considerable amount of research has focused on language development in DNS, with investigators primarily noting delays rather than deviance. Although there is general consensus that language is more impaired than are other cognitive abilities in individuals with DNS, and that differences between linguistic and nonlinguistic cognitive development tend to increase with chronological age, there is some controversy regarding the nature of the language deficit in DNS (cf. Chapman, 1993; Fowler, 1993). The literature indicates, however, that production deficits tend to exceed comprehension deficits, and that grammar appears to be disproportionately affected (Beeghly & Cicchetti, 1987; Beeghly, Weiss-Perry, & Cicchetti, 1990; Chapman, 1995; Fowler, 1990; Miller, 1987, 1992).

In contrast, there has been relatively little research published on early stages of language development in WMS. One study found that the performance of children with WMS on language items on the Bayley Scales of Infant Intelligence exceeded their performance on nonlanguage items, whereas the reverse was true for children with DNS (Mervis & Bertrand, in press). Similarly, a study of language and symbolic gesture in two young children with WMS uncovered deviant relations between language and symbolic gesture that are consistent with the unusual relation between language and cognition in older individuals with WMS (Thal, Bates, & Bellugi, 1989). Studies also reported different relations between linguistic development and purportedly linked nonlinguistic cognitive development in children with WMS (e.g., lack of pointing before first referential object word; Goodman, 1994, 1995; Mervis & Bertrand, in press). These studies all involved small groups of children and yielded results that were not always consistent. One recent longitudinal study found considerable variability in language acquisition in three children with WMS (Mervis et al., 1995). Although such longitudinal analyses of language acquisition are informative, they typically involve small samples. Larger samples are needed to identify more clearly global patterns of language development in WMS and to overcome problems with variability, which often plague small samples. This study, using a cross-sectional design, is the first to involve large numbers of children with WMS and DNS to address these issues.

There are a number of possibilities for what the trajectories of language development could be like in WMS and DNS: (a) Consistent with the striking differences in the steady state, in which children with WMS display far more sophisticated mastery of language than do their counterparts with DNS, we might expect a developmental trajectory in which children with WMS are, from the outset, more adept at language acquisition than are children with DNS; (b) alternatively, based on comparable levels of general cognitive impairment, we might speculate that children with WMS and DNS are equivalently delayed in language acquisition; (c) finally, due to the complex and multifaceted nature of language, differences in language development between children with WMS and children with DNS may occur across linguistic domains, within linguistic domains, or along boundaries that divide linguistic domains. This study sought to address these possibilities and the questions raised earlier: What happens during language development to take these two groups to such very different linguistic endpoints? How do their patterns of language development compare?

METHODS

Instrumentation

All data for this study were collected using the MacArthur Communicative Development Inventory (CDI), a widely used parental report measure of language development (Fenson et al., 1993, 1994).

The CDI has two scales: a Words and Gestures scale, which assesses the onset of communication skills (for normally developing children between 8 and 16 months of age), and a Words and Sentences scale, which assesses later developing communication skills, including grammatical development (for normally developing children between 16 and 30 months of age). Both scales were utilized in this study.

Words and Gestures scale.   Part 1 of the Words and Gestures scale consists of a checklist of 396 words that have been found to be the first to appear in the receptive and expressive vocabularies of normally developing English-speaking children between the ages of 8 and 16 months (Fenson et al., 1993). Next to each word item, the parent is asked to indicate if their child (a) "understands" the word, or (b) "understands and says" the word. The checklist is divided into 19 semantic categories: sound effects, animal names, vehicle names, toys, food items, articles of clothing, body parts, furniture, household objects, outside things and places to go, people, routines and games, verbs, words for time, adjectives, pronouns, question words, prepositions, and quantifiers.

In Part 2 of the Words and Gestures scale, the child's use of intentional gestures (e.g., pointing, showing) and referential/representational gestures (e.g., putting telephone to ear) is assessed. Gestures of this type are of interest because they have been found to correlate with the onset of language comprehension, language production, or both in normally developing children.

Words and Sentences scale.   Part 1 of the Words and Sentences scale consists of a checklist of 689 words that typically are produced by normally developing English-speaking children between the ages of 16 and 30 months (this includes 396 words from the Words and Gestures scale). Next to each word item, the parent is asked to indicate if their child "says" the word. The same 19 semantic categories found on the Words and Gestures scale are represented on the Words and Sentences scale, with two additional categories for auxiliary verbs (i.e., "helping verbs") and conjunctions.

Part 2 of the Words and Sentences scale assesses the acquisition of grammar. Specifically, parents are asked if their child has begun to combine words; possible answers include *not yet, sometimes,* and *often.* If the parents indicate that their child has begun to combine words, they are then asked to provide examples of the three longest sentences they have recently heard their child say. In addition, parents are provided with a checklist of nouns and verbs in both regular and irregular inflected forms to assess the onset of inflectional morphology. Finally, grammatical complexity is assessed by presenting 37 sentence pairs, each of which represents a minimal contrast in grammatical complexity, that are typical examples of early multiword combinations. For example, some pairs index the attainment of bound morphemes (e.g., "two shoe" vs. "two shoe*s*"; "doggie kiss me" vs. "doggie kiss*ed* me"), some index free morphemes (e.g., "baby crying" vs. "baby *is* crying"; "cookie mommy" vs. "cookie *for* mommy"), and some index sentence embeddings and noun phrases (e.g., "don't read book" vs. "don't *want you* read *that* book"; "want cookies" vs. "want cookies *and milk*"). The parent simply marks "the one that sounds *most* like the way your child talks right now." The analyses presented in this study address the production checklist, examples of the child's longest utterances, and the grammatical complexity measure, as well as a parental report measure of mean length of utterance (MLU).

For both the Words and Gestures scale and the Words and Sentences scale, normative data also are provided for *associations* between the various dimensions of language development assessed by the CDI. This enables an examination of one dimension of language development in the context of another (e.g., word production in the context of gesture production; grammatical complexity in the context of word production). Naturally, there will be variability in the extent to which these dimensions are associated in different children; furthermore, the strength of associations are likely to vary at different time points in development. By providing normative information about these associations at different time points in language development, the CDI enables one to look for potential dissociations between domains of language, dissociations which not only indicate extremes of normal language development but which are particularly likely to be found in atypical populations such as children with WMS and DNS. The CDI provides this normative information in the form of "dissociation percentiles," which indicate where a given child "ranks" compared to the normative CDI sample. For example, for "word production relative to word comprehension," a child who scores in the 80th percentile is producing more words than are 80% of the children in the CDI normative sample who were comprehending the same number of words as he or she was (indicating high production relative to comprehension); accordingly, a child who scores in the 20th percentile is only producing more words than are 20% of the children in the CDI normative sample who were comprehending the same number of words as he or she was (indicating low production relative to comprehension). The more extreme the dissociation percentile (whether high or low), the larger the dissociation between the two domains, with the 50th percentile indicating no dissociation whatsoever relative to the normative sample.

Participants

The participants, 54 children with WMS and 39 children with DNS, were part of an ongoing longitudinal investigation of language acquisition. The WMS group was comprised of 30 boys and 24 girls, and the DNS group was comprised of 23 boys and 16 girls. For the datapoints reported in this study, participants ranged in age from 12 months to 76 months. Participants were recruited through the Williams Syndrome Association and the Down Syndrome Association (through advertisements in the national and regional newsletters), as well as through medical and other professional contacts. Because of the nature of the study, diagnostic information was acquired through parental report. Participants with DNS were included if parents indicated that diagnosis had been confirmed by chromosomal analysis. Participants with WMS were included if they had been diagnosed with WMS and did not evidence any confounding developmental abnormalities. Many of the children were administered both the Words and Gestures scale and the Words and Sentences scale of the CDI. This article presents cross-sectional data from the children's first datapoints on each scale, resulting in 74 datapoints for children with WMS and 58 datapoints for children with DNS.

Procedure

Through initial contact with parents, the child's approximate level of language development was ascertained to determine the appropriate CDI scale to administer. If parents indicated their child was producing fewer than 50 words and was not yet combining words, the Words and Gestures form was sent. If parents indicated that their child was producing more than 50 words or was combining words, the Words and Sentences form was sent. If it was not clear what level of language development the child had reached, parents were asked to complete both scales. Parents were mailed the CDI along with a self-addressed, postage-paid envelope for its return.

Instructions for completing the CDI were stated clearly on the form itself, and a cover letter accompanied the questionnaire and provided the telephone number of a researcher who assisted parents with any questions or comments regarding the questionnaire.

RESULTS

Whole-Sample Results Across Both Scales

As a first pass through the data, pooling all datapoints across both forms of the CDI enabled an examination of the sample as a whole. This is important because different patterns of results on the two forms potentially could be caused by sampling effects due to having the more advanced children receive the Words and Sentences scale. Because of differences between the forms, the only variable on which datapoints could be compared across forms was language age-equivalent scores based on the normative data for the CDI. After excluding datapoints for which a child had both the Words and Gestures scale and the Words and Sentences scale administered at the same age, our sample for this analysis contained 69 datapoints for children with WMS and 54 datapoints for children with DNS (9 datapoints were excluded, 5 for children with WMS and 4 for children with DNS, with the higher score retained for each child). Table 1 indicates characteristics of the sample.

A one-way analysis of variance (ANOVA) yielded no differences between the two syndrome groups overall in age, $F(1, 122) = 0.896$, *ns*. There was a trend for the children with WMS to produce larger absolute numbers of words, $F(1, 122) = 3.4, p = .07$; however, this could be related to the fact that there were more children with WMS than with DNS who completed the Words and Sentences scale, which has a higher ceiling for the number of words produced (maximum is 689 vs. 396 for the Words and Gestures scale). Thus, language age equivalence, based on the CDI normative sample, is a more appropriate anchor on which to compare the two groups. Analysis by one-way ANOVA yielded no difference between the two groups in overall language age equivalence, $F(1, 122) = 0.954$, *ns*. The individual datapoints depicted in Figure 1 illustrate that, overall, the two syndrome groups appear to produce similar numbers of words throughout the age range sampled here. It is important to note that although there is variability, these children are, on average, 20 months behind their normally developing peers with regard to expressive language.

Following the initial analysis of all datapoints combined, the two scales were analyzed separately to examine the more detailed information about language development that the CDI provides. Unless otherwise indicated, analyses were conducted using one-way ANOVA, with syndrome as the independent variable.

TABLE 1
Sample Characteristics: Both Communicative Developmental Inventories Scales Combined

Variable	Williams Syndrome[a]		Down Syndrome[b]	
	M	SD	M	SD
Age (months)	41	14	39	11
Word production	217	222	150	172
Language age (in months)	19.5	6.8	18.4	5.2
Language delay (in months)	21.5	12.4	20.3	8.9

Note. All comparisons not significant (at $p = .05$).
[a]$n = 69$; [b]$n = 54$.

Words and Gestures Scale: The Onset of Symbolic Communication

Overall findings.   A total of 66 datapoints initially were obtained for the Words and Gestures scale (34 for children with WMS and 32 for children with DNS). After excluding those children who were producing more than 300 words, considered to be the ceiling for this scale, 60 datapoints remained (32 WMS and 28 DNS). Table 2 describes characteristics of the sample both before and after this exclusion.

The analyses discussed here included only children producing 300 or fewer words on the CDI Words and Gestures scale. No significant group differences were found with regard to age, number of words comprehended, or number of words produced, $F(1, 59) = 0.37, 1.80$, and 0.07, respectively, *ns.* Group differences emerged, however, with regard to total number of gestures, $F(1, 59) = 9.9, p < .01$.

Language Production over Whole Sample

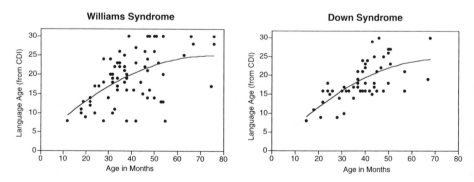

FIGURE 1   Word production across whole sample (both Communicative Development Inventory [CDI] forms combined). Language age is based on CDI normative data for word production.

TABLE 2
Sample Characteristics: Words and Gestures Scale

| | All Participants | | | | Production < 300 Words | | | |
| | Williams Syndrome[a] | | Down Syndrome[b] | | Williams Syndrome[b] | | Down Syndrome[c] | |
Variable	M	SD	M	SD	M	SD	M	SD
Age (months)	34	11.2	34	9.7	34	11.5	32	9.1
Word comprehension	173	115**	224	118	163	111	201	107
Word production	77	101	93	119	61	82	56	69.0
Gesture production	35	15*	47	14	34	14*	45	14.0
% Comprehension/Production	63	29.3	60	26	63	29.3	60	26
% Comprehension/Gesture	57	30.5*	79	20.2	55	30.5*	77	20.9
% Production/Gesture	56	32.7*	81	21.1	55	33*	80	22.1

Note: [a]$n = 34$. [b]$n = 32$. [c]$n = 28$.
$*p < .05$. $**p < .10$.

The children with DNS produced significantly more gestures than did the children with WMS (see Figure 2). The mean language age for the WMS group was 14.5 months, and the mean language age for the DNS group was 15.4 months, $F(1, 59) = 0.70$, *ns*. It is important to note that both groups of children were delayed relative to normal children, falling well below the 10th percentile according to the CDI normative sample (Figure 3).

Relation between components of early language development.   The relations among comprehension, production, and gesture in children with WMS and DNS also are informative because they may yield clues to mechanisms that may differentiate children with the two syndromes, either from one another or from normal children. As mentioned earlier, the CDI provides normative data for indexes of dissociation among these three components of early language, in the form of percentile scores that indicate where a given child ranks relative to the CDI normative sample. In addition to enabling one to look for potential dissociations among domains of language development, these percentile scores allow for an examination of the relations among various language parameters intraindividually, rather than relying on sample means.

Three dissociation percentile scores were examined for the Words and Gestures scale: (a) word production level given the child's word comprehension, (b) gesture level given the child's word comprehension, and (c) gesture level given the child's word production. Table 2 provides the means and standard deviations for these variables (some children, two with DNS and five with WMS, had missing values

Words and Gestures Scale Overall Results

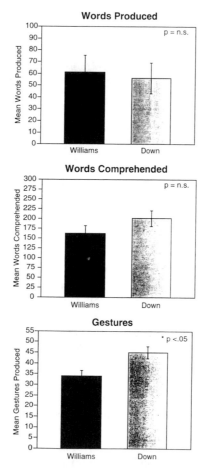

FIGURE 2   Mean words produced (top), words comprehended (middle), and gestures produced (bottom) for
children who completed the Communicative Development Inventory's Words and Gestures form.

for the production/comprehension variable because the dissociation percentiles
cannot be derived reliably for children near the floor or ceiling of the normative
tables). Results indicated that relative to normally developing children, on
average, children with WMS and DNS had similar relations between word
comprehension and word production, $F(1, 52) = 0.151$, *ns.* That is, relative to
normal children at the same comprehension levels, the WMS group was, on

Total Words Comprehended (Words and Gestures Scale)

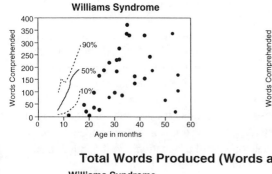
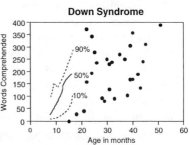

Total Words Produced (Words and Gestures Scale)

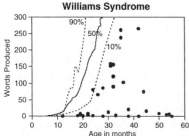
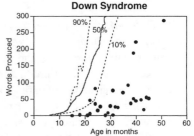

FIGURE 3 Individual datapoints from children who completed the Communicative Development Inventory's (CDI) Words and Gestures form. Words comprehended are depicted in the top two figures, words produced in bottom two figures. Solid and dashed lines indicate percentiles based on CDI normative data.

average, at the 63rd percentile for word production, and the DNS group was at the 60th percentile. Two-tailed binomial tests indicated that many more children in the WMS group were above the 50th percentile than would be expected by chance (21 of 27 were above the 50th percentile, $p = .004$), and somewhat more children in the DNS group were above the 50th percentile than would be expected by chance (18 of 26 were above the 50th percentile, $p = .05$). A chi-square analysis revealed no significant difference between groups on this parameter, $\chi^2(1, N = 53) = 0.5$, ns.

The relation between word comprehension and gestures, and between word production and gestures was different for the two syndrome groups, however. Results indicated that relative to normally developing children, children with DNS, on average, had significantly more gestures given their word comprehension and word production levels than did children with WMS, $F(1, 59) = 10.2$ and 11.3, respectively, $p < .01$, for both analyses. Furthermore, the children with DNS in this sample gestured more than most normal children do at similar comprehension and word production levels. The DNS group was, on average, at the 77th percentile for gestures relative to normal children at the same comprehension levels, and at the 80th percentile relative to children at the same production levels, whereas the WMS group was at the 55th percentile for gestures relative to normal children at the same comprehension and production levels. Two-tailed binomial tests indicated that many more children in the DNS group were above the 50th percentile on these variables than would be expected by chance (25 of 28 were above the 50th percentile, $p < .0001$), whereas no more children in the WMS group were above or below the 50th percentile than would be expected by chance (14 of 32 were below the 50th percentile, $p = ns$). A chi-square analysis revealed significant differences between groups on these parameters, $\chi^2(1, N = 60) = 8.03$ for both analyses, $p < .01$. Figure 4 depicts the relations among word production, word comprehension, and gesture for the two syndrome groups.

Differences between children producing fewer than 50 words and children producing more than 50 words. Because of the relatively large word production range in the samples, it is instructive to look at children in the earliest stages of word production (< 50 words) separately from those who have larger productive vocabularies (> 50 words). Productive vocabulary of 50 words was used as a cutoff because prior to this lexical level most children are at the one-word stage, which is considered to be a fairly homogeneous stage of language development (e.g., Nelson, 1973). As it turns out, results were different in the two

Relationships among Comprehension, Production, and Gesture

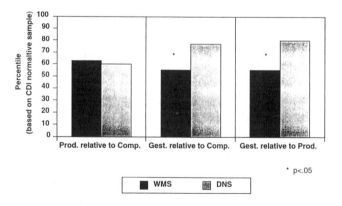

FIGURE 4   Relations among word comprehension, word production, and gesture production for Words and Gestures form. Percentile indicates mean dissociation percentile score based on Communicative Development Inventory (CDI) normative sample. Higher percentile scores indicate children were producing more words (or gestures) than were children in the CDI normative sample at the same levels of word comprehension (or word production). The 50th percentile is the mean for the CDI normative sample.

subsamples and were different from the sample as a whole. Table 3 lists characteristics of the two subsamples.

In the subsample of children with productive vocabularies of fewer than 50 words, those with DNS tended to comprehend more, $F(1, 36) = 3.8$, $p = .06$; produced significantly more words, $F(1, 36) = 14.4$, $p < .001$; and gestured more, $F(1, 36) = 8.6$, $p < .01$, than did the children with WMS. In contrast, in the subsample of children with productive vocabularies of more than 50 words, word comprehension and word production were not different in the two syndrome groups, $F(1, 22) = 0.846$ and 0.577, respectively, ns; and the participants with DNS still gestured significantly more than did those with WMS, $F(1, 22) = 13.1$, $p < .01$ (see Figure 5). These differential findings in the children producing fewer than 50 words versus those producing more than 50 words may have been influenced in part by the presence of a number of datapoints for children with WMS in our sample from older children who were still in the very first stages of language development. It is possible that these older children did not, in fact, have "classic" WMS (i.e., deletion of one copy of the elastin gene), or were more affected (i.e., may have a larger deletion). Studies are under way to tease apart such variability in the phenotypic presentation of WMS. Nevertheless, these findings suggest the possibility that in the earliest stages of language acquisition, children with DNS may have an advantage over children with WMS, an advantage that attenuates as the children acquire larger vocabularies (and subsequently begin to develop grammar). This finding, if replicated, would be extraordinary because it represents a complete reversal of the later linguistic profile of individuals with WMS and DNS.

TABLE 3

Words and Gestures Scale: Participants Producing Fewer versus Greater Than 50 Words

| | Production < 50 Words | | | | Production > 50 Words | | | |
| | Williams Syndrome[a] | | Down Syndrome[b] | | Williams Syndrome[c] | | Down Syndrome[d] | |
Variable	M	SD	M	SD	M	SD	M	SD
Age (months)	34.6	14.4	28.8	8.14	33	5.7**	38.5	7.5
Word comprehension	96	82.2*	154	96.7	260	65.9	286	67.2
Word production	5.3	6.1*	21.2	17.2	143	70.8	118.6	83.3
Gesture production	27	13*	40	15	44	8.4*	55	4.6
% Comprehension/Production	51.5	30.7	51.8	27.8	83	11.6	76	12.4
% Comprehension/Gesture	55	30.8**	72	23.3	57	31.3*	87	11.6
% Production/Gesture	55	33.2**	75	25.8	55	34*	90	6.9

[a]$n = 19$. [b]$n = 18$. [c]$n = 13$. [d]$n = 10$.
*$p < .05$. **$p < .10$.

Words and Gestures Scale: Children Producing Greater vs. Less than 50 Words

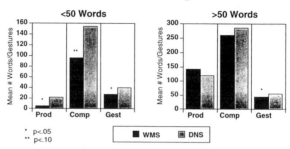

FIGURE 5   Mean levels of word production, word comprehension, and gesture production for children producing fewer than 50 words (left panel) and more than 50 words (right panel) on the Communicative Development Inventory's Words and Gestures form.

Summary of findings from Words and Gestures scale of the CDI.

Taken together, the current findings indicate there are minimal differences between children with WMS and children with DNS early in language development, with the notable exception of gestures, in which the communicative abilities of children with DNS outstrip those of children with WMS. At this earlier stage of communicative development, if anything, children with DNS may have an overall advantage over children with WMS, an advantage that fades as productive vocabulary increases. Although there is considerable variability, both groups of children are significantly delayed in their language development. We now turn to the next stage in language acquisition, the development of grammar. As we will see, it is here where the relative advantage shifts.

Words and Sentences Scale: The Emergence of Grammar

Overall findings, word production.   A total of 58 datapoints initially were obtained for the Words and Sentences scale (35 for children with WMS and 23 for children with DNS). After excluding those children who were producing more than 600 words, considered to be the ceiling for this scale, 48 datapoints remained (27 WMS and 21 DNS). Table 4 describes characteristics of the sample both before and after this exclusion.

Before excluding datapoints from those children at ceiling on the scale, results indicated that the children with WMS produced significantly more words than did those with DNS, $F(1, 57) = 4.41$, $p < .05$. Without these datapoints, this difference diminished to a trend, $F(1, 47) = 2.12$, $p = .15$. The children who completed this form of the CDI were, on average, 15 months older than those who completed the

TABLE 4
Sample Characteristics: Words and Sentences Scale

| | All Participants | | | | Production < 600 Words | | | |
| | Williams Syndrome[a] | | Down Syndrome[b] | | Williams Syndrome[c] | | Down Syndrome[d] | |
Variable	M	SD	M	SD	M	SD	M	SD
Age (months)	47	13.5	47	8.7	45	13	46.0	7.7
Word production	366	208*	252	195	280	152	215	159
Grammar complexity	13	14*	3	7.8	7	9.1*	1.2	2.2
% Production/Complexity	52	23.7*	32	22.2	52	23.7*	32	22.2
Mean length of utterance	6.2	4*	3.4	2.3	4.9	2.4*	2.9	.84
% Production/Mean length of utterance	64	26.3*	47	30.8	64	26.3*	47	30.8

[a]$n = 35$. [b]$n = 23$. [c]$n = 27$. [d]$n = 21$.
*$p < .05$.

Words and Gestures form, and they were producing, on average, 200 more words. The mean language age for the WMS group was 22.7 months, and the mean language age for the DNS group was 21.0 months, $F(1, 47) = 2.5$, ns. Thus, this more linguistically advanced group was still quite delayed in language development, with both syndrome groups falling well outside typical developmental limits. The analyses discussed next utilized those children producing 600 or fewer words on the CDI Words and Sentences scale. When the children at ceiling were included, the differences that emerged in grammatical development were magnified.

Grammatical development.   The CDI provides several measures of grammatical development. As described earlier, grammatical complexity is indexed by a checklist of 37 pairs of contrasting phrases for which the parent is asked to indicate "which sounds the most like what the child is producing now." The score on this measure of complexity is the total number of word pairs for which it is indicated the child currently is saying the more complex phrase of the pair. This measure of grammatical complexity has been shown to correlate strongly with laboratory measures of MLU in normally developing children ($r = .88$ at 20 months, $r = .76$ at 24 months; Fenson et al., 1994). As depicted in Figure 6, the children with WMS achieved significantly higher scores on this grammatical complexity measure of the CDI than did those with DNS, $F(1, 47) = 7.9, p < .01$.

Examining a child's MLU has a long history in the child language literature and has been used widely as an indicator of a child's level of grammar (Brown, 1973; Miller, 1981). Accordingly, another index of grammatical development on the CDI is the mean length in morphemes of the three longest utterances (M3L) that the

Words and Sentences Scale Overall Results

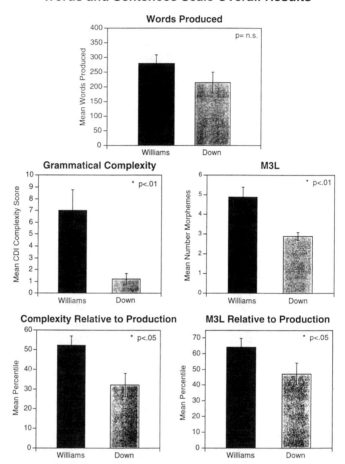

FIGURE 6   Mean levels of word production (top panel), grammatical complexity (middle left panel), and MLU (middle right panel) for children who completed the Communicative Development Inventory's (CDI) Words and Sentences form. Bottom two panels depict mean percentile dissociation scores for grammatical complexity relative to word production (left) and MLU relative to word production (right). Higher percentile scores indicate children had more grammatical complexity in their language (or longer MLUs) than did children in the CDI normative sample at the same levels of word production. The 50th percentile is the mean for the CDI normative sample.

child has produced recently according to the parent (see Fenson et al., 1994, for a discussion of this measure as an index of MLU). In our sample of children with WMS and DNS, strong differences in the M3L emerged (see Figure 6). Children with WMS produced significantly longer utterances than did their DNS counterparts, $F(1, 43) = 12.9, p < .001$, complementing the finding of more complexity in the speech of children with WMS as compared to children with DNS. Sample sentences from matched participants with WMS and DNS (see Figure 7) highlight these differences.

Relation between word production and grammar.   The   differences   in grammar between children with WMS and children with DNS are striking. Nevertheless, because of the trend for children with WMS to say more words than do those with DNS, it could be argued that this difference is what accounts for the difference in grammatical complexity and phrase length. Fortunately, the CDI provides normative data for indexes of dissociation between word production and the complexity measure, and between word production and M3L. As with the dissociation measures for the Words and Gestures scale, these variables allow for an intraindividual comparison of word production and grammar, which is more appropriate than using group means. Two such variables were used for examining grammatical development on the Words and Sentences scale, each expressed in the form of a percentile score: (a) sentence complexity given the child's word production and (b) M3L given the child's word production. As described earlier, the

Examples of 3 Longest Sentences

Williams Syndrome Age: 3 years; 3 months	Down Syndrome Age: 3 years; 10 months	Williams Syndrome Age: 3 years; 5 months	Down Syndrome Age: 4 years; 2 months
Production		Production	
610 Words	601 Words	434 Words	426 Words
Mamma, need *to* pick *up* toy*s*, vacuum floor.	Gonna go car.	Karen read *a* book *with* Daddy.	Baby go bye-bye.
I go *my* room get *one* book bring *out here*.	Matt want bottle.	Karen go *on* turtle *in the* pool.	Stop baby don't.
Please *have some* grape*s* *in my* cup *right now*.	Here-ya-go / Hold me.	*I* like *a* bottle please.	Three, four, five.

FIGURE 7   Sample sentences from children matched for word production on the Communicative Development Inventory's Words and Sentences form highlight differences between children with WMS and children with DNS in grammatical complexity and MLU.

dissociation percentiles indicate where a given child ranks compared to the normative CDI sample.

Table 4 provides the means and standard deviations for the dissociation variables, which are depicted graphically in Figure 6. As with the Words and Gestures scale, some children had missing values for these variables (7 children with DNS and 4 children with WMS for production/complexity, 1 child with DNS and 3 children with WMS for production/M3L) because the percentiles cannot be derived reliably for those near the floor or ceiling of the normative tables. Results indicated that relative to normally developing children, children with WMS displayed more grammatical complexity, $F(1, 36) = 6.9$, $p < .05$, and had a longer M3L, $F(1, 42) = 4.1, p < .05$, for their level of word production than did children with DNS (Figure 6). In fact, the children with WMS were, on average, no different than normally developing children with regards to the relation between the numbers of words they produced and their grammatical development; if anything, they tended to produce longer utterances than do most normally developing children at their lexical levels (16 of 23 children with WMS were above the 50th percentile for M3L relative to word production, two-tailed binomial probability = .06; 9 of 20 children with DNS were above the 50th percentile, $p = ns$; $\chi^2(1, N = 43) = 2.65$, $p = .10$. In contrast, the children with DNS were, on average, quite different from normally developing children in this regard; if anything, their speech was marked by far less grammatical complexity than is that of most normally developing children at their lexical levels (11 of 14 children with DNS were below the 50th percentile for grammatical complexity relative to word production, two-tailed binomial probability = .04; 13 of 23 children with WMS were above the 50th percentile, $p = ns$; $\chi^2(1, N = 37) = 4.37, p < .05$.

Combining words: An additional index of language development.
Combining words is a critical stage of language development in normal children, although little is known about this important linguistic milestone in atypically developing populations. The CDI assesses word combinations by having parents indicate if their child is combining words *often, sometimes,* or *not yet.* To create "dissociation percentiles" from the CDI normative database, percentile ranks for word production were generated for each "level" of word combinations (E. Bates, personal communication, January 18, 1994). In other words, a child who was combining words sometimes received a percentile rank based on how his or her word production level compared to the normative children who also were combining words sometimes. A high percentile rank indicated the child was producing more words than most normal children do when they are at the point where they are only combining words sometimes (i.e., the child may be considered to be a linguistically "late" combiner); conversely, a low percentile rank indicated that the

child was producing fewer words than most normal children do when they are at the point where they are combining words sometimes (i.e., the child may be considered to be a linguistically "precocious" combiner). Although these measures are admittedly rough, they enabled an examination of this important index of language development.

As it turned out, however, no differences were revealed in the relation between word combinations and word production levels in children with WMS and DNS, $F(1, 47) = 1.5$, ns. On average, children with WMS were at the 52nd percentile relative to normally developing children, whereas children with DNS were at the 42nd percentile. Two-tailed binomial tests indicated that fo r both groups, no more children were above or below the 50th percentile than expected by chance (16 of 27 children with WMS were above the 50th percentile, $p = ns$; 9 of 21 children with DNS were above the 50th percentile, $p = ns$); a chi-square analysis also revealed no significant difference between groups on this parameter, $\chi^2(1, N = 48) = 1.27$, ns.

Summary of findings with Words and Sentences scale of the CDI.　　In the group of older and more linguistically advanced children, those with WMS were producing more words than were those with DNS. This finding could be an extension of the results from the Words and Gestures scale, which indicated progressive improvement once language gets under way in children with WMS. It is important to note, however, when higher production levels were controlled for individually using normatively based dissociation percentile scores, significant differences in grammatical development persisted. Regardless of the number of words produced, children with WMS displayed grammatical skills far superior to their counterparts with DNS. Moreover, once they reached this level of linguistic development, the children with WMS appeared to display a normal grammatical developmental trajectory relative to word production, whereas the children with DNS continued to evidence delayed grammatical development (see Figure 8). It is quite intriguing that despite their relative language delay, children with WMS not only surpass children with DNS in grammatical development, but they may actually begin achieving grammatical milestones at a normal rate. Equally intriguing is the strong dissociation between lexical and grammatical development in children with DNS, suggesting a deviant pattern of language development that has not been reported for other groups. These differential patterns are explored in more detail.

DISCUSSION

In this study, we sought to gain information regarding the emerging linguistic abilities of children with WMS as compared to children with DNS against a large sample of normative data acquired through the CDI. The data reveals that, despite

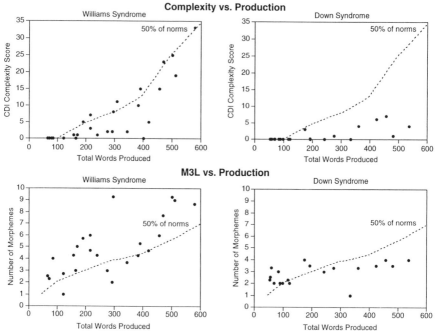

FIGURE 8   Individual datapoints from children who completed the Communicative Development Inventory's (CDI) Words and Sentences form. Grammatical complexity plotted against word production is depicted in the top two figures, MLU is plotted against word production in the bottom two figures. Dashed lines indicate the 50th percentile based on CDI normative data.

variability, initially both groups of children are delayed equally in the acquisition of words (an average delay of 2 years for both groups). First words appear in these children at about the same time that nonretarded children begin to combine words that they already have in their lexicon. This equivalently delayed language acquisition in children with WMS and DNS is surprising because it is not at all predictive of the later differences these two syndrome groups evidence in linguistic abilities.

Despite equivalent language delay, two intriguing differences emerged between groups: an early gesture advantage for the DNS group, and a later grammatical advantage for the WMS group. The proclivity of the children with DNS for gesturing was a very robust finding. A preference for gestural expression over verbal expression in children with DNS was noted previously in the literature (see Miller, 1987, for a brief discussion). However, because sign language is a communicative modality that is taught widely to young children with DNS (Miller, 1987, 1992), gestures on the CDI perhaps could have been confounded with the use of signs in this study. Nevertheless, it is possible that their apparent "overgesturing" may be a compensatory strategy used by the children with DNS for their delayed word production. Furthermore, that children with DNS may be relatively good at extracting sensory detail from the visual communicative context may relate to findings of significantly better visuospatial short-term memory in adolescents with DNS as compared to age- and IQ-matched adolescents with WMS (Wang & Bellugi, 1994).

In contrast, several investigators noted that children with WMS appear to be selectively "agestural"; they do not evidence the communicative gestures that normally developing children do prior to the onset of first words (Mervis & Bertrand, in press), and they display significantly fewer gestures during free play than do age-matched children with DNS and language-matched normal controls (Goodman, 1994, 1995). Furthermore, Thal et al. (1989) reported that two young children with WMS displayed dissociations in symbolic gesture that were unlike anything observed in normal children or children with specific language delay. That our study failed to find evidence of impoverished gesturing by children with WMS could be due to the way in which the CDI assesses gesturing, which may not be as sensitive as observational or laboratory measures. For example, the CDI assesses the number of gestures the children have in their "gestural lexicon," rather than the frequency of use of gestures.

Whereas children with DNS may compensate for their poverty of spoken language by the use of gestures, children with WMS may compensate by their affective style, tending to be overly engaging with social partners. For example, Bertrand, Mervis, Rice, and Adamson (1993) noted that children with WMS spend an inordinate amount of time focused on an adult partner's face, relative to normally developing children. Older children and adolescents with WMS similarly are captivated by social partners; their narratives are rich and complex, containing a variety of devices for engaging the listener (Bellugi, Jones, Harrison, Rossen, & Klima, 1995; Reilly et al., 1991). Individuals with WMS are not merely adept at "reading" affect from a social partner, however; recent studies demonstrate that both children and adults with WMS are able to infer another's emotions or mental state without the aid of affective prosodic or facial cues (Karmiloff-Smith et al., 1995; Singer, Delehanty, Reilly, & Bellugi, 1993). Whatever reasons may underlie the differences in gesture between individuals with WMS and those with DNS, a better understanding of the relation between language development and gesture (an area currently under investigation by many researchers) will help to elucidate the significance of these differences.

Regarding the early grammatical abilities of children with WMS, because our research found remarkably preserved grammatical skills in adolescents with WMS, we speculated how early in language development this advantage/preservation would evidence itself. This study provides evidence to support the preservation of early grammatical skills for children with WMS who have advanced beyond the earliest stages of language development, in marked contrast with their counterparts with DNS, who are much slower to develop grammar. Thus, even when no advantage was found in the total number of words produced by children with WMS, they were clearly superior to the children with DNS in their grammatical achievements. It is worth noting that the differences in language acquisition between children with WMS and those with DNS could have emerged at any point, including first words. The fact that grammatical development is what differentiates the two groups is an extremely provocative finding given their differing linguistic profiles evidenced later in life. It is also quite surprising that in the domain of language we observe an early profile of marked delay in children with WMS, which is not predictive of the rich and complex linguistic abilities seen later in development. Further studies of language development throughout childhood are under way to link this early profile with the adolescent and adult profile (Jones, Rossen, & Bellugi, 1995; Jones et al., 1993; Singer, Jones, & Bellugi, 1995).

Another trend in early language development that was noted by researchers and parents of children with WMS is that some of the children seem to say more than they actually comprehend. Although this study did not completely replicate these findings (the children with WMS in our sample were, on average, in the 63rd percentile for word production relative to word comprehension), we acquired numerous anecdotes from parents that do attest to this phenomenon. In fact, a number of parents indicated that on the CDI Words and Gestures form, in addition to the word checklist columns *understands* and *understands and says,* they need a separate column for *says, but does not understand!* Further investigation of this possibility clearly is needed.

Although this study contributes to existing knowledge about language acquisition in atypical populations by providing extensive information about language development in large samples of children with contrasting genetic disorders, there are several limitations that must be kept in mind. First, the cross-sectional nature of the study is able to uncover patterns of language development in the two populations, but it is not able to uncover developmental trajectories. Longitudinal studies, currently under way in our laboratory, will complement the findings presented herein and will enable us to better address developmental trajectories in the two syndrome groups. Second, the fact that these data are based on parental report rather than experimental observations could introduce some bias, particularly if parents have a tendency to overestimate their child's linguistic capabilities. Numerous studies, however, documented the validity of the CDI for assessing language development through parent report (see Fenson et al., 1994), and any parental bias that did exist would not be expected to differ between syndrome groups. Third, although the mailing procedure by which the data were collected enabled us to amass the largest sample of children with WMS ever studied, this technique has inherent limitations such as lack of control over accuracy of the data and homogeneity of the sample. We believe, however, that these limitations are offset by the large sample sizes, which are quite unusual for studies of such rare genetic syndromes. In fact, this study provides the largest sample of children with WMS in this developmental range that has ever been studied, providing crucial information that complements ongoing observational studies in our lab and in others. Furthermore, the basic developmental trends identified in this study are compatible with other observational studies (e.g., Chapman, 1995; Goodman, 1994, 1995; Mervis & Bertrand, in press; Mervis et al., 1995).

A final note pertains to unavoidable sampling issues facing a cross-sectional study such as this one. In determining where to "dive in" to our assay of language development in a syndrome as rare as WMS, we distributed the CDI to as many parents as we could contact. When we examined our returns, there appeared overall to be more variability in the WMS group than in the DNS group. This could be due to differences in base rates of the syndromes, such that a fuller range of the WMS population was sampled than of the DNS population. The WMS sample was drawn from a national sample, whereas the DNS sample was drawn from a local sample, which could also confer more variability on the WMS sample. Finally, although both syndromes have clear clinical manifestations, it is only in the past year that a genetic probe for WMS has become clinically available, which enables children to be identified as having WMS at an earlier age than was possible when we completed the collection of data for this study. Because of this, it is possible that some children in our sample may not have classic WMS; studies of variability in the phenotypic expression of WMS are currently under way, and they should help address sampling issues in the future. Longitudinal studies with matched samples of individuals with WMS and DNS are also under way to confirm and expand our findings.

CONCLUSIONS

This study represents one of the largest investigations to date of emerging language in two genetically based neurodevelopmental disorders, and it provides the largest group of young children with WMS ever studied. Despite striking differences in the linguistic abilities of adolescents and adults with WMS and DNS, the results presented here indicate that both syndrome groups are equally delayed in the onset of language. Early in language development, the groups are differentiated primarily by a proclivity for gesture production by the children with DNS. Later in language development, the groups are cleaved by grammatical development, where the children with WMS display a significant advantage over children with DNS. That individuals with WMS may display normally developing language with the advent of grammar, whereas those with DNS display what could almost be termed "agrammaticism," highlights the importance of grammar for human language and raises intriguing questions about genetic influences on brain and language development. This study is one of the first to examine these broader issues of language development in children with WMS as compared to children with DNS. Longitudinal studies are under way to assist in identifying developmental trajectories for patterns that may differentiate language acquisition processes in the two syndromes. The relation between gestures and words in WMS and DNS also is being examined in more detail, as are characteristics of the early lexicon in children with WMS and DNS as compared to normally developing children. Expanding these investigations to include other atypical populations, such as autistic children and children with focal lesions, will provide further opportunities to view variation within and across components of early language, thereby enhancing our understanding of language development and its neural underpinnings.

ACKNOWLEDGMENTS

This research was supported in part by grants from the National Institutes of Health to Ursula Bellugi (RO1 HD 26022 and 1 P01 HD 33113–01) and to Elizabeth Bates (P50 NS22343 and P01 DC01289), a grant from the Oak Tree Philanthropic Foundation to Ursula Bellugi, and a grant from the March of Dimes Foundation to the Salk Institute.

Special thanks to the parents of children with Williams syndrome and Down syndrome who participated in this study, as well as to the Williams Syndrome Association and the Down Syndrome Association. Our thanks also to Judy Goodman, Valerie Loewe, Paul Wang, Judy Reilly, and Edward S. Klima for their help and valuable comments.

REFERENCES

Beeghly, M., & Cicchetti, D. (1987). An organizational approach to symbolic development in children with Down syndrome. In D. Cicchetti & M. Beeghly (Eds.), *Atypical symbolic development* (pp. 5–30). San Francisco: Jossey-Bass.

Beeghly, M., Weiss-Perry, B., & Cicchetti, D. (1990). Beyond sensorimotor functioning: Early communicative and play development of children with Down syndrome. In D. Cicchetti & M. Beeghly (Eds.), *Children with Down syndrome: A developmental perspective* (pp. 329–368). New York: Cambridge University Press.

Bellugi, U., Bihrle, A., Jernigan, T., Trauner, D., & Doherty, S. (1990). Neuropsychological, neurological, and neuroanatomical profile of Williams syndrome. *American Journal of Medical Genetics, S6*, 115–125.

Bellugi, U., Bihrle, A., Neville, H., Jernigan, T., & Doherty, S. (1992). Language, cognition and brain organization in a neurodevelopmental disorder. In M. Gunnar & C. Nelson (Eds.), *Developmental behavioral neuroscience: The Minnesota Symposia on Child Psychology* (Vol. 24, pp. 201–232). Hillsdale, NJ: Lawrence Erlbaum Associates, Inc.

Bellugi, U., Jones, W., Harrison, D., Rossen, M. L., & Klima, E. S. (1995, March). *Discourse in two genetically-based syndromes with contrasting brain anomalies.* Paper presented at the meeting of the Society for Research in Child Development, Indianapolis, IN.

Bellugi, U., Wang, P., & Jernigan, T. (1994). Williams syndrome: An unusual neuropsychological profile. In S. Broman & J. Grafman (Eds.), *Atypical cognitive deficits in developmental disorders: Implications for brain function* (pp. 23–56). Hillsdale, NJ: Lawrence Erlbaum Associates, Inc.

Bertrand, J., Mervis, C. B., Rice, C. E., & Adamson, L. (1993, March). *Development of joint attention by a toddler with Williams syndrome.* Paper presented at the Conference on Research and Theory in Mental Retardation and Developmental Disabilities, Gatlinburg, TN.

Brown, R. (1973). *A first language: The early stages.* Cambridge, MA: Harvard University Press.

Chapman, R. S. (1993, July). *Longitudinal change in language production of children and adolescents with Down syndrome.* Paper presented at the Sixth International Congress for the Study of Child Language, Trieste, Italy.

Chapman, R. S. (1995). Language development in children and adolescents with Down syndrome. In P. Fletcher & B. MacWhinney (Eds.), *The handbook of child language* (pp. 641–663). Cambridge, MA: Blackwell.

Ewart, A. K., Morris, C. A., Atkinson, D., Weishan, J., Sternes, K., Spallone, P., Stock, A. D., Leppert, M., & Keating, M. T. (1993). Hemizygosity at the elastin locus in a developmental disorder, Williams syndrome. *Nature Genetics, 5,* 11–16.

Fenson, L., Dale, P., Reznick, S., Bates, E., Thal, D. & Pethick, S. (1994). Variability in early communicative development. *Monographs of the Society for Research in Child Development, 59*(5, Serial No. 242).

Fenson, L., Dale, P., Reznick, S., Thal, D., Bates, E., Hartung, J., Pethick, S., & Reilly, J. (1993). *MacArthur Communicative Development Inventories: Technical manual.* San Diego, CA: Singular Publishing Group.

Fowler, A. E. (1990). Language abilities in children with Down syndrome: Evidence for a specific syntactic delay. In D. Cicchetti & M. Beeghly (Eds.), *Children with Down syndrome: A developmental perspective* (pp. 302–328). New York: Cambridge University Press.

Fowler, A. E. (1993, July). *Phonological limits on reading and memory in young adults with Down syndrome.* Paper presented at the Sixth International Congress for the Study of Child Language, Trieste, Italy.

Goodman, J. (1994). Language acquisition and purported cognitive correlates: Clues from Williams syndrome. *Dissertation Abstracts International, 54*(01), 4417B.

Goodman, J. (1995). Language acquisition in children with Williams syndrome [Abstract]. *Genetic Counseling, 6,* 167–168.

Jernigan, T. L., Bellugi, E., Sowell, E., Doherty, S., & Hesselink, J. R. (1993). Cerebral morphological distinctions between Williams and Down syndromes. *Archives of Neurology, 50,* 186–191.

Jones, W., Rossen, M. L., & Bellugi, U (1995). Distinct developmental trajectories of cognition in Williams syndrome [Abstract]. *Genetic Counseling, 6,* 178–179.

Jones, W., Singer, N., Rossen, M., & Bellugi, U. (1993, November). *Fractionations of higher cognitive functions in Williams syndrome: Developmental trajectories.* Paper presented at the annual meeting of the American Speech–Language–Hearing Association, Anaheim, CA.

Karmiloff-Smith, A., Klima, E. S., Bellugi, U., Grant, J., & Baron-Cohen, S. (1995). Is there a social module? Language, face processing, and theory of mind in subjects with Williams syndrome. *Journal of Cognitive Neuroscience, 7,* 196–208.

Mervis, C. B., & Bertrand, J. (in press). Relations between cognition and language: A developmental perspective. In L. B. Adamson & M. A. Romski (Eds.), *Research on communication and language disorders: Contributions to theories of language development.* New York: Paul Brookes.

Mervis, C. B., Bertrand, J., Robinson, B. F., Armstrong, S. C., Klein, B. P., Turner, N. D., Baker, D. E., & Reinberg, J. (1995, April). *Early language development of children with Williams syndrome.* Paper presented at the biennial meeting of the Society for Research in Child Development, Indianapolis, IN.

Miller, J. F. (1981). *Assessing language production in children.* Baltimore: University Park Press.

Miller, J. F. (1987). Language and communication characteristics of children with Down syndrome. In S. P. Pueschel, C. Tingey, J. E. Rynders, A. C. Crocker, & D. M. Crutcher (Eds.), *New perspectives on Down syndrome* (pp. 233–262). Baltimore: Paul Brookes.

Miller, J. F. (1992). Development of speech and language in children with Down Syndrome. In I. T. Lott & E. E. McCoy (Eds.), *Down syndrome: Advances in medical care* (pp. 39–50). New York: Wiley-Liss.

Morris, C. A. (1995). The search for the genetic etiology of Williams syndrome and supravalvular aortic stenosis [Abstract]. *Genetic Counseling, 6,* 153–155.

Nelson, K. (1973). Structure and strategy in learning to talk. *Monographs of the Society for Research in Child Development, 38*(1–2, Serial No. 149).

Reilly, J. S., Klima, E. S., & Bellugi, U. (1991). Once more with feeling: Affect and language in atypical populations. *Developmental Psychopathology, 2,* 367–391.

Singer, N. G., Delehanty, S. G., Reilly, J. S., & Bellugi, U. (1993, March). *Development of emotional inferences in Williams syndrome.* Paper presented at the biennial meeting of the Society for Research in Child Development, New Orleans, LA.

Singer, N. G., Jones, W., & Bellugi, U. (1995, March). *Trajectories of language and cognitive development in children with Williams and Down syndromes.* Paper presented at the meeting of the California Speech–Hearing Association, San Diego, CA.

Thal, D., Bates, E., & Bellugi, U. (1989). Language and cognition in two children with Williams syndrome. *Journal of Speech and Hearing Research, 32,* 489–500.

Udwin, O., & Yule, W. (1990). Expressive language of children with Williams syndrome. *American Journal of Medical Genetics, S6:* 108–114.

Wang, P. P., & Bellugi, U. (1993). Williams syndrome, Down syndrome, and cognitive neuroscience. *American Journal of Diseases of Children, 147,* 1246–1251.

Wang, P. P., & Bellugi, U. (1994). Evidence from two genetic syndromes for a dissociation between verbal and visual–spatial short-term memory. *Journal of Clinical and Experimental Neuropsychology, 16,* 317–322.

Wang, P. P., Hesselink, J. R., Jernigan, T. L., Doherty, S., & Bellugi, U. (1992). The specific neurobehavioral profile of Williams syndrome is associated with neocerebellar hemispheric preservation. *Neurology, 42,* 1999–2002.

DEVELOPMENTAL NEUROPSYCHOLOGY, *13*(3), 371–396

Early Language Development in Children With Prenatal Exposure to Stimulant Drugs

Suzanne Dixon
University of California, San Diego

Donna Thal
San Diego State University
University of California, San Diego

Julie Potrykus
Children's Hospital Research Center, San Diego

Tracie Bullock Dickson
University of Maryland

Jill Jacoby
San Diego State University

Early language development was assessed in 60 children of substance-abusing mothers (CSAMs) born at term and without other pre- or postnatal complications. The MacArthur Communicative Developmental Inventory was used in 2 studies: laboratory measures of a subset of children in Study 2 replicated and extended the results of Study 1. Results showed significant delays in all aspects of language measured for a sizable proportion of the CSAMs. Neither type of drug nor general developmental status predicted language ability. The small number of children in birth homes showed the best performance on all language measures; those in foster care,

---

Requests for reprints should be sent to Suzanne Dixon, University of California, San Diego, San Diego, CA 92093.

including relative care, showed the worst. In both studies, older CSAMs did more poorly than younger ones.

Prenatal use of the stimulant drugs cocaine and methamphetamine affects from 5% to 12% of pregnancies nationwide (Chasnoff, Landress, & Barrett, 1990; Dominguez, Vila-Coro, Slopis, & Bohan, 1991; J. L. Mills & Robins, 1993; National Institute of Drug Abuse, 1989). The central nervous system appears to be a particular target of these drugs for some neonates (Chasnoff, Bussey, Savich, & Stack, 1986; Dixon & Bejar, 1989; Volpe, 1992), and the long-term developmental consequences of this exposure are only beginning to be known. Early reports of temperament difficulties (Kaltenbach, Nathanson, & Finnigan, 1989), poor play organization (Howard, Beckwith, Rodning, & Kropewske, 1989), and behavior problems (Billing, Erickson, Sleneroth, & Zetterstrom, 1985; Singer, Farkas, & Kliegman, 1992) in children of substance-abusing mothers (CSAMs)[1] have suggested underlying difficulties with behavioral organization that could adversely affect cognitive and linguistic development (Bentz, Hansen, McEvoy, Steward, & Banon, 1993; Fried, O'Connell, & Watkinson, 1992; Howard, 1989; McEvoy & Dixon, 1993). Assessments of general development at 2 years of age suggest that a subgroup may be vulnerable to delays and that lower developmental quotients are related to smaller head circumference (Chasnoff, Griffith, Freier, & Murray, 1992). This suggests a neurologic basis for these delays. Griffith, Chasnoff, Gillogby, and Fria (1990) reported delays in average verbal reasoning in a group of 2-year-old CSAMs who were compared to non-drug-exposed controls of the same age from the same community. The differences increased at the 3-year assessment of this same group, with increasing delays in the verbal domain in spite of IQ measures in the normal range (Griffith, Azuma, & Chasnoff, 1994). These data suggest that particular patterns of developmental disorder, similar to those seen in children with specific language impairment, may occur with higher than normal frequency in CSAMs. A similar finding was noted by Dutch investigators (van Baar & de Graaf, 1994). A Canadian study also demonstrated language delay in a carefully matched sample of adopted cocaine-exposed children (Nulman et al., 1994). At the least, these results suggest that early language and cognitive development needs to be examined carefully in this group of children. Clinical work is compatible with this hypothesis; several centers have noted increasing numbers of children presenting with language delay who have drug exposure as a prenatal factor.

The frequent association between early language delay and later learning difficulties in children with specific language impairment (Bishop & Adams, 1990;

---

[1]We use the acronym *CSAMs* to refer to children with prenatal exposure to the stimulant drugs cocaine, methamphetamine, or both.

Bishop & Edmundson, 1987; Silva, McGee, & Williams, 1983) suggests the careful evaluation of language in children with prenatal exposure to stimulant drugs may identify a subgroup of children who need more in-depth learning evaluations and educational support.

In this article we report two studies of such children. In the first study, we used the MacArthur Communicative Development Inventory (CDI) to examine language and gesture in a sample of CSAMs. The children in Study 1 were seen clinically in the first 3 years of life. In the second study, we used a combination of the same parental report and laboratory measures of language and gesture on a small subset of CSAMs chosen for stable homes of rearing and for the absence of other known adverse influences on development. Our goal was to provide preliminary descriptions of several aspects of language development using a cross-sectional design.

STUDY 1

Method

Participants

Sixty children with English as their only language and with prenatal stimulant drug exposure (cocaine or methamphetamine) were identified in several ways from the clinical log of the first author. Some had positive toxicology assessments at birth and were asked later to participate in developmental studies of language and cognition based on the presence of this risk factor. Some of these families participated for a single datapoint; others were inducted into a longitudinal study. Only one CDI result per child is reported here, the second in cases of multiple assessments. Other children with the same risk factor were seen in the Special Babies clinic at the University of California, San Diego Medical Center. Children with previously identified developmental difficulties or with other risk conditions were excluded. Of this sample, 38% were non-Hispanic Whites, 48% were African American, and the rest were of mixed ethnicity.

All children had a general physical examination, including anthropometric evaluations. A history that included medical, developmental, demographic, and social factors was taken; and children were reviewed for the presence of other factors that might adversely affect development. Participants were excluded if any additional risk factors were present. These included prematurity, congenital syphilis, perinatal anoxia, fetal alcohol syndrome, severe sepsis, postnatal hospitalization, child abuse, chronic illness, or other potentially handicapping conditions. Most children (84%) were in foster or adoptive care and had been placed there at birth. The remainder remained with their birth mothers, who were in recovery. No children were included who lived in homes with ongoing substance abuse.

Procedure

Language assessment. The child's primary care provider, a parent or guardian, was asked to complete the CDI: Words and Gestures (henceforth referred to as the Infant form) for children between the ages of 8 and 16 months, and the CDI: Words and Sentences (henceforth referred to as the Toddler form) for children over 16 months (Fenson et al., 1993). The CDI is a parental report instrument designed to elicit information about language development in children between 8 and 30 months of age. The Infant form assesses vocabulary comprehension, vocabulary production, and gesture production; the Toddler form assesses vocabulary production and, in those children who combine words, utterance length and early grammar. The CDI has been standardized on more than 1,800 normal children and has been used widely in research on normal and atypical populations, including those from a range of socioeconomic statuses (Bates & Thal, 1991; Bates, Thal, Whitesell, Fenson, & Oakes, 1989; Dale, 1991; Dale, Bates, Reznick, & Morisset, 1989; Fenson et al., 1993; Thal, Marchman, et al., 1991). The ethnicity of the norming population was comparable to the 1990 Census (Bureau of the Census, 1991) figures. However, significantly fewer mothers in the CDI sample had not completed high school, suggesting that the norms should be applied with caution to children from low-education and low-income families.

For children whose parents completed the Infant form, the number of words produced, number of words comprehended, and number of gestures produced were calculated. For children whose parents completed the Toddler form, the number of words produced, number of children producing word combinations, mean of the three longest utterances produced (M3L), and a grammatical complexity score were calculated. All scores were converted to percentiles to allow for across-age comparisons and comparison to the norming group (Fenson et al., 1993).

Clinical evaluation. A developmental assessment was completed on 32 children using the Revised Developmental Screening Inventory (Knobloch, Stevens, & Malone, 1980) and on 28 children using the Bayley Scales of Infant Development (Bayley, 1969). The Revised Developmental Screening Inventory contains both linguistic and nonlinguistic measures and specifies a classification of development as *normal, questionable,* or *abnormal;* however, language level does not enter into this summary classification. This three-part scale was used here. Scoring of the Bayley Mental Developmental Index was modified to classify children in these same categories in the following way: 85 = normal, 70–85 = questionable, below 70 = abnormal. Long-term foster care and adoptive home placements were classified together. Permanent placement before 6 weeks with the birth parent(s) was classified as a birth home of rearing. Stable placement with relatives and nonrelative foster care were noted in the other cases.

The type of drug exposure was determined by a review of the medical record regarding positive maternal toxicology during pregnancy, at delivery in the mother or the infant, or both. Although it was assumed that most, if not all, children were exposed to nicotine and alcohol as well as the stimulant drugs, children with alcohol as the primary drug of exposure and children who had features of fetal alcohol syndrome were excluded from this study.

The results from the group as a whole are described first. Then the group is divided into three age cohorts: those between 8 and 16 months old, those 17 to 24 months, and those 25 to 30 months of age. Children who were 8 to 16 months old were evaluated using the CDI Infant form. The rest of the children were evaluated with the CDI Toddler form.

Overall this sample represents the experience of a specialist clinician with children born at term who presented with the risk condition of prenatal stimulant drug exposure (CSAMs) but with no other biomedical factors that might impinge on development and no other previously identified developmental concerns.

Results

Sample Characteristics

The mean age for the whole group was 20.8 months (see Table 1), ranging from 8 to 30 months, and there were equivalent numbers of boys and girls. Children with prenatal amphetamine exposure constituted 43% of the sample, and those with cocaine exposure constituted the rest. About a fourth of the children with prenatal exposure to cocaine also were exposed to heroin. The exposure history was equivalent in all three age cohorts. Developmental status was judged to be normal in 73% of the sample, 10% had abnormal development, and 17% had results in the questionable range. Developmental status was not related to the specific drug to which the children had been exposed or to the homes in which they were being reared.

Most of the participants were not living with their birth families. Half the children resided in adoptive homes, 37% were in a fostering arrangement (17%, or about half the children in foster care, were with relatives), and 13% were with their birth mothers.

A higher proportion of the children in birth homes were exposed to amphetamine (62%), whereas only 20% of those in relative care had this exposure as opposed to cocaine; however, this difference was not significant. The age, sex, and general developmental status did not differ significantly across the place of residence.

TABLE 1
Characteristics of Sample Population in Study 1 by Age Group

	All	8–16 months	17–24 months	25–30 months
N	60	19	19	22
Age (months)	20.8 ± 6.8	11.8 ± 1.2	21.8 ± 1.9	27.6 ± 1.8
% normal development	73.3	68.4	94.7	59.1
% out-of-home placement	86.7	79.9	89.5	90.9
% amphetamine exposure	48.3	42.1	47.4	40.9

Language Development

Table 2 presents the language percentile scores for the CSAMs group as a whole and broken down into the three age groups. The word production levels for 23% of the children were so low that they did not meet the minimum (5th percentile) for percentile assignment. As a result, percentile scores could not be assigned to these children. This proportion was similar in the two younger cohorts (14 children in the 8- to 16-month-old group and 16 children in the 17- to 24-month-old group). This number was considerably higher in the oldest cohort, comprising nearly a third of this group. For CSAMs who produced enough words to allow scoring of the CDI, the mean percentile for word production was near the average of the norming sample, but there was greater variation.

8 to 16 months.   For children in the youngest cohort who met the minimum for percentile assignment, word production, word comprehension, and gesture production, percentiles were near the mean for the norming group. However, 21% of this group did not meet the minimum criterion for word production, 10% did not meet the criterion for word comprehension, and 5% fell below the 5th percentile for gesture production, suggesting serious delay for some of the children in this age group. Comprehension and production percentiles were correlated significantly (r = .55, p < .04), suggesting the language delays seen in these children reflect difficulty with comprehension as well as production.

17 to 30 months.   Two subgroups of children received the Toddler form. As noted earlier, a larger proportion of the older (25–30 month) cohort failed to meet the percentile assignment criterion. In addition, for those in the older group whose vocabulary was large enough to be assigned a percentile rank, scores were lower than were those for children in the 17- to 24-month age group.

Approximately a fourth of the 17- to 24-month-old cohort did not reach the percentile assignment criterion for M3L. For the remaining children, M3L was comparable to that of the norming group. For the oldest cohort, nearly half did not

TABLE 2
Scores on the MacArthur Communicative Development Inventory in Study 1 by Age Group

		Age		
	All	8–16 months	17–24 months	25–30 months
Production				
Mean percentile	41.9 ± 26.1	49.0 ± 29.4	43.5 ± 24.1	32.9 ± 23.7
% below 5th percentile	23.3	21.1	15.8	31.8
Comprehension				
Mean percentile	na	43.9 ± 28.6	na	na
		(n = 17)		
% below 5th percentile		10.5		
Gestures—Total				
Mean percentile	na	46.5 ± 34.4	na	na
		(n = 18)		
% below 5th percentile		5.3		
Mean length of three longest utterances				
Mean percentile	39.8 ± 26.4	na	50.4 ± 22.0	27.4 ± 26.6
	(n = 45)		(n = 14)	(n = 12)
% below 5th percentile	25.0		26.3	45.5
Sentence complexity				
Mean percentile	31.4 ± 24.1	na	43.0 ± 21.4	21.4 ± 22.1
	(n = 41)		(n = 19)	(n = 22)
% below 5th percentile	24.0		26.3	45.5

Note. Scores are the mean percentile for the group of children who scored above the 5th percentile. Percentage of children with scores below the 5th percentile are immediately below each score. Different *n*s reflect differing numbers of participants scoring below the 5th percentile. *na* = not applicable.

meet the 5th percentile for M3L, and the average performance for those who did was near the lowest quartile. Relative sentence complexity measures were similar to the M3L: the 17- to 24-month-old cohort was close to the norming group mean, and the older cohort was near the lower quartile. Relative M3L, as a percentile ranking, also was related significantly negatively to age, regression $F(1, 24) = 6.32$, $p = .02$. The relative length of utterance was shorter for the oldest cohort, and the correlation of this measure with age was negative and significant ($r = -0.46$, $p = .04$).

This negative relation with age was examined using a regression analysis on the language measures versus age across all age groups. Word production percentile showed a negative relation with age, regression $F(1, 44) = 3.48$; $p = .06$, indicating a trend toward significantly lower performance in the older group.

The general lower language competency in the drug-exposed group as a whole can be characterized by the quartile splits (see Figure 1). In word production, 50% of the population were at, below, or in the first quartile, whereas only 8% were in

MacArthur CDI:Toddler
Vocabulary Production

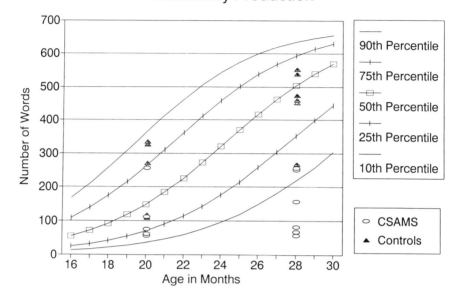

FIGURE 1   Percentage of children with prenatal exposure to stimulant drugs who fell within the first (lowest 25%), second (25th to 50th percentile), third (50th to 75th percentile), and fourth (highest 25%) quartiles on the norms for the MacArthur Communicative Development Inventory.

the top quartile. The M3L distributions showed that 61% of the sample were at or below the lowest quartile, and only 8% were in the highest. Although lower scores were seen in all three cohorts, they were most dramatic in the oldest group. Not one child in the 25- to 30-month-old group scored in the highest quartile on any language measure; 64% were in or below the 1st quartile on word production, and 82% were at that level in M3L and sentence complexity.

Some atypical relations between aspects of language measures were seen in the older cohort. In that group, only three CSAMs produced fewer than 50 words, and two did not combine words, appearing to be significantly delayed in all areas of language. However, of the 19 children who produced more than 50 words in this age group, there were still 6 (32%) who did not combine words. Using a more conservative vocabulary level of 75 words as the cutoff for expecting children to combine, the proportion of CSAMs who did not combine still did not decrease substantially. Five, or 26% of the children in the oldest cohort, did not produce word combinations at this vocabulary level. In contrast, in the norming sample, over 97% of children combined words at this age, and nearly 80% of all children did so at a vocabulary level of 75 words. The overall percentage of noncombiners among the CSAMs in this age and vocabulary range exceeded expectations by more than sixfold.

Association Between Language and Demographic Variables

Analysis of variance was used to compare the age-based groups on the type of drug to which they had been exposed. No significant relation was found between particular drug of exposure and any measure of language, including expressive vocabulary (raw score or percentile), M3L, and sentence complexity (across the whole age range or within any age subgroup). Analysis of groups by developmental status also revealed no significant difference for production vocabulary (in the whole group or in any age cohort) or for gesture production (in the youngest age group).

The home of rearing was associated significantly with the CDI results in the two older groups. To obtain a better understanding of this relation, the children were redivided by home of rearing rather than age. Analyses were redone for all of the demographic variables and language variables using analysis of variance for continuous variables and chi-square for categorical variables. These results are presented in Table 3.

As can be seen in the top of Table 3, there was no significant relation between home of rearing and any of the other demographic variables including age, drug of exposure, sex, or developmental status, although only a small number of children (8) were in the birth home, and nearly two thirds of this group had amphetamine exposure. There was a clear and significant relation between home placement and language scores. Specifically, the sentence complexity scores varied significantly in various homes of rearing, $F(3, 40) = 2.71, p = .05$], and M3L showed a similar trend, $F(3, 25) = 2.80, p = .06$. Post hoc analyses ($p < .05$) showed that children in the birth homes did significantly better than did those in the out-of-home placements.

Although the difference between groups was not significant for word production, the direction of the effect was the same. Of the 30 children in adoptive care, 6, or 20%, fell below the 5th percentile in vocabulary. The average performance of the rest was at about the 30th percentile. Of the 10 children in relative care, 4, or 40%, scored below the 5th percentile in vocabulary, and the expressive language level of the rest was near average. Of the 12 children in foster care, a fourth had unscorable vocabulary levels, and the rest had a vocabulary near the mean. Eight children were with their birth parent(s). Only 1 fell below the 5th percentile in vocabulary. Mean vocabulary was above the 50th percentile for the rest of the birth-home group.

Because the effect for home of rearing originally was identified in the two older cohorts, the effects of home placement was reanalyzed for each of those groups separately. Within the oldest cohort (25–30 months), but not the middle cohort

TABLE 3
Home of Rearing and Demographic Factors and Language Scores on the MacArthur
Communicative Development Inventory (CDI)

	Home of Rearing				
	Adoptive	Relative	Foster	Birth	p value
Demographic variables					
N	30	10	12	8	
Age 21.8 ± 6.7	20.7 ± 6.5	19.6 ± 7.0	18.9 ± 7.7	ns	
% amphetamine	50.0	20.0	33.0	62.5	ns
% female	63.0	25.0	41.7	50.0	ns
Development					
% normal	80.0	80.0	50.0	75.0	ns
% questionable	16.0	10.0	16.7	25.0	ns
% abnormal	3.3	10.0	33.0	0.0	ns
Language variables					
N	24	6	9	7	
Word production	33.4 ± 23.5	47.4 ± 31.5	52.5 ± 28.9	52.5 ± 21.1	ns
% below 5th percentile	20.0	40.0	25.0	12.5	
CDI Toddler form only					
n	15	2	5	4	
M3L	31.5 ± 23.1	58.0 ± 24.0	35.4 ± 22.9	67.4 ± 28.7	<.06
% below 5th percentile	23.0	80.0	25.0	0.0	
Sentence complexity	27.3 ± 24.6	20.7 ± 17.7	39.7 ± 22.5	56.3 ± 18.0	<.006
% below 5th percentile	22.0	7.0	8.0	0.0	

Note. Language scores are the mean percentile for the group of children who scored above the 5th percentile. Percentage of children with scores below the 5th percentile are immediately below each score. M3L = mean length of utterances. ns = not significant.

(17–24 months), the associations were similar to those of the group as a whole. M3L and home of rearing were associated, $F(3, 11) = 9.50, p = .005$, as was sentence complexity, $F(3, 21) = 5.98, p = .005$, in this oldest cohort. Post hoc analyses showed that children in the birth homes did significantly better in these two measures than did the other groups. Thus, the effect for home of rearing on language appears to come predominantly from the 25- to 30-month, the oldest, cohort.

Reporting biases in both directions were possible here, with birth mothers possibly being less experienced with child observation or overreporting their own child's competency. Foster parents, including relatives, may have underreported because of multiple time demands limiting observation, or conversely, may have been more accurate because of experience and specific concerns regarding development.

Discussion

These results suggest that language is a vulnerable area of development in a significant proportion of CSAMs. About 5 times the expected number fell below the 5th percentile on several measures of language at all ages. An atypically large proportion of children between 8 and 16 months of age also fell below the 5th percentile for language comprehension and gesture production, and this suggests they are at risk for later language delay (see Thal, Bates, Goodman, & Jahn-Samilo, this issue).

Children between 25 and 30 months of age showed poorer relative performance than did younger children, and they seemed to have difficulty developing word combinations. This was evident even in children who had vocabulary sizes at which one would expect to see the emergence of word combinations. In addition, for the older group, M3L and grammatical complexity was poorer than for those in the norming population. These data, in conjunction with other studies that reported increased delay with increased age in CSAMs (Griffith et al., 1994; van Baar & de Graaf, 1994) suggest the possibility that, at the stage of development of grammar and more complex sentence structures, many children with stimulant drug exposure have an especially hard time. Longitudinal studies are needed to determine if the findings in this study are due to subtle sample differences that could affect language performance, alone or in combination with other factors.

Home of rearing was the only demographic variable associated with language development, and only in children older than 25 months, the period during which grammar emerges. Although home placements for children with prenatal exposure to stimulant drugs were neither random nor systematic, this observation raises questions about the role home environment played in our results. Out-of-home placement, particularly foster care, may provide less consistent support for language development. Alternatively, mothers who were allowed to keep their drug-exposed babies may have had less severe addiction, resulting in less exposure and lower risk for the child. Mothers in stable recovery also may have been more focused on their child's development, either supporting it optimally or inflating their perception of the behavior. An additional, and quite different, explanation also is possible. Perhaps the home environment has an influence on the effectiveness of parental report, and the results reported in this article reflect reporting bias rather than the true language abilities of the children. Further studies that include behavioral as well as parent report measures across different homes of rearing are necessary to disentangle these possibilities. We look at these factors in Study 2.

STUDY 2

In the second study we evaluated the language development of a subset of children, comparing the MacArthur CDI information with detailed laboratory observations of language and gesture. This served to replicate and expand the results of Study 1.

Method

Participants

Twelve children with documented prenatal exposure to cocaine, methamphetamine, or both were identified from the clinical files of the first author as described previously. Six of the children were 20 months old, and 6 were 28 months old. All 12 were in stable, long-term foster or adoptive middle-class homes as indicated by a Hollingshead score of 3 or above (Hollingshead, 1965). This intentionally biased the sample toward optimal language development, minimizing the impact of the chaotic environments and changes often experienced by CSAMs. The clinical records of these children were reviewed as described in Study 1, and children were excluded from this study using the same criteria. Judgment of normal development was derived from the Revised Developmental Screening Inventory (Knobloch et al., 1980) and from a developmental history questionnaire completed by the caretaker at the time of the experimental observation. The questionnaire requested information about the presence of major health problems, frequent ear infections, and hearing problems. Children with such conditions were excluded.

Each CSAM was matched to a normal control for age, sex, ethnicity, and socioeconomic status based on the home of rearing. All control participants were selected randomly from the pool of subjects jointly used by developmental researchers at San Diego State University and the University of California, San Diego. That pool contained a large number of subjects across the entire middle-class range obtained through ads in local family newspapers and recruited at an annual family health fair sponsored by a local children's hospital. Judgments of normal development for this control group were determined by the developmental history questionnaire completed by the caretaker at the time of the experimental observation.

Procedure

Language and symbolic gesture use were assessed using a combination of parental report (the CDI Toddler form) and laboratory behavioral measures described in the next section of this article. The CDI was administered and scored as described previously.

All laboratory sessions were videotaped using a professional videocassette recorder (Mitsubishi, model VB–1000) and two video cameras (Panasonic, model

WV–3260) mounted on pan/tilt heads (Panasonic, model WV–PH10). A body microphone (Shure Brothers, Inc., wireless transmitter, model L1–W) was placed in a child-size vest designed especially for developmental studies and was worn by each child during the experimental sessions. Adult utterances were recorded with an omnidirectional wall microphone (Realistic, model PZ–M). All data were coded blindly off the tapes after the recorded sessions.

Spontaneous Language Samples. All sessions began with a 10-min warm-up of free play with a set of toys designed to entice young children to interact with adults in the laboratory setting, followed by a play session with the experimenter using a different set of toys also selected to stimulate a representative sample of language. A second language sample of 10 min was recorded during a parent–child play session with another set of language-stimulating toys. These samples (totaling 30 min) were used for analyses of vocabulary production, mean length of utterance (MLU), and phonology.

Up to 100 consecutive intelligible utterances were transcribed by four research assistants skilled in phonetic transcription using the International Phonetic Alphabet. Two 5-min portions of each language sample were transcribed independently by a second transcriber to assess reliability. Point-to-point agreement was 96% (range = 80–95) for words and 93% (range = 79%–98%) for the number of consonant sounds produced. The number of different words produced and MLU were determined using the Code for the Human Analysis of Transcripts (MacWhinney & Snow, 1990). Phonetic inventories for consonants in word-initial and word-final position were identified for each child by visual examination of each transcription corpus, and the mean number of phonemes was determined.

Spontaneous Naming and Recognitory Gesture Production. A semistructured task in which 10 toys were presented to the child, one at a time, in a randomized order was used to assess production of word and gesture labels. If the child did not spontaneously name the object within 30 sec, the examiner asked the child what the toy was called. In addition, if the child did not produce a typical representational (i.e., recognitory) gesture, the examiner asked the child to show what she or he could do with the toy. The items used in this task included a toy telephone, car, airplane, doll, spoon, toothbrush, flower, hat, cup, and dog—the same exemplars used in the gesture imitation task described later in this article. Scores for this task were the number of vocal labels and the number of recognitory gestures produced.

Comprehension books. A two-way, forced-choice, picture-identification task was used to sample comprehension of single words including nouns, verbs, and modifiers. This task has been used with normal children between 16 and 28 months of age and has been validated against data from the parental report (Bates et al., 1989; Thal & Bates, 1988). For this task the child was seated across the table from the examiner who held two 8-in. × 11-in. pictures in front of the child and instructed him or her to look at both and to show or point to a particular object, action, or attribute. Scores were the percentage correct of the total number of items in the test.

Comprehension commands.　This measure assessed comprehension of two-word combinations. Each participant was asked to carry out both typical and atypical actions such as "Kiss the doll" (typical) or "Kiss the ball" (atypical). In each condition, five requests to carry out an action with an object were presented to each participant in random order. Trials were always presented in pairs with the typical command administered first. Two scores were obtained for this test: the number of typical commands completed and the number of atypical commands completed.

Single gesture imitation.　The ability to imitate representational gestures was assessed in a task in which the experimenter modeled individual gestures that were carried out with realistic toy objects or with a plain wooden or plastic block (placeholder). The placeholder condition was included because it provided a more decontextualized format than did realistic objects and could be used to infer that the gestures actually were representational. This has been used in a number of studies of normal and delayed toddlers (Bates et al., 1989; Thal & Bates, 1988; Thal, Tobias, & Morrison, 1991). After an initial practice trial to familiarize the child with the requirements of the task, 10 object–gesture pairs with both realistic toys or placeholders were presented in random order with the exception that the same concept with a realistic and placeholder object never occurred in immediate sequence. Thus, if "car" was presented with a realistic toy car, the next presentation would not be "car" with a placeholder object. Each action was modeled up to five times to elicit imitation. Children were reinforced for all gestures produced regardless of correctness. Separate scores were calculated for the number of correct imitations produced with a realistic object and with a placeholder object.

Spontaneous gesture production.　This was assessed using the spontaneous naming task described previously in the discussion concerning language production measures.

Data Analysis

Permutation tests for two independent samples (Siegel & Castellan, 1988) were used to test the significance of differences between the experimental and control groups for the CDI Toddler form, spontaneous naming, production of spontaneous gesture labels, imitation of single recognitory gestures with real objects and with placeholders, vocabulary comprehension, and comprehension of multiword commands specifying typical and atypical relations. The other measures were analyzed using the Mann–Whitney U test.

Results

Parental Report of Language Production

The MacArthur CDI.   The number of different words produced was lower in both CSAM age cohorts than in the control cohort, but the difference reached significance only for the 28-month-olds (see Table 4). In addition, there was no significant difference in the mean number of words produced by the older and younger CSAMs. That is, the older CSAMs did not show the larger vocabulary size usually seen in the 3rd year of life and demonstrated by the older control group here. The mean percentile on word production for the older CSAMs was significantly lower than that of the control group ($p < .003$). The difference between the 20-month-old CSAMs and control groups was not significant. As expected, there was a significant difference ($p < .001$) between the younger and older CSAMs in mean percentile, with the 28-month-olds achieving lower percentiles than did the 20-month-olds.

Differences between groups also were seen for the production of early word combinations. Only two of the six 20-month-old CSAMs combined words, whereas five of the six controls did. Due to the variability of this skill at 20 months, neither group should be seen as atypical. However, at 28 months, 97% of the children in the norming group for the CDI made word combinations at least sometimes (Fenson et al., 1993), and all control children combined words at that age. Among the 28-month-old CSAMs, only two of six produced word combinations. Of the four noncombiners, three had vocabularies larger than 50 words, the vocabulary level at which word combinations are expected to emerge (Bates, Bretherton, & Snyder, 1988). This replicates the findings with 25- to 30-month-old CSAMs in Study 1.

Figure 2 shows the distribution of the CSAMs plotted against the CDI norms for word production. The 20-month-old CSAMs score within the normal range for age, although they do cluster in the lower third of the distribution, with one exception. The 28-month-old CSAMs, on the other hand, cluster below the 10th percentile, although there is variability across the group.

Finally, the complexity of these early utterances, at least as reflected on the M3L produced, was significantly lower than was that of controls for both groups of CSAMs ($p < .01$). Thus, the longest utterances produced were shorter in the CSAMs compared to controls. These data also look similar to those from the larger pool of participants described in Study 1, with poorer performance in the CSAMs, particularly in the older group.

TABLE 4
Language Scores on the MacArthur Communicative Development Inventory for Children
with Prenatal Exposure to Stimulant Drugs and Normal Controls—Study 2

	Age and Group			
	20 Months		28 Months	
	CSAMs	Controls	CSAMs	Controls
Number of different words produced	109 ± 79	202 ± 115	157 ± 90***	462 ± 102
Word production: Percentiles	38[a] ± 21	51 ± 18	8 ± 6**	47 ± 21
Mean length of three longest utterances	1.2 ± 1.2**	3.3 ± 1.6	0.8 ± 1.3**	5.7 ± 2.1

Note. Asterisks are placed above the scores for which there is a significant difference between groups. CSAM = children of substance-abusing mothers.
[a]Significantly higher than 28-month CSAMs, $p < .001$.
**$p < .01$. ***$p < .001$.

Laboratory Observations

The laboratory measures replicated the CDI data. CSAMs scored lower than did normal controls in several aspects of language, as seen in Table 5.

Spontaneous-language samples.   Although both groups of CSAMs produced fewer words than did their controls, only the 28-month-old group produced significantly fewer. The MLU produced by the CSAMs was shorter, and, again, the 28-month-old CSAMs were significantly lower than were controls (see Table 5).

With regard to phonological development, there was no significant difference between the 20-month groups in the number of different consonants produced in word-initial position. In addition, the types of sounds produced were the same across the two groups and contained all single consonants used by normal children in this age range (Stoel-Gammon, 1983). The 28-month CSAMs, on the other hand, produced significantly fewer different consonants in the word-initial position than did controls, and fewer consonants than were used by normal children in this age range (Dyson, 1988).

Neither 20-month-old CSAMs nor controls used many word-final consonants, and there was no significant difference between the groups, a result that is typical of normal children in this age range. The number of final consonants of the 28-month-old CSAMs, however, was restricted severely compared to expectations (Dyson, 1988) and was significantly smaller than that of normal controls.

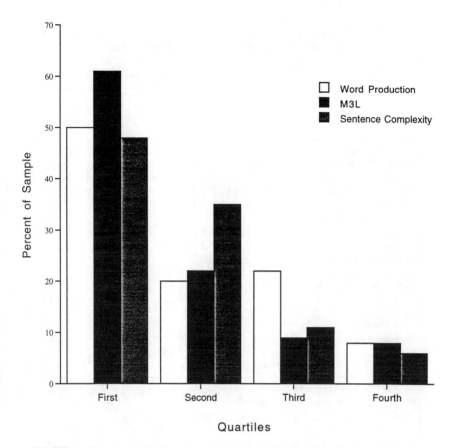

FIGURE 2 Number of words produced by 20- and 28-month-old children with prenatal exposure to stimulant drugs and age-matched controls plotted against the quartiles and median of the normative sample for the MacArthur Communicative Development Inventory.

Spontaneous naming. Results of the spontaneous naming paralleled the CDI Toddler form and language sample data. The 20-month-old CSAM group did not differ significantly from controls on the number of words produced, whereas the 28-month-old CSAM cohort produced significantly fewer words than did controls ($p < .001$).

Comprehension book. A significant difference was found between both 20- and 28-month-old CSAMs and their controls for comprehension of words on the comprehension book ($p < .01$ for both ages). In the 20-month-olds, it appeared that control participants responded to the task but did not perform better than expected by chance in this forced-choice task. The CSAMs, however, did not respond readily

TABLE 5
Scores From Laboratory Measures of Language and Gesture for Children With Prenatal
Exposure to Stimulant Drugs and Normal Controls

	Age and Group			
	20 Months		28 Months	
	CSAMs	Controls	CSAMs	Controls
Language production				
Number of different words (language sample)	29 ± 14	50 ± 23	24 ± 20*	102 ± 34
Mean length of utterance	1.16 ± 1.3	1.32 ± 0.3	1.16 ± 0.18**	2.18 ± 0.53
Spontaneous naming	3.9 ± 2.4	5.8 ± 3.19	2.7 ± 2.8*	9.1 ± 1.2
Number of different phonemes				
Word initial	5.50 ± 3.45	8.16 ± 4.07	4.16 ± 3.87**	11.50 ± 1.87
Word final	1.00 ± 1.26	2.33 ± 2.10	0.83 ± 1.69**	7.16 ± 2.23
Language comprehension				
Single words (% correct)	18 ± 23*	57 ± 28	43 ± 31**	79 ± 9
Commands (number followed)				
Typical	3.0 ± 1.5	2.7 ± 1.2	2.3 ± 1.5**	4.3 ± 1.2
Atypical	1.2 ± 1.0*	2.0 ± 2.1	2.0 ± 2.1*	3.5 ± 1.0
Gesture production				
Spontaneous imitation	6.2 ± 1.8	7.9 ± 1.7	6.5 ± 2.6*	8.5 ± 1.9
Expected	8.0 ± 2.4	8.87 ± 3.6	7.8 ± 2.8	9.0 ± 3.3
Unexpected	6.5 ± 1.9	7.4 ± 2.4	6.0 ± 2.8*	8.3 ± 3.4

Note. Asterisks are placed above the scores for which there is a significant difference between groups. CSAM = children of substance-abusing mothers.
*$p < .05$. **$p < .01$.

to the task and showed difficulty in pointing to pictures at all. At 28 months of age, the picture was different: Controls were able to do the task and demonstrated good comprehension of the words, whereas the CSAMs responded at chance levels, performance more typical of children under 2.

Comprehension commands.   In the condition in which children were asked to perform a typical action with an object (e.g., "kiss the doll"), the only significant difference was between the 28-month-old CSAMs and controls ($p < .01$), with the CSAMs completing fewer of the requested actions. For the atypical condition (e.g., "kiss the ball"), both 20- and 28-month CSAMs performed significantly more poorly than did controls ($p < .01$ for both). In other words, at both ages, CSAMs were significantly poorer than were their normal peers in the comprehension of phrases that required processing of at least two words in an atypical situation. When asked to perform these more cognitively complex tasks, such as comprehending commands that lacked support from the nature of the toys or that were unexpected based on previous experience, they performed more poorly than did controls.

Discussion

A more careful look at a small subset of prenatally drug-exposed children in the laboratory replicated and extended the findings in the larger sample described earlier. Although most of this subset demonstrated language competency within the normal range, a significant number clustered at the lower ranges in expressive vocabulary, complex gestures, and comprehension. The particular hurdle of sentence construction was delayed in this group in comparison to norms. For example, most normal children combine some words by 28 months (Bates et al., 1988; Bates, Dale, & Thal, 1994) or at vocabulary levels of 50 to 75 words (Fenson et al., 1993). A substantial portion of the group of children with prenatal exposure to stimulant drugs described in this study did not. Furthermore, the length of the utterances produced was shorter than was the length of utterances produced by children of the same age and socioeconomic status who had no prenatal drug exposure. This was seen on the parental report and in the laboratory.

The comparable findings using the CDI and behavioral measures suggests that the CDI questionnaire does a good job of characterizing language in children with prenatal exposure to stimulant drugs who are being raised in stable, middle-class home environments. Parents or guardians in these homes were able to report accurately language functioning in this group. Further studies are necessary to determine if this is the case for children in less stable home environments, children who have lived in a number of different foster homes, or children in homes with significant stressors (including ongoing drug use), for example.

As in Study 1, the older cohort in Study 2 did more poorly than the younger one. Although these data are cross-sectional, they replicate the CDI data reported in Study 1 in which a large proportion of children with prenatal exposure to stimulant drugs were delayed in language at the point in development at which normal children begin to acquire grammar. Similarly, more complex gestures and cognitively challenging comprehension tasks emerged more slowly in this group. This suggests there may be some particular difficulty in organizing language and accessing it in the service of reasoning. This finding may have implications for long-term language and learning.

In the second study, the confounds of changes in placement, growing up in a household with continuing substance abuse, or chaotic lifestyle were minimized. Children in this study were in early, stable placements with largely middle-class families who were invested strongly in supporting the developmental progress of these children. Although environmental factors certainly could still have been influencing early language development, these were minimized in this group. In this sense they are comparable to a Canadian sample of children in stable adoptive placements since birth who also demonstrated comparable delays in both expressive and receptive language measures in spite of normal global developmental competency (Nulman et al., 1994). This atypical circumstance (i.e., not in lower socioeconomic status homes with continuing substance abuse) was similar in both age cohorts of this sample. The poorer performance in the older cohort does not seem to be explained by more pernicious environmental factors, at least as a major influence along any apparent social, economic, or interactional dimensions. There appears to be a core difficulty in the developmental tasks needed for early language acquisition, particularly at the juncture of early grammar.

GENERAL DISCUSSION

Both studies reported here indicate that language development is atypical in some children with prenatal stimulant drug exposure. Expressive vocabulary levels appeared to be worse in older toddlers, with relative performance at the lowest quartile in both studies. Comprehension and communicative gestures also appeared to emerge later in the CSAM group. After the 2nd year, word combinations appeared to be shorter and less complex than were those produced by comparison children. Phonology also was delayed in a large proportion of the children. Thus, every aspect of language appeared to be lower in the CSAMs, although the majority demonstrated general developmental levels within the broad normal range. Both the CDI and laboratory measures were consistent in demonstrating these findings.

Our findings are consistent with observations made by others. Griffith et al. (1994), in tracking well-matched high-risk groups of children in the context of an intervention program for addicted women, reported increasing disparity in verbal IQ measures and language competence in the drug-exposed group as they entered the preschool years. Van Baar (1990) showed that early language, especially comprehension, appeared to be impaired in a drug-exposed group in comparison to children without that exposure. Reporting on the same group at school age, van Baar and de Graaf (1994) showed that language skills became increasingly poor compared to the skills of normal controls, from 18 to 24 months in their drug-exposed group, with general cognitive measures, especially verbal tasks, also showing relative decrement at ages 4 and 5. Nulman et al. (1994) demonstrated similar language delays in a group of 23 cocaine-exposed children adopted at birth in comparison to a carefully matched control group and suggested these findings indicate a primary neurotoxicity that affects both receptive and expressive language components. Their work is synchronous with the findings in Study 2, in which the postnatal environment is stable. Fried et al. (1992) also reported altered language development at 60 and 72 months of age in a group of children and demonstrated a relation to prenatal exposure to the legal stimulant drug nicotine. That report also stressed the need to look at various components of language and cognition in assessing behavioral teratology, a strategy that we employed in this study, rather than focusing on global summary scores of general development using standardized tests. Our observation of lower levels on specific language measures in older toddlers is consistent with these other published studies in which ratings of global intellectual competencies as measured by standard tests are normed.

The late-2nd and 3rd years of life appear to present special difficulties for this group of children. At the point of the emergence of grammar and the use of language to elicit unexpected mental linkages, the CSAM group appeared to have more difficulties. In addition, even at vocabulary levels at which word combinations typically emerge, the CSAM group lagged behind. This disjunction in the usual pattern of language development raises questions about what mental processes may be atypical in this group.

General cognitive delays, although present in a few of the CSAMs, do not appear to account for the specific language delays observed in this study. As in the Chicago (Azuma & Chasnoff, 1993, Griffith et al., 1990) and Toronto (Nulman et al., 1994) studies, the language and verbal capacities of CSAMs seem to be selectively affected. Chaotic life experience and lack of verbal stimulation have been implicated in delayed language development in other groups of children with prenatal exposure to stimulant drugs. Our Study 1 also suggests that the home of rearing may have some influence on development, but this factor does not account for the lower levels of performance of the older groups in both studies. Although the children described here also had additional life stressors, most (including all in Study 2) were in stable rearing environments, as were those children reported by Nulman et al. A study by van Baar and de Graaf (1994) also implicated stability of environment in the late-preschooler period as providing a minor contribution to general cognitive and linguistic measures. It is important to note that in our study, even children in stable adoptive placements and without major perinatal or postnatal adverse conditions demonstrated significant lags in several aspects of language development.

Adopted children, as a group, are at a higher risk for behavioral and developmental difficulties, but these differences have been reported primarily for school-age populations, those with multiple or late foster placements, or those with nutritional compromise (Dalby, Fox, & Haslam, 1982; Jerome, 1993; Kotsopoulos, Cote, & Joseph, 1988). However, in the current clinical and social situations, studies of children in stable adoptive placements are the best feasible approach to examining the behavioral teratology of cocaine use, which in itself is a complex syndrome of multiple exposures and other adverse risk conditions (J. L. Mills & Robins, 1993; Neuspiel & Hamel, 1991).

One possible explanation for the consistent reports of language delay in some children with prenatal exposure to stimulant drugs is that those brain centers concerned with the organization of experience (i.e., "executive function") may be relatively impaired. This impairment may be seen functionally as difficulty organizing linguistic structures into meaningful utterances. Previous studies (Goldman-Rakic, Isseroff, Schwartz, & Bugbee, 1983; McEvoy & Dixon, 1993; Struthers & Hansen, 1993) demonstrated that CSAMs have difficulties on measures of executive function. Play disorganization in children with prenatal drug exposure has been described by others (Howard et al., 1989; Rodning, Beckwith, & Howard, 1989a, 1989b). This language delay may be another functional consequence of these other organizational difficulties. Indeed, play organization and language skill have been linked in other work (Bretherton et al., 1981).

Cocaine and methamphetamine affect the neurotransmitters and centers that are important in organizing attention and arousal (Wiggins, 1992). Dopamine and serotonin levels appear to be altered for at least weeks to months in infants after stimulant-drug exposure (Davidson-Ward et al., 1989). Additional prenatal changes in this neurochemical milieu may alter these abilities over the long term, and language difficulties may be one of the consequences of this exposure, serving as a window into more general cognitive processes of attention and organization.

Neurostructural changes caused by in utero fetal and placental vasoconstriction also may influence the task of organizing language. We and others (Chasnoff et al., 1986; Dixon & Bejar, 1989; Dominguez et al., 1991; Volpe, 1992) showed the propensity of stimulant drugs to result in small, and occasionally large, areas of cerebral injury. Microcephaly present at birth appears not to exhibit catch-up as semantic growth does in this population. The injury appears to be concentrated in the central cerebral regions and the frontal lobes, areas associated with the organization and coordination of behavior and attention. Structural–functional relations in the developing brain are poorly established at this time. However, in a rat model, subtle changes in brain structure after prenatal cocaine use was associated with behavioral change. Also, there is increasing recognition that these frontal lobe functions are active and can be identified in early childhood (Welsh & Pennington, 1988). In addition, the localization of frontal cerebral activity changes substantially during the period of language acquisition (Mills, Coffey, & Neville, 1994). These observations suggest that subtle neurostructural changes in CSAMs may occur and that these may result in an atypical pattern of language development.

All these mechanisms, and perhaps others, may be operative in explaining some of the differences in language in the drug-exposed groups. This study cannot specify any etiology for certain. Neuspiel (1994) described various mechanisms for the associations between prenatal drug exposure and development, and the complexity of the interactions between them. Azuma and Chasnoff (1993) also described the direct and indirect pathways that may alter linguistic and cognitive development in CSAMs, including some environmental issues that also were implicated here. We accept the complexity of this situation, particularly in most clinical samples. This work suggests that neurologic factors play a role in the vulnerability in this group of children. However, these studies are small and need further replication and expansion. Results must be appraised with that limitation in mind. Large prospective studies would be of help in accounting for some of the life experience differences of this group. A major social policy issue must be addressed through such efforts to see whether early out-of-home placement or intense support of addicted birth mothers results in improved outcome for such children. Early intervention services and stability at home are likely to improve outcome, but this needs specific study. Finally, there may be vulnerable subgroups within this population that need further definition to target prevention and intervention activities.

The MacArthur CDI appears to be an appropriate instrument for evaluating language in CSAMs in stable home environments, recording the same story from parents and guardians that the more detailed laboratory observations tell. The specific assessment of language appears to be clinically important in this group because general measures of development may not identify children with language delays. Children with early language delays, particularly of the type that include delays in gesture and comprehension, as described here (Thal et al., 1991), are at greater risk for continuing language and learning difficulties than are those with only expressive language delays. Even without other risk factors (which often confound the clinical picture and add to the risk) or demonstrated delays in other areas of development, children with prenatal stimulant drug exposure should be monitored carefully for delays or atypical features in early language development. Intervention programs serving this group of youngsters should have a strong emphasis on early communicative skills and ongoing evaluation of language into school age.

ACKNOWLEDGMENTS

The work was supported in part by grant P50 DC01289 and DC00089 from the National Institutes of Health.

REFERENCES

Azuma, S., & Chasnoff, I. J. (1993). Outcome of children prenatally exposed to cocaine and other drugs: A path analysis of three-year data. *Pediatrics, 92,* 396–402.

Bates, E., Bretherton, I., & Snyder, L. (1988). *From first words to grammar: Individual differences and dissociable mechanisms.* New York: Cambridge University Press.

Bates, E., Dale, P., & Thal, D. (1994). Individual differences and their implications for theories of language development. In P. Fletcher & B. MacWhinney (Eds.), *The handbook of child language* (pp. 96–142). Oxford, England: Oxford University Press.

Bates, E., & Thal, D. (1991). Associations and dissociations in child language development. In J. Miller (Ed.)., *Research on child language disorders: A decade of progress.* Austin, TX: Pro-Ed.

Bates, E., Thal, D., Whitesell, K., Fenson, L. & Oakes, L. (1989). Integrating language and gesture in infancy. *Developmental Psychology, 25,* 1004–1019.

Bayley, N. (1969). *Bayley Scales of Infant Development*. New York: Psychological Corporation.

Bentz, K., Hansen, R., McEvoy, R., Steward, M., & Banon, K. (1993). Cognitive functions of preschool children exposed to drugs prenatally [Abstract]. *Journal of Developmental and Behavioral Pediatrics, 14,* 4.

Billing, L., Erickson, M., Sleneroth, G., & Zetterstrom, R. (1985). Preschool children of amphetamine-addicted mothers: Somatic and psychomotor development. *Acta Paediatrica Scandinavica, 74,* 179–184.

Bishop, D., & Adams, C. (1990). A prospective study of the relationship between specific language impairment, phonological disorders and reading retardation. *Child Psychology and Psychiatry, 31,* 1027–1050.

Bishop, D., & Edmundson, A. (1987). Language-impaired 4-year-olds: Distinguishing transient from persistent impairment. *Journal of Speech and Hearing Research, 52,* 156–173.

Bretherton, I., Bates, E., McNew, S., Shore, C., Williamson, C., & Smith, M. (1981). Comprehension and production of symbols in infancy: An experimental study. *Developmental Psychology, 17,* 728–736.

Bureau of the Census (1991). *General population characteristics* (Vol. 1). Washington, DC: U.S. Government Printing Office.

Chasnoff, I., Bussey, M. E., Savich, R., & Stack, C. (1986). Perinatal cerebral infarction and maternal cocaine use. *Journal of Pediatrics, 108,* 456–459.

Chasnoff, I., Griffith, D. R., Freier, C., & Murray, J. (1992). Cocaine/polydrug use in pregnancy: Two year follow-up. *Pediatrics, 89,* 284–289.

Chasnoff, I., Landress, H. J., & Barrett, M. E. (1990). The prevalence of illegal drug use or alcohol use during pregnancy and discrepancies in mandatory reporting in Pinellas County, Florida. *New England Journal of Medicine, 322,* 1202–1206.

Dalby, J. T., Fox, L., Haslam, R. H. A. (1982). Adoption and foster care rates in pediatric disorders. *Journal of Developmental and Behavioral Pediatrics, 3,* 61–68.

Dale, P. (1991). The validity of a parent report measure of vocabulary and syntax at 24 months. *Journal of Speech and Hearing Science, 34,* 565–571.

Dale, P., Bates, E., Reznick, S., & Morisset, C. (1989). The validity of a parent report instrument of child language at 20 months. *Journal of Child Language, 16,* 239–249.

Davidson-Ward, S. L., Bautista, D. B., Buckley, S., Schuetz, S., Wachsman, L., Bean, K., & Warburton, D. (1989). Circulating catecholamines and adenoreceptors in infants of cocaine-abusing mothers [Abstract]. *Pediatric Research, 34,* 81.

Dixon, S., & Bejar, R. (1989). Echoencephalographic findings in neonates associated with maternal cocaine and methamphetamine use: Incidence and clinical correlates. *Journal of Pediatrics, 115,* 770–778.

Dominguez, R., Vila-Coro, A. A., Slopis, J. M., & Bohan, T. P. (1991). Brain and ocular abnormalities in infants with in-utero exposure to cocaine and other street drugs. *American Journal of Diseases of Children, 145,* 688–695.

Dyson, A. T. (1988). Phonetic inventories of 2- and 3-year-old children. *Journal of Speech and Hearing Disease, 53,* 89–93.

Fenson, L., Dale, P., Reznick, J. S., Thal, D., Bates, E., Pethick, S., Hartung, J., & Reilly, J. (1993). *MacArthur Communicative Development Inventories: User's guide and manual.* San Diego, CA: Singular Publishing Group.

Fried, P., O'Connell, C., & Watkinson, B. (1992). 60- and 72-month follow-up of children prenatally exposed to marijuana, cigarettes and alcohol: Cognitive and language assessment. *Developmental and Behavioral Pediatrics, 13,* 383–391.

Goldman-Rakic, P. S., Isseroff, A., Schwartz, M. L., & Bugbee, N. M. (1983). The neurobiology of cognitive development. In P. H. Mussen (Ed.), *Handbook of child psychology* (pp. 281–344). New York: Wiley.

Griffith, D., Azuma, S., & Chasnoff, I. J. (1994). Three-year outcome of children exposed prenatally to drugs. *Journal of the American Academy of Child Psychiatry, 33,* 20–27.

Griffith, D., Chasnoff, I. J., Gillogby, K., & Fria, C. (1990). Developmental follow-up of cocaine-exposed infants through age 3-years. *Infant Behavior and Development, 13,* 126(A).

Hollingshead, A. (1965). *Two-factor index of social position.* New Haven, CT: Yale University Press.

Howard, J. (1989). Cocaine and its effects on the child and newborn. *Developmental Medicine and Child Neurology, 31,* 255–263.

Howard, J., Beckwith, L., Rodning, C., & Kropewske, V. (1989). The development of young children of substance-abusing parents. *Zero to Three, 9,* 8–12.

Jerome, L. (1993). A comparison of the demography, clinical profile and treatment of adopted and nonadopted children at a children's mental health centre. *Canadian Journal of Psychiatry, 38,* 290–294.

Kaltenbach, K., Nathanson, L., & Finnigan, L. (1989). Temperament characteristics of infants born to drug-dependent women. *Pediatric Research, 25,* 73.

Knobloch, H., Stevens, F., & Malone, A. (1980). *The Revised Developmental Screening Inventory.* Houston, TX: Gesell Developmental Test Materials.

Kotsopoulos, S., Cote, A., & Joseph, L. (1988). Psychiatric disorders in adopted children. *Journal of American Orthopsychiatry, 58,* 608–610.

MacWhinney, B., & Snow, C. (1990). The CHILDES project: An update. *Journal of Child Language, 17,* 457–472.

McEvoy, R., & Dixon, S. (1993, March). *Executive function in children with prenatal drug exposure.* Paper presented at the 60th annual meeting of the Society for Research in Child Development, New Orleans, LA.

Mills, D., Coffey, S., & Neville, H. J. (1994). Changes in cerebral organization in infancy during primary language acquisition. In G. Dawson & K. Fischer (Eds.), *Human behavior and the developing brain* (pp. 427–455). New York: Guilford.

Mills, J. L., & Robins, L. N. (1993). Effects of in-utero exposure to street drugs. *American Journal of Health, 83*(Suppl. 1), 10–20.

National Institute of Drug Abuse. (1989). *National household survey on drug abuse: Population estimates* (Rep. No. 89–1636). Rockville, MD: U.S. Department of Health and Human Services.

Neuspiel, D. (1994). Behavior in cocaine exposed infants and children: Association versus causality. *Drug and Alcohol Dependence, 36,* 101–107.

Neuspiel, D., & Hamel, S. (1991). Cocaine and infant behavior. *Journal of Developmental and Behavioral Pediatrics, 12,* 55–64.

Nulman, I., Rovet, J., Altmann, D., Bradley, C., Einarson, T., & Koren, G. (1994). Neurodevelopment of adopted children exposed in utero to cocaine. *Canadian Medical Association Journal, 151,* 1591–1597.

Rodning, C., Beckwith, L., & Howard, J. (1989a). Characteristics of attachment organization and play organization in prenatally drug-exposed toddlers. *Developmental Psychopathology, 1,* 277–289.

Rodning, C., Beckwith, L., & Howard, J. (1989b). Prenatal exposure to drugs: Behavioral distortions reflecting CNS impairment. *Neurotoxicology, 10,* 629–634.

Siegel, S., & Castellan, C. (1988). *Nonparametric statistics for the behavioral sciences.* New York: McGraw-Hill.

Silva, P., McGee, R., & Williams, S. (1983). Developmental language delay from 3 to 7 years and its significance for low intelligence and reading difficulties at age seven. *Developmental Medicine and Child Neurology, 25,* 783–793.

Singer, L., Farkas, K., & Kliegman, R. (1992). Childhood medical and behavioral consequences of maternal cocaine use. *Journal of Pediatrics, 17,* 389–406.

Stoel-Gammon, C. (1983). Phonetic inventories at 15–24 months: A longitudinal study. *Journal of Speech and Hearing Research, 28,* 505–512.

Struthers, J. M., & Hansen, R. (1993). Visual recognition memory in drug-exposed infants. *Developmental and Behavioral Pediatrics, 13,* 108–111.

Thal, D., & Bates, E. (1988). Language and gesture in late talkers. *Journal of Speech and Hearing Research, 31,* 115–123.

Thal, D., Marchman, V., Stiles, J., Aram, D., Trauner, D., Nass, R., & Bates, E. (1991). Early lexical development in children with focal brain injury. *Brain and Language, 40,* 491–527.

Thal, D., Tobias, S., & Morrison, D. (1991). Language and gesture in late talkers: A one-year follow-up. *Journal of Speech and Hearing Research, 34,* 604–612.

van Baar, A. (1990). Development of infants of drug dependent mothers. *Journal of Child Psychology and Psychiatry, 31,* 911–920.

van Baar, A., & de Graaf, B. M. (1994). Cognitive development at preschool-age of infants of drug-dependent mothers. *Developmental Medicine and Child Neurology, 36,* 1063–1075.

Volpe, J. J. (1992). Effect of cocaine use on the fetus. *New England Journal of Medicine, 327,* 399–407.

Welsh, M., & Pennington, B. (1988). Assessing frontal lobe functioning in children: Views from developmental psychology. *Developmental Neuropsychology, 4,* 199–230.

Wiggins, R. C. (1992). Pharmacokinetics of cocaine in pregnancy and effects on fetal maturation. *Clinical Pharmacokinetics, 22,* 85–93.

DEVELOPMENTAL NEUROPSYCHOLOGY, *13*(3), 397–445

Language Comprehension and Cerebral Specialization From 13 to 20 Months

Debra L. Mills
University of California, San Diego

Sharon Coffey-Corina
University of Washington

Helen J. Neville
University of Oregon

The purpose of this study was to examine developmental changes in the organization of brain activity linked to comprehension of single words in 13- to 20-month-old infants. Event-related potentials (ERPs) were recorded as children listened to a series of words whose meanings were understood by the child, words whose meanings the child did not understand, and backward words. The results were consistent with a previous study suggesting that ERPs differed as a function of word meaning within 200 ms after word onset. At 13 to 17 months, ERP differences between comprehended and unknown words were bilateral and broadly distributed over anterior and posterior regions. In contrast, at 20 months of age these effects were limited to temporal and parietal regions of the left hemisphere. The results are discussed in relation to the general effects of maturation, the maturation of language-relevant brain systems, and the development of brain systems linked to level of ability independent of chronological age. We offer the working hypothesis that the neurophysiological changes that give rise to certain ERP effects reported here are linked to the remarkable changes in early lexical development that typically occur between 13 and 20 months, whereas others produce more general maturational effects.

Requests for reprints should be sent to Debra L. Mills, Department of Cognitive Science, 0515, University of California, San Diego, La Jolla, CA 92093–0515.

At maturity, the human brain is highly differentiated in its functional organization. Different brain regions mediate different aspects of sensory, language, and nonlanguage cognitive processing. Within the language domain, evidence from neuroimaging studies, including positron emission tomography (Peterson, Fox, Posner, Mintun, & Raichle, 1988; Peterson, Fox, Snyder, & Raichle, 1990; Posner, Peterson, Fox, & Raichle, 1989), functional magnetic resonance imaging (Neville et al., 1994, 1995), and electrophysiological evidence (Neville, Mills, & Lawson, 1992; Neville, Nicol, Barss, Forster, & Garrett, 1991; Osterhout & Holcomb, 1990), suggest that different brain systems are involved in processing different aspects of language. Much less is known about the extent to which different neural systems are specialized for processing different types of information in normal infants and children. In this research, the broad goals were to examine how specializations for language-relevant brain systems arise during the course of primary language acquisition.

LESION STUDIES

Much of what is known about the development of cerebral specialization for language stems from retrospective studies of patients who sustained unilateral or focal brain injury at different points in development (Basser, 1962; Hecaen, 1983; Lenneberg, 1967; see Stromswold, 1995, for a review). These studies suggest that brain injury sustained in early childhood does not have the same sequelae as does injury to the same brain region occurring in an adult. In children, aphasia that results from unilateral injury tends to be less severe and less persistent than comparable damage occurring in an adult. Moreover, damage to either the left or right hemisphere may lead to aphasia in young children. Based on these findings, Lenneberg proposed that initially the two cerebral hemispheres are equipotential for language and that the left hemisphere specialization for language does not become stabilized until after puberty.

The equipotentiality position lost favor in the 1970s and was criticized based on both methodological concerns and over interpretations of the findings (e.g., Kinsbourne & Hiscock, 1983). For example, damage to the right hemisphere resulting in aphasia in a young child may have been due to a number of factors including representation of language in the right hemisphere for that particular child. Neuroanatomical (Witelson & Pallie, 1973) and electrophysiological evidence from infants (Molfese & Molfese, 1979) suggested that lateral differences in structure exist before birth and that asymmetries in neural activity linked to language processing occur in infancy, although the functional significance of these early asymmetries has not yet been determined. The idea that lateralization develops at all was called into question (Kinsbourne & Hiscock, 1977). Evidence against the equipotentiality hypothesis also emerged from studies of children with hemispherectomies (Dennis & Kohn, 1975; Dennis & Whitaker, 1976; Vargha-Khadem,

Isaacs, Papaleloudi, Polkey, & Wilson, 1991) and from children with focal brain injury (Aram, Ekelman, & Whitaker, 1986, 1987; Vargha-Khadem, O'Gorman, & Watters, 1985). These studies suggested that different patterns of impairment result from left- versus right-hemisphere damage and that these impairments can be persistent, although subtle.

In two prospective studies of infants with focal brain injury (Bates et al., this issue; Thal et al., 1991), the authors concluded that although there is some early differentiation of neural systems that mediate different aspects of language processing at an early age, these brain systems do not map onto those described in the adult literature. They found that children with unilateral damage to the right hemisphere were at greater risk for delays in word comprehension, whereas children with damage to the left-temporal regions were at risk for delays in productive vocabulary and grammar. In summary, the lesion literature is inconsistent with some studies providing evidence of a left-hemisphere bias for language from birth, whereas other studies suggest that the right hemisphere may play an important role in early language acquisition. This study addressed these issues by examining changes in the lateral and anterior–posterior distribution of brain activity linked to language processing during the first 2 years of life.

EFFECTS OF ALTERED EARLY EXPERIENCE

Another important approach in studying brain development has been to study adults who had altered early sensory or language experience. The results from studies of deaf adults (Neville, 1991a, 1991b; Neville et al., 1992) suggest the development of cerebral specializations for different aspects of language are differentially vulnerable to altered early sensory and language experience. Moreover, these studies suggest the functional specialization of these systems may develop along with increasing levels of language abilities. Prospective studies of school-age normal and language-impaired children further support these hypotheses (Holcomb, Coffey, & Neville, 1992; Neville, Coffey, Holcomb, & Tallal, 1993). In this study, we further tested the hypothesis that the specialization of language-relevant brain systems is, at least in part, driven by increasing levels of language abilities.

NORMAL DEVELOPMENT AND EVENT-RELATED
POTENTIAL STUDIES

It is important to chart the developmental time course of the differentiation of language-relevant brain systems during primary language acquisition in normal[1] infants. The use of event-related brain potentials (ERPs) recorded from the scalp is

---

[1]Here the term *normal development* is used to describe variability in rates of word learning in healthy monolingual hearing infants. It is not intended to reflect a cultural standard of behavior.

one of the few noninvasive techniques currently available for the study of neural events associated with sensory and cognitive processing in healthy human infants (e.g., Dehaene-Lambertz & Dehaene, 1994; Karrer & Ackles, 1987; Kurtzberg, 1985; Mills, Coffey, & Neville, 1994; Mills, Coffey-Corina, & Neville, 1993; Molfese, 1989, 1990; C. Nelson & Collins, 1991). The purpose of this study was twofold; first, to examine patterns of neural activity linked to comprehension of single words in 13- to 20-month-old normal infants and, second, to determine which changes in the organization of brain activity occur as a function of changes in lexical development.

LANGUAGE ACQUISITION: COMPREHENSION VERSUS PRODUCTION

In normal infants, the ability to produce words increases dramatically between 13 and 20 months (Bates, Bretherton, & Snyder, 1988; Fenson et al., 1993). During this time, vocabulary size tends to increase gradually at first and then accelerates rapidly (e.g., Benedict, 1979; Bloom, 1973; Fenson et al., 1993; Goldfield & Reznick, 1990; K. Nelson, 1973). For example, a child may take several months to produce the first 50 words and thereafter may begin acquiring several new words per day (see Barrett, 1995, for a review). Some research suggests that the way the child uses single words also changes at the time of the vocabulary spurt (K. Nelson, 1973). Prior to the vocabulary burst (i.e., fewer than 50 words produced), spoken words tend to be context bound and primarily consist of nouns, affect expressions, and vocal routines such as *Hi* and *Bye* (e.g., Bates et al., 1988; Dore, 1985; K. Nelson, 1983). After the vocabulary burst, words tend to be used in a more referential manner and in a variety of different contexts, may specify relations such as possession or location, and come from a variety of different lexical categories (e.g., Bates et al., 1988; Werner & Kaplan, 1963).

The co-occurrence of a spurt in the size of the child's expressive vocabulary with qualitative changes in the way words are used led some researchers to suggest that reorganizational processes lead to the increase in production, including the attainment of nominal insight, that is, the idea that all things have names (Dore, 1978; McShane, 1979); changes in the ability to form conceptual categories (Gopnik & Meltzoff, 1986); and knowledge of linguistic constraints, that is, semantically and syntactically imposed limits on the potential meanings for novel words (Markman, 1991). According to this perspective, before the vocabulary burst, new words are acquired slowly and require many pairings of the new word and its referent. After the vocabulary spurt, the underlying reorganizational process allows the child to acquire new words rapidly with minimal exposure.

The majority of these studies focused on changes in expressive vocabulary. Changes in comprehension are more difficult to measure and are less frequently studied (Golinkoff & Hirsh-Pasek, 1995; Hirsh-Pasek & Golinkoff, 1993). Fenson et al. (1993) and Fenson, Dale, Reznick, Bates, and Thal (1994) used a parental report checklist to study the development of early language comprehension. That study suggested that, like production, the size of a child's receptive vocabulary progresses slowly at first and then grows rapidly. The increase in receptive vocabulary may occur at a somewhat earlier age than does the spurt in productive vocabulary. For example, on average, a 12-month-old understands approximately 50 words, but this number may double or triple in just 2 to 3 months (e.g., Barrett, 1995; Benedict, 1979; Fenson et al., 1993, in press).

Is the spurt in productive vocabulary driven by underlying changes in comprehension? A recent study of language comprehension abilities in 13- to 18-months-olds argued against the hypothesis that the naming explosion is the result of concomitant changes in comprehension abilities (Woodward, Markman, & Fitzsimmons, 1994). In that study, both 13- and 18-month-olds showed comprehension of a novel word after minimal exposure. The results suggest the ability to rapidly acquire new word meanings occurs well before the naming explosion. However, only one novel label was trained. Thus, it was not clear whether the child acquired a new auditory specific to the target or merely chose the target because it had been named recently. A more recent study using a preferential looking paradigm, taught two novel object–word pairs to control for this possibility (Schafer & Plunkett, 1996). The results support the finding that infants in the 13-to 17-month age range can acquire new receptive labels with minimal exposure. If rapid word learning does reflect changes in underlying conceptual abilities, it is unlikely the subsequent burst in productive vocabulary is due to the same underlying processes that mediate comprehension. These findings suggest the activation of different systems may underlie the reported spurts in comprehension versus production. For example, changes in productive abilities may be linked to changes in memory or articulatory factors (Woodward et al., 1994), whereas increases in comprehension abilities are more likely to be the results of conceptual changes. Recent neurobiological evidence from infants with focal brain injury (Bates et al., this issue) support the hypothesis that different neural systems may meditate the acquisition of comprehension versus the production of single words. However, neural network modeling research suggests that it is not necessary to posit different neural systems to account for these disparities in comprehension and production (Plunkett, 1993, 1995).

This research addresses two questions: (a) What changes in brain organization, if any, precede, accompany, or follow the reported vocabulary bursts? and (b) What are the relative roles of comprehension and production abilities in setting up changes in the specialization of these language systems? To address this issue directly, it is important to study changes in brain organization linked to word processing in infants before and after the reported vocabulary bursts, and to examine the effects of language production abilities on brain organization for children who show similar comprehension abilities.

ERP STUDIES OF LANGUAGE ACQUISITION

The use of ERPs is ideally suited to studying changes in language comprehension. ERPs do not require an overt response from the infant and, therefore, bypass some of the motivational and performance-related limitations of behavioral testing. Previously we reported on changes in cerebral specialization linked to language comprehension and production abilities in normal 20-month-old infants (Mills et al., 1993). In that study, ERPs were recorded to words whose meanings the children comprehended and produced, unknown words and backward words. The results suggest that by 20 months of age there is a considerable degree of specialization for processing different types of words both within and between the two hemispheres. A positive component peaking within the first 100 ms, P100, displayed a left-greater-than-right asymmetry to both comprehended and unknown words. The P100 is thought to index the processing of sensory information, and the asymmetry may reflect an initial left-hemisphere bias for processing language stimuli. Later ERP components, that is, negative deflections occurring at 200 ms (N200) and 350 ms (N350), discriminated between comprehended and unknown words over temporal and parietal regions of the left hemisphere. In contrast, ERP differences between comprehended and backward words were bilateral.

Differential activation of neural activity elicited to comprehended, unknown, and backward words also was illustrated by differences in the lateral and anterior–posterior distribution of ERPs to the different types of words. Words that were comprehended and produced by the child elicited N200 and N350 responses that were bilateral and were largest over temporal and parietal regions. Unknown words elicited highly asymmetrical (right greater) N200 and N350 responses that were equipotential over anterior and posterior regions. In contrast, the N200 and N350 responses were absent or attenuated to backward words, which elicited a broad positivity in this time window. These results suggest that by at least 20 months of age specialized brain systems mediate the processing of words that are comprehended and produced by the child, and that these systems are distinct from those activated to words the child does not understand, and from backward words.

To assess the effects of differences in language production abilities on the patterns of activity described, the children were separated into two groups based on the number of words they produced, and they were designated as either high producers or low producers. Both groups showed differences in the N200 response to comprehended and unknown words that were limited to temporal and parietal regions of the left hemisphere. However, the two groups showed marked differences in the amplitude and distribution of ERPs to comprehended words. Group differences were obtained in the amplitude and distribution of the N200, the latency and responsiveness of the N350, and the distribution of a broad negative wave, the N600–900. More generally, the results suggested the ERPs elicited by words that were comprehended and produced became more focally distributed with increasing language production abilities. It was our working hypothesis that these group differences in ERP responses reflect changes in the organization of language-relevant neural systems linked to the level of language abilities.

In this study we further tested these hypotheses with a group of younger infants, from 13 to 17 months of age, who varied in language comprehension abilities. This period in development is characterized by a considerable degree of variability in the number of words children understand, with estimates ranging from zero for some children to several hundred for others (Fenson et al., 1993, in press). In addition, this is the period during which most children say their first words. In this study we used the size of the child's receptive vocabulary to assign children into two groups who were matched for chronological age but who varied in language abilities. ERPs were recorded as the children listened to words whose meanings they comprehended, words whose meanings they did not comprehend, and backward words. Based on our previous study with 20-month-old infants, we predicted that specific ERP components would be sensitive to word meanings and that increasing levels of language comprehension abilities would be associated with increased specializations of neural systems subserving language processing.

METHOD

Participants

Children were recruited for the study through advertisements in local newspapers, posters displayed in the area, requests at play groups, and referrals from parents whose children had participated in previous studies. Only full-term, healthy infants with monolingual experience with English participated in the study. Thirty-nine children aged 13.0 to 17.5 months participated in the study. Data from 16 girls and 12 boys were retained for analysis (mean age = 14.5 months). Data from an additional 11 children (5 girls and 6 boys) were not used because the children refused to keep the electrocap on for the duration of the session or because there was too much eye or body movement artifact in the data, that is, there were fewer than 10 artifact-free trials per condition.

Language Assessment

Within 1 week prior to participating in the electrophysiological portion of the study, each child was seen for language testing. The behavioral session was used both to estimate each child's level of speech and language abilities and to determine which words to present during the electrophysiological testing session. All behavioral sessions were videotaped.

MacArthur Communicative Development Inventories (CDI).   Parental estimates of language comprehension and production abilities for single words were obtained using the MacArthur CDI: Words and Gestures (Fenson et al., 1993). The CDI includes a checklist of 396 items organized within a variety of different lexical categories (e.g., common nouns organized by semantic category, verbs, adjectives, and question words). The inventory is structured such that parents can indicate which words their child understands and which words their child both understands and says. The CDI was normed on over 1,000 children from 6 to 30 months of age, and its reliability and validity have been well established for use with children in this age range (Bates et al., 1988; Bretherton, McNew, Snyder, & Bates, 1983; Fenson et al., 1989).

Vocabulary checklist rating scales.   Parents were asked to give confidence ratings for 120 words that frequently are comprehended by children in this age range as determined from the norms on the CDI. Parents rated each word on a 4-point scale ranging from 1 (*very confident the child does not know and/or say the word*) to 4 (*very confident the child does know and/or say the word in a variety of contexts and with a variety of different exemplars*). Separate ratings were given for comprehension and production.

Comprehension book.   This task was used as a validation measure to ensure that the children understood the meanings of the 10 words chosen as "comprehended" words for presentation during the ERP session. The task consisted of a simple, two-way, forced-choice picture–word matching test. For each item, the child was asked to point to one of two pictures (colored line drawings) that matched the word spoken by the experimenter. This comprehension measure has been validated against the data from the normed language inventories (Bates, Thal, Whitesell, Fenson, & Oakes, 1989; Thal & Bates, 1988a, 1988b). All behavioral sessions were videotaped.

Experimental Stimuli

The stimuli were selected from 120 words (from the Vocabulary Checklist Rating Scale) naturally spoken by a woman. The words had been digitized at 16 Khz and stored on an IBM PC computer. Each word was edited for precise time of onset to allow for synchronization with the digitization of the ERPs. These words were used to construct a stimulus list for each child prior to ERP testing. When possible, we used a standard list of words across children. Three types of words were used: words the child comprehended or, if the child had started to talk, words the child both comprehended and produced (comprehended words, $n = 10$); words the child did not comprehend or produce (unknown words, $n = 10$); and words the child comprehended and produced that were presented backward (backward words, n = 10). The comprehended (or produced) words were selected from the words the child correctly identified in comprehension books and words that received the highest parental rating (4) for comprehension alone or for both comprehension and production on the vocabulary checklist rating scales. Six of the children correctly identified fewer than 10 items on the comprehension book task, and five other children either could not or would not engage in this task at all. For four of these children, a set of objects was used successfully in place of the pictures. For the other seven, the rating scale alone was used to select the 10 comprehended words presented during ERP testing. Examples of commonly used words were *nose, ball, dog, cat,* and *bear.* The unknown words were words assigned a rating of 1 by parents; that is, they were confident their child did *not* understand or produce the words. To ensure that the unknown words were not comprehended by the child, the unknown words were selected from a list of low-probability words (e.g., *pint, tone, fade,* and *staff*). The comprehended and unknown words were matched on word length (duration in milliseconds) and number of syllables. The backward words consisted of the same list of words as the comprehended words except the digitized files were played backward.

An editing program was used to ensure that the onset and offset time was the same for forward and backward words. The backward words were used as control responses to complex auditory stimuli with some of the same physical characteristics of speech. The words varied in length from 562 ms to 688 ms (mean comprehended and backward = 599, mean unknown = 598 ms) and were presented at intensities that ranged from 61 to 71 dB SPL (mean comprehended and backward = 66.9, mean unknown = 66.6).

Electrophysiological Testing

Electrode placement.   The electroencephalogram (EEG) was recorded using tin electrodes (Electro-Cap International) from sites over frontal (F7 and F8), anterior temporal (50% of the distance from F7/8 and T3/4), temporal (33% of the distance from T3/4 to C3/4), parietal (50% of the distance between T3/4 and P3/4), and occipital (O1 and O2) regions of the left and right hemispheres. In addition, the electrocculogram was recorded from electrodes placed over (Fp1) and under the eye to reject trials on which blinks and vertical eye movement occurred, and from left- and right-frontal electrodes to reject trials on which horizontal eye movement occurred. Impedances were kept below 5 Khoms and were balanced (within 1 Khom) across the left and right hemispheres at any given position. All electrodes were referenced to linked mastoids. The EEG was amplified by Grass model 7P511 amplifiers with a bandpass of 0.1 to 100 Hz and sampled continuously every 8 ms. Averages of the EEG were conducted using 2-sec epochs, that is, 100 ms prestimulus and 1900 ms poststimulus. All electrophysiological sessions were videotaped.

Artifact rejection.   Visual inspection of the data for eye and muscle artifact was conducted offline on a trial-by-trial basis. Assessment of responses from electrodes both over and under the eye allows for the discrimination of potentials generated by the eye (which are opposite in polarity above and below the eye) from events generated by the brain (which are the same in polarity). It is our experience that this distinction is critical for obtaining artifact-free data, especially in infants and toddlers. The percentage of trials rejected due to eye and movement artifact ranged from 28% to 76%, with a mean of 54%. That is, there were between 14 and 32 artifact-free trials per experimental condition (M = 28). There were no significant differences in the percentage of trials rejected for the different experimental conditions, different language groups, or for girls versus boys.

Testing.   Ten comprehended, 10 unknown, and 10 backward words were used. Each word was presented six times, for a total of 180 trials. Because both eye and muscle movement create artifact in the EEG, it was difficult to obtain artifact-free data from children in this age range. A considerable amount of time and effort was spent developing a procedure that would maintain the children's interest (i.e., keep them sitting still) long enough to collect enough usable data. During testing the children sat on their parent's lap and listened to words. The words were presented from a speaker located behind a moving puppet in a puppet theater. The procedure was designed to give the appearance that the puppet was "talking." However, the movements were not synchronized to the word presentations. To maintain the children's interest, a variety of puppets was used. Also, a reinforcement procedure was adopted. After the child sat still and watched the puppet for approximately 10 trials, the experimenter activated a battery-operated toy attached to the front of the puppet theater and praised the child. Development of the procedure made a dramatic improvement in the attainment of artifact-free data.

Measurement of ERP Components

ERP component amplitudes were quantified by computer with reference to the 100 ms prestimulus baseline. Peak amplitudes and latencies (for the maximum negative or positive point in a specified time window) were measured according to the following criteria: P100 as the most positive deflection between 50 and 175 ms, N200 as the most negative deflection between 125 and 250 ms, and N375 as the most negative deflection between 275 and 450 ms; mean area measures were also obtained for each of the windows described. In addition, the N600–1200 was defined and measured as the mean negative amplitude between 600 and 1200 ms.

BEHAVIORAL RESULTS

Table 1 provides a summary of the children's performance on measures of language comprehension and production. The behavioral data were analyzed for differences between girls and boys and two language groups (high and low comprehenders), in separate one-way analyses of variance (ANOVAs) on each of the measures of language comprehension and production. In addition, Pearson product–moment correlations were conducted to examine age trends on each of the behavioral language tests. The ANOVAs and correlations were conducted using BMDP program 3D in the 7.0 release (Dixon, 1992).

Language Comprehension

Two parental report measures, the CDI (Fenson et al., 1993) and a vocabulary checklist rating scale provided measures of language comprehension. There were no significant differences on these measures as a function of sex (Table 1). Surprisingly, there were no significant correlations with age. That is, there were no differences in the absolute numbers of words comprehended or produced from the 13- to 17-month-olds. Across the entire sample, the median scores for both comprehension and production was somewhat higher, by 10 to 20 percentile points, than the median scores for children in the same age range on the CDI. The scores from the CDI were used to separate the children into two groups based on language comprehension abilities. A median split was conducted such that the children who comprehended 150 words or more on the CDI were assigned to the "high-comprehension" group. Children who scored below this level were assigned to the "low-comprehension" group. The high-comprehension group consisted of 9 girls and 5 boys. The low-comprehension group consisted of 7 girls and 7 boys. The means and standard errors for the two groups are shown in Table 1. The high and low comprehenders also differed on a second measure of comprehension, the vocabulary checklist rating scale, $F(1, 25) = 4.71, p = .0001$.

Language Production

The CDI and vocabulary checklist rating scale also provided measures of language production abilities. There were no significant differences in production abilities linked to sex or age on either of these measures (Table 1). The high comprehenders also tended to produce more words than did the low comprehenders: CDI measure, $F(1, 25) = 4.04, p = .0004$; rating scale, $F(1, 25) = 3.60, p = .0014$. However, there

TABLE 1
Behavioral Test Scores As a Function of Gender and Comprehension Group

Participants	Mean Age in Months	MacArthur Communicative Development Inventory		Rating Scale	
		Number Comprehended	Number Produced	Number Comprehended	Number Produced
All 28	14.6	154	42	42	14
se	.29	16.61	7.81	4.33	2.75
Range	13.0–17.2	9–333	1–148	0–76	0–46
Girls (n = 16)	14.8	163	44	45	17
se	.40	24.27	10.06	6.19	4.20
Range	13–17	9–342	1–106	0–76	0–46
Boys (n = 12)	14.4	139	38	38	10
se	.42	19.50	12.85	5.79	2.60
Range	13–17	35–269	5–149	4–70	0–26
High comprehenders (n = 14)	14.5	220[a]	66*	58*	22*
se	.37	17.21	11.11	11.08	4.33
Range	13–17	151–342	7–149	40–76	0–46
Low comprehenders (n = 14)	14.7	88	16	27	6
se	.45	11.08	4.67	5.51	1.76
Range	13–17	9–133	0–53	0–70	0–21

[a]Groups are different by definition.
*Differences between high and low comprehenders were significant at $p < .01$.

was considerable variability in production abilities for both the high and low comprehenders. The relative effects of comprehension and production are discussed later.

ERP RESULTS

13- to 17-Month-Olds

ERPs were averaged separately for words whose meanings were comprehended by the child, words whose meanings the child did not comprehend, and backward words. The data for each ERP component were analyzed separately in mixed-model ANOVAs on two levels of group (high-comprehension vocabulary and low-comprehension vocabulary), three levels of word type (comprehended, unknown, and backward), two levels of hemisphere (left and right), and five levels of electrode site (frontal, anterior temporal, temporal, parietal, and occipital). The BMDP 4V program from the BMDP release 7.0 (Dixon, 1992) package was used to conduct the primary ANOVAs and planned comparisons. The Greenhouse–Geisser correction for repeated measures was applied to all measures with more than 1 degree of freedom. The Newman–Keuls test was used for post hoc comparisons (Winer, 1962). The mean square error terms used for the post hoc tests were from the appropriate factor in the main ANOVA. Preliminary analyses revealed no significant main effects or interactions with sex on any of the components, therefore sex was removed as a factor in the analyses. The main effects and interactions for the entire sample are presented first, followed by group effects due to differences in language comprehension and production abilities. Although both peak amplitude and mean area measures were taken, only the peak amplitude measures are reported here unless the area measures yielded different results. Results from the primary ANOVAs and planned comparisons are presented in Tables 1 to 3. The post hoc tests are described in the text. All post hoc effects reported were significant at the .05 level unless specified otherwise.

ERP Waveforms

Figures 1 and 2 display the ERPs averaged across all 28 participants to the words that were comprehended, unknown, and backward. The different types of words elicited a series of positive and negative deflections that varied in morphology and distribution across the scalp. A positive peak at approximately 100 ms (P100) was elicited to all stimuli, followed by two negative peaks at 200 ms (N200) and 375 ms (N375) that were elicited only by the comprehended words. Both the N200 and N375 were absent or attenuated to the unknown and backward words. Subsequently, a broad negative wave with an anterior distribution was evident from 600 to 1200 ms (N600–1200) to all stimuli.

ERP Sensitivity to Word Type

Effects of Word Meaning on ERP Latencies

The latency of the P100 to comprehended words (104 ms) was earlier than to unknown words (115 ms), which was earlier than to backward words (126 ms; see Table 2). The P100 latencies to both comprehended and unknown words tended to be earlier from the right than from the left hemisphere, whereas backward words showed the opposite pattern (Table 2, Word Type × Hemisphere). There were no main effects or interactions for the latencies of the N200 or N350.

Effects of Word Meaning on ERP Amplitudes

P100.   For all three types of words, the amplitude of the P100 was larger from anterior than posterior regions (Table 2). There were no main effects of word type.[1]

All 28 13–17 MONTH OLDS

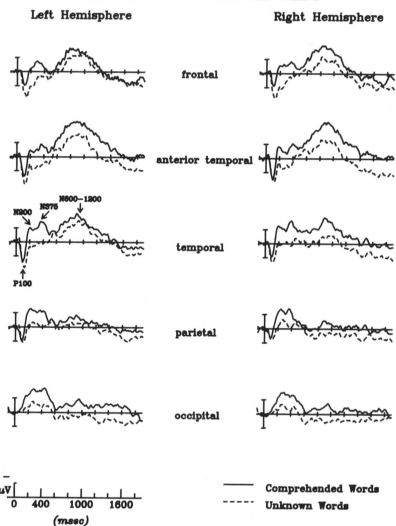

FIGURE 1   Event-related potentials to comprehended and unknown words for all 13- to 17-month-olds over frontal, anterior temporal, temporal, parietal, and occipital regions of the left and right hemispheres.

TABLE 2
Analysis of Variance for P100 Peak Amplitude and Latency for Comprehended, Unknown, and Backward Words

P100		Peak Latency	Peak Amplitude
Source	df	F	F
Word type (W)	2,52	1.17	10.41**
Hemisphere (H)	1,26	0.58	0.34
Electrode site	4,104	38.02**	5.40**
W × H	2,52	1.65	3.67*
Planned comparisons			
Comp × Unk	1,26	5.37*	0.88
Comp × Back	1,26	20.43**	0.28
Unk × Back	1,26	5.15*	2.50

Note. Comp = comprehended words; unk = unknown words; back = backward words; P100 = positive component peaking within the first 100 ms.
*$p < .05$. **$p < .01$.

However, the P100 was larger to unknown than to backward words over left-frontal and left-anterior temporal regions (Newman–Keuls, $p = .05$).

N200.   Across all three word types, the peak amplitudes of the N200 tended to be larger from posterior than from anterior regions (Figures 1 and 2). The lateral distribution of the N200 differed for words (comprehended and unknown) versus nonwords (backward; see Table 3, Word Type × Hemisphere × Electrode Site). The N200 amplitudes to comprehended and unknown words were slightly larger from the right than from the left hemisphere at sites over frontal, anterior temporal, and temporal regions (Figure 3). In contrast, the N200 to backward words showed the opposite trend.

The N200 amplitudes also were modulated by word meaning (Figures 1 and 2, Table 3). The N200 to comprehended words were larger than to unknown and backward words (planned comparisons). N200 amplitude differences to comprehended versus

---

[1]Visual inspection of the ERPs suggested marked amplitude differences between comprehended and unknown words over the frontal regions (see Figure 1). A separate ANOVA conducted for the frontal regions failed to reach significance for word type (comprehended vs. unknown) at the frontal lead, $F(1, 26) = 2.22$, $p = .15$. Examination of the individual participants showed that the P100 to unknown words was larger than to comprehended words at the frontal leads in six participants. The amplitude differences ranged from 15 to 20 μv for each participant and thus were large enough to be visible in the grand average. However, these differences were not present in a sufficient number of participants to yield significant α results.

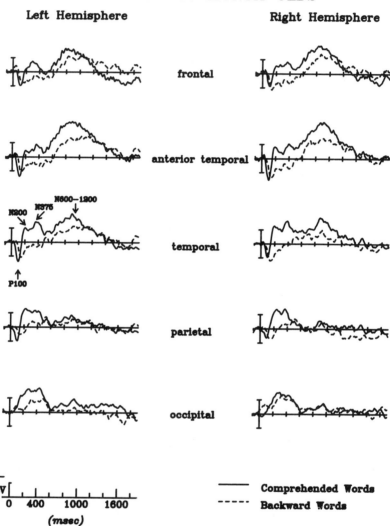

FIGURE 2   Event-related potentials to comprehended and backward words for all 13- to 17-month-olds over frontal, anterior temporal, temporal, parietal, and occipital regions of the left and right hemispheres.

412

TABLE 3
Analysis of Variance for N200 Peak Amplitude and Mean Area for Comprehended,
Unknown, and Backward Words

N200		Peak Amplitude	Mean Area
Source	df	F	F
Word type (W)	2,52	15.21**	11.24**
Hemisphere (H)	1,26	0.73	0.54
Electrode site (E)	4,104	7.60**	19.25**
W x E	8,208	2.42*	0.83
W x H x E	8,208	1.5	3.00*
Planned comparisons			
Comp x Unk			
W	1,26	12.13**	20.49**
E	4,104	5.84**	14.12**
H x E	4,104	0.83	3.37*
Comp x Back			
W	1,26	25.66**	14.66**
W x E	4,104	2.87*	3.91*
Unk x Back			
W	1,26	0.01	0.00
W x E	1,26	1.89	2.41*
W x H x E	4,104	1.33	5.17**

Note. Comp = comprehended words; unk = unknown words; back = backward words; N200 = negative deflection occurring at 200 ms.
*$p < .05$. **$p < .01$.

unknown words were broadly distributed over frontal, anterior temporal, temporal, parietal, and occipital regions, and over both the left and right hemispheres (Newman–Keuls, for all sites anterior to occiput, $p = .01$; occipital areas, $p = .05$). The N200 was larger to comprehended than to backward words over all areas anterior to the occiput, Newman–Keuls, $p = .01$ (main effects, Table 3). Post hoc tests revealed that over the occipital regions, differences were significant for the left hemisphere but not for the right hemisphere. There were no main effects of N200 peak amplitude differences between unknown and backward words. However, there were differences in the lateral distribution of the N200 words (both comprehended and unknown) versus backward words as described previously (Table 3 and Figure 3).

N375.   For all three types of words, the N375 peak amplitude tended to be larger from over posterior than from over anterior regions (Figures 1 and 2 and Table 4). Planned comparisons showed that the N375 to comprehended words was larger than to unknown and backward words. Moreover, these differences were observed at all electrode sites (Newman–Keuls, for all sites anterior to the occiput,

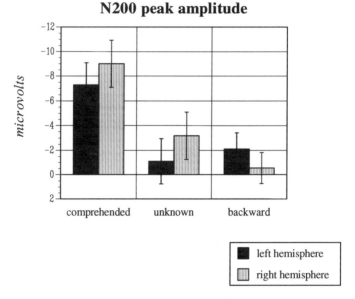

13-17 month olds all 28s

N200 peak amplitude

FIGURE 3 N200 peak amplitudes to comprehended, unknown and backward words for all 13-to 17-month-olds. This figure shows that both comprehended and unknown words displayed N200 responses that were larger over the right than over the left hemisphere over regions anterior to the parietal regions. Backward words did not show significant hemisphere effects.

$p = .01$; occipital areas, $p = .05$). The N375 peak amplitudes did not differ for unknown and backward words.

N600–1200 mean area.   Subsequent to the N375, there was a broad negative wave from approximately 600 to 1200 ms, N600–1200, that displayed a frontal distribution. The N600–1200 was larger to comprehended words than to unknown words but did not differ for comprehended versus backward words, or for unknown versus backward words (Table 5).

Summary of ERP Sensitivity to Word Type

All three types of words elicited a positive component at 100 ms (i.e., P100) that was larger from anterior than from posterior regions. P100 latencies distinguished between all three types of words. Comprehended and unknown words were characterized by two negative components at 200 and 375 ms (i.e., N200 and N375) that were

TABLE 4
Analysis of Variance Tables for N375 Peak Amplitude and Mean Area for Comprehended,
Unknown, and Backward Words

N375		Peak Amplitude	Mean Area
Source	df	F	F
Word type (W)	2,52	9.76**	8.38**
Electrode site	4,104	5.97**	9.53**
Planned comparisons			
Comp x Unk			
W	1,26	14.8**	12.22**
Comp x Back			
W	1,26	11.45**	11.06**
Unk x Back			
W	1,26	0.32	0.04

Note. Comp = comprehended words; unk = unknown words; back = backward words; N375 =
negative deflection occurring at 375 ms.
  *$p < .05$. **$p < .01$.

larger over posterior than over anterior regions and were absent or attenuated to
backward words. Comprehended words were discriminated from unknown and backward words over frontal, anterior temporal, temporal, parietal, and occipital regions of
both the left and right hemispheres. There also were differences in ERPs between unknown
and backward words. The P100 peak latency was earlier and, over anterior regions, its
amplitude was larger to unknown than to backward words. In addition, the N200 to
unknown and backward words displayed different lateral distributions over anterior
regions in the window from 125 to 250 ms.

ERP Sensitivity to Language Comprehension Abilities

In this section, the effects of group differences in language comprehension abilities
(i.e., high comprehenders and low comprehenders) on the latency amplitude and
distribution of ERPs to the different types of words are reported for each of the ERP
components (Figures 4 and 5, Tables 6, 7, 8, and 9). ERPs to backward words were
not different for the two groups. The following results compare the two groups for
differences in ERPs to comprehended and unknown words.

Effects of Comprehension Abilities on ERP Latencies

There were no group differences in the latencies of the P100, the N350, or for
the duration of the N600–1200. The peak latency of the N200 was earlier for the

13–17 month olds

High Comprehenders N=14

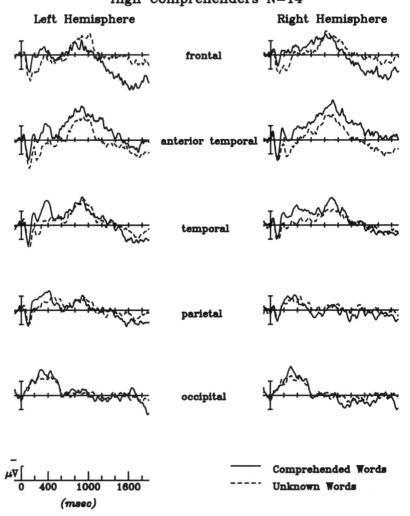

FIGURE 4 Event-related potentials to comprehended and unknown words for 13- to 17-month-old high comprehenders.

TABLE 5
Analysis of Variance for N600–1200 Mean Area for Comprehended,
Unknown, and Backward Words

N600–1200		Mean Area
Source	df	F
Word type	2,52	2.67 (p = .08)
Electrode site	4,104	13.59**
Planned comparisons		
Comp x Unk	1,26	4.96*
Comp x Back	1,26	1.86
Unk x Back	1,26	1.06

Note. Comp = comprehended words; unk = unknown words; back = backward words;
N600–1200 = negative deflection occurring between 600 and 1200 ms.
*$p < .05$; **$p < .01$.

TABLE 6
Analysis of Variance for P100 Peak Amplitude and Latency for High Versus
Low Producers

P100		Peak Amplitude
Source	df	F
Language group (L)	1,26	2.24
L x Hemisphere	4,104	3.57 (p = .07)
Planned comparisons		
High comprehenders		
Hemisphere	1,13	12.81**
Low comprehenders		
Hemisphere	1,13	0.00

Note. P100 = positive component peaking within the first 100 ms.
*$p < .05$. **$p < .01$.

high comprehenders (197 ms) than for the low comprehenders (216 ms). Group
differences in the N200 latency were most prominent over posterior regions of the
left hemisphere (Table 7, Language Group × Word Type × Electrode Site, Language
Group × Word Type × Hemisphere).

Effects of Comprehension Abilities on ERP Amplitudes

There were no main effects of language group. However, there were several
interactions with word type and distribution. These effects are discussed for each
of the components.

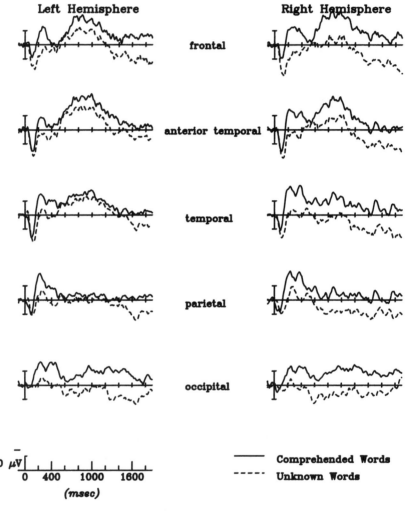

13–17 month olds
Low Comprehenders N=14

FIGURE 5   Event-related potentials to comprehended and unknown words for 13- to 17-month-old low comprehenders.

TABLE 7
Analysis of Variance Tables for N200 Peak Amplitude and Mean Area for High Versus Low Producers

N200		Peak Latency	Peak Amplitude	Mean Area
Source	df	F	F	F
Language group (L)	1,26	4.34*	0.15	2.33
L x W x H	1,26	7.48*	1.07	0.79
L x W x E	4,104	3.08*	3.15*	1.65
Planned comparisons				
High comprehenders				
Word type (W)	1,13	0.83	5.97*	5.83*
Hemisphere (H)	4,22	0.17	3.52 ($p = .08$)	4.22 ($p = .06$)
Electrode site (E)	4,52	0.71	4.07*	10.28*
W x E	4,52	1.25	7.37*	2.53*
H x E	4,52	2.97*	0.07	1.30
W x H	1,13	6.63*	0.31	0.73
Low comprehenders				
W	1,13	0.03	23.52**	14.92**
E	4,52	0.49	2.85	5.09*

Note. N200 = negative deflection occurring at 200 ms.
*$p < .05$. **$p < .01$.

TABLE 8
ANOVA for N375 Peak Amplitude and Mean Area for High Versus Low Producers

N375		Peak Amplitude	Mean Area
Source	df	F	F
L x H x E	4,104	1.57	2.95*
Planned comparisons			
High comprehenders			
Word type (W)	1,13	4.17 ($p = .06$)	2.48
Electrode site (E)	4,152	3.37	5.26*
Low comprehenders			
Word type	1.13	11.94**	11.30**

Note. N375 = negative deflection occurring at 375 ms.
*$p < .05$. **$p < .01$.

TABLE 9
Analysis of Variance Tables for N600–1200 Mean Area for
Comprehended, Unknown, and Backward Words

N600–1200		Mean Area
Source	df	F
Language age	1,26	3.48*
Planned comparisons		
High comprehenders		
Word type	1,13	0.16
Low comprehenders		
Word type	1,13	5.26*

Note. N600–1200 = negative deflection occurring between 600 and 1200 ms.
*p < .05. **p < .01.

P100. The P100 displayed a Language Group × Hemisphere interaction that approached significance (Table 6). Because results from 20-month-olds on this paradigm showed an asymmetrical, left-greater-than-right P100 to comprehended and unknown words, we pursued this interaction further. For the high-comprehension group, like our results for the 20-month-olds (Mills et al., 1993), the peak amplitude of the P100 was larger from the left than from the right hemisphere for both comprehended and unknown words (Figure 6). For the low comprehenders the P100 amplitude was bilaterally distributed. Neither group showed significant P100 amplitude differences between comprehended and unknown words.[2]

N200. There were no significant differences in the overall amplitudes of the N200 for the high and low comprehenders (Table 7). However, examination of the interactions with word type and electrode type showed that the low comprehenders displayed broadly distributed N200 differences to comprehended and unknown words (Figure 7, Table 7, and Newman–Keuls, p = .01 for frontal, temporal, parietal, and occipital regions). In contrast, the high comprehenders showed a more limited distribution of N200 responsiveness to the different types of words. For the high comprehenders the N200 was larger to comprehended than to unknown words over

---

[2]However, visual inspection of the data suggested that for the low comprehenders the P100 was larger to unknown words than to comprehended words over the frontal area. These differences were not significant for word type at frontal for low comprehenders: $F(1, 13) = .89, p = .36$. The apparent P100 amplitude differences can be attributed to four participants in this group who displayed frontal P100 responses that were larger (by 15 to 20 μv) to unknown words than to comprehended words.

P100 Peak Amplitude
13-17 Month Olds (N=28)

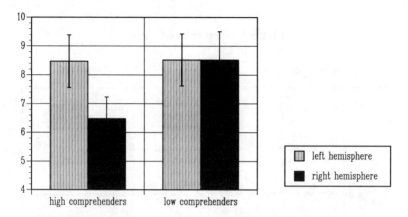

FIGURE 6   P100 peak amplitudes over the left and right hemispheres for the 13-
to 17-month-old high and low comprehenders. High comprehenders show a left-
greater-than-right asymmetry. In contrast, low comprehenders show symmetrical
P100 responses. Peak amplitudes were averaged over anterior and posterior regions.

sites anterior to the parietal areas (Newman–Keuls, $p = .01$ for frontal and anterior
temporal regions; $p = .05$ for temporal and left, but not right, parietal regions).

N375.   The two groups differed in the distribution of the N375 responsiveness between comprehended and unknown words (Table 8). As for the N200, the
low comprehenders showed larger N375 responses to comprehended than to
unknown words over all electrode sites (Newman–Keuls, temporal region = .01,
frontal, anterior temporal, parietal, and occipital regions $p = .05$), whereas for the
high producers these effects were limited to anterior temporal and temporal
regions ($p = .05$).

N600–1200.   Figures 4 and 5 illustrate apparent group differences in the
N600–1200 to comprehended and unknown words. However, the effect of language
group on the N600–1200 differences to comprehended and unknown words only
approached significance (Table 9). Newman–Keuls tests showed that the
N600–1200 was larger to comprehended than to unknown words only for the low
producers ($p = .05$).

13-17 month olds
N200 Peak Amplitude

High Comprehenders

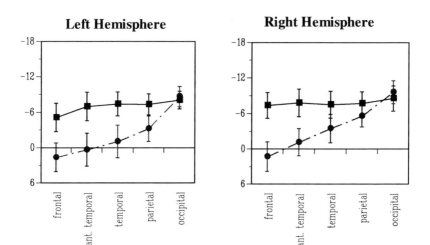

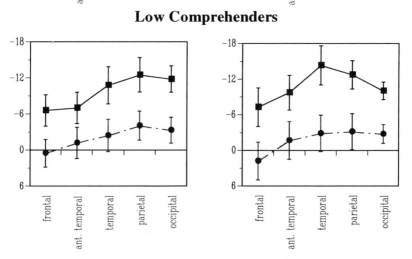

FIGURE 7 N200 peak amplitudes for the 13- to 17-month-old high and low comprehenders over frontal, anterior temporal, temporal, parietal, and occipital regions of the left and right hemispheres.

Summary of ERP Sensitivity to Language Comprehension Abilities

For the high-comprehension group, the P100 displayed a left-greater-than-right asymmetry, which was consistent with the left-hemisphere asymmetry previously reported for 20-month-olds (Mills et al., 1993). In contrast, the P100 amplitude was symmetrical for the low-comprehension group. The latency of the N200 to comprehended words was earlier for the high than for the low comprehenders. Indeed, for the high comprehenders it was the same as previously reported for the 20-month-olds (197 ms). In addition, a marked difference between the groups was in the distribution of the N200 and N350 responsiveness to comprehended versus unknown words. Whereas the low comprehenders displayed differences between known and unknown words over all sites within both hemispheres, word differences in the high comprehenders occurred over frontal, anterior temporal, temporal, and left parietal regions but were absent over right parietal and both occipital regions.

ERP Sensitivity to Language Production Abilities

Because the high and low comprehenders also differed in language production abilities, it was of interest to examine ERP effects on productive vocabulary independent of comprehension abilities. Separate analyses were conducted on a subset of children (n = 14) who were matched for language comprehension but differed in productive vocabulary size, that is, fewer than 50 words (M = 20, range = 7–32) and more than 50 words (M = 65, range = 50–97). The analyses revealed no significant ERP effects linked to productive vocabulary size independent of comprehension abilities.

Summary of ERP Effects at 13 to 17 Months

Word Type

ERPs differed as a function of word meaning by at least 200 ms after word onset. ERP amplitude differences between comprehended and unknown words were bilaterally distributed over frontal, anterior temporal, temporal, parietal, and occipital regions. ERP differences between unknown and backward words were shown in the amplitude and latency of the P100, and in the distribution of the N200.

Language Comprehension Abilities

Consistent with our previous findings, when group differences were observed the high comprehenders displayed ERPs that were earlier and more focally distributed than were those of the low comprehenders. Group differences in ERPs were shown in the lateral distribution of the P100 to comprehended words; the latency of the N200; and the distribution of N200, N350, and N600–1200 responsiveness to comprehended and unknown words.

Language Production Abilities

There were no significant group differences linked to the size of the child's productive vocabulary when receptive vocabulary size was held constant.

13- to 20-Month Comparisons

One of the main goals of this research was to examine changes in the organization of language-relevant brain systems that occur as children pass through different ages and attain new language milestones and to compare these with changes linked to level of ability when age is held constant. To this end it was important to compare the patterns of brain activity observed in the 13- to 17-month-old children with those previously reported in 20-month-olds (Mills et al., 1993). A comparison of the results from these two studies suggests that between 13 and 20 months of age there are marked changes in the organization of neural activity linked to language processing. In this section we briefly review the patterns of ERPs displayed by the 20-month-olds from the previous study for each of the components and compare their data with our sample of 13- to 17-month-olds.

20-Month-Old participants

A complete description of the 20-month-old participants is available in Mills et al. (1993). Briefly, the participants were 16 girls and 8 boys (mean age = 20.5 months, range = 19.50–21.75 months). The children produced a mean of 184 (range = 33–531) words as determined by the CDI. It was not possible to obtain a measure of the number of words comprehended because comprehension is not measured separately from production on the CDI at 20 months and older. There were no effects of sex on the organization of ERPs to the different types of words.

Procedure

The procedure was the same as described for the 13- to 17-month-olds, with the exception that recordings from over anterior temporal regions were not available for the 20-month-olds. Therefore, the anterior temporal sites recorded from the 13- to 17-month-olds were not included in the analyses for the age comparisons.

Comparisons between the 13- to 17-month-olds and the 20-month-olds were conducted using mixed-model ANOVAs with repeated measures with two levels of age groups (13 to 17 months and 20 months), three levels of word type (comprehended, unknown, and backward), two levels of hemisphere (left and right) and four levels of electrode site (frontal, temporal, parietal, and occipital regions).

For both the 13- to 17-month-olds and the 20-month-olds, the P100 was measured as the most positive peak between 50 and 175 ms. To accurately measure the N200, N350, and N600–900 it was necessary to set slightly different time windows for the two groups (N200: 125–250 ms at 20 months, 125 –275 at 13–17 months; N350: 275–450 at 20 months, 300–450 at 13–17 months; N600–900: 600–900 ms at 20 months, 600–1200 at 13–17 months). The ANOVA values for the age effects and interactions with age are presented in Tables 10, 11, 12, and 13. ERPs to comprehended, unknown, and backward words for the 20-month-olds are presented in Figures 8 and 9.

TABLE 10
Analysis of Variance for P100 Peak Amplitude and Latency for 13–17
Versus 20-Month-Olds

P100		Peak Latency	Peak Amplitude
Source	df	F	F
Age (A)	1,50	7.22**	0.05
A x H x E	3,150	0.25	3.24*

Note. H = hemisphere; E = electrode site; P100 = positive component peaking within first 100 ms.
*p < .05. **p < .01.

TABLE 11
Analysis of Variance for N200 Peak Latency and Peak Amplitude for
13–17 Versus 20-Month-Olds

N200		Peak Latency	
Source	df	F	F
Age (A)	1,50	5.82*	0.65
A x W	2,200	0.62	4.46**
A x E	3,150	0.39	3.24*
A x W x H	2,100	3.43*	1.38
A x H x W x E	6,300	0.82	2.22*

Note: W = word type; H = hemisphere; E = electrode site; N200 = negative deflection occurring at 200 ms.
*p < .05. **p < .01.

TABLE 12
Analysis of Variance for N350 Peak Latency and Peak Amplitude for
13–17 Versus 20-Month-Olds

N350		Peak Latency	
Source	df	F	
Age (A)	1,50	26.42**	0.51
A x W	2,100	4.34*	2.01
A x E	3,150	1.99	2.94 ($p = .06$)
A x H x E	2,100	1.05	2.82*

Note. W = word type; H = hemisphere; E = electrode site; N350 = negative deflection occurring at 350 ms.
*$p < .05$. **$p < .01$.

Age-Related Differences in ERP Latencies

The latencies of the P100, N200, and N350 were earlier (by 10 to 25 ms) for the 20-month-olds than for the 13- to 17-month-olds (Tables 10 and 11). The P100 showed the age differences in latencies for comprehended, unknown, and backward words. In contrast, the N200 showed latency differences only for the comprehended words. The N350 latencies, and duration of the N600–900, showed age differences for the comprehended and unknown words but not for the backward words.

Age-Related Differences in ERP Amplitudes

There were no overall amplitude differences for any of the components; however, there were interactions with word type and distributions for the N200, N350, and N600–900.

P100. For the 20-month-olds, the P100 displayed a left-greater-than-right asymmetry for comprehended and unknown words. For the 13- to 17-month-olds, the P100 was symmetrical for the group as a whole (Table 10). However, as noted earlier, the 13- to 17-month-old high comprehenders also showed a left-greater-than-right asymmetry.

N200. The anterior–posterior distribution of the N200 differed between 13 and 20 months (Figure 10; Table 11, Electrode Site × Age). For the 13- to 17

All 24 20—MONTH OLDS

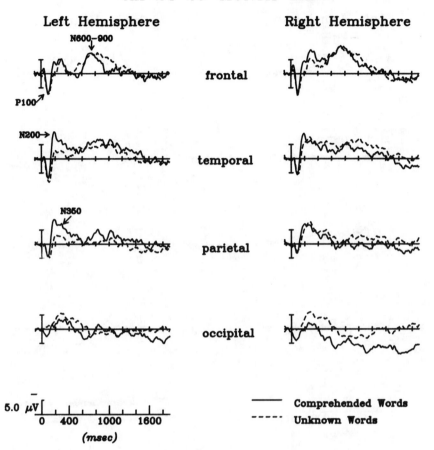

FIGURE 8   Event-related potentials to comprehended and unknown words for 20-month-olds.

month-olds the amplitude of the N200 tended to be larger from posterior than from anterior regions (Table 3, electrode site), whereas for the 20-month-olds the N200 was largest over temporal and parietal regions (Mills et al., 1993). Simple effects for each word type showed that the N200 to the unknown words was on average 4 μv larger for the 20-month-olds than for the 13- to 17-month-olds (Table 11).

Of particular interest were age-related changes in ERP differences to comprehended and unknown words. The distribution of the N200 responsiveness to comprehended and unknown words showed marked differences in distribution between words (Figure 10; Table 11). For the 13- to 17-month-olds the distribution

All 24 20-MONTH OLDS

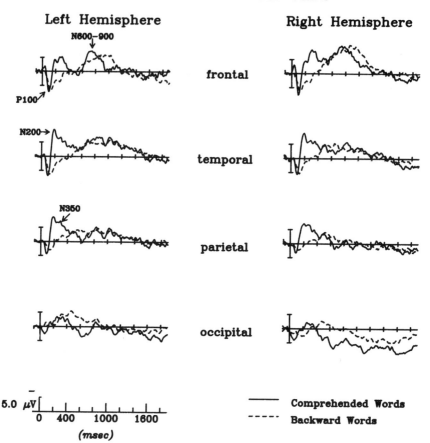

FIGURE 9   Event-related potentials to comprehended and backward words for 20-month-olds.

of the N200 differences to comprehended and unknown words was distributed broadly over anterior and posterior regions of both the left and right hemispheres (see earlier discussion). In contrast, the 20-month-olds showed N200 amplitude differences only over temporal and parietal regions of the left hemisphere (Mills et al., 1993).

Both age groups showed bilateral N200 differences to comprehended versus backward words. However, only the 20-month-olds showed N200 amplitude differences between unknown and backward words. These age-related differences can be accounted for primarily by larger N200 responses to unknown words for the

N200 Peak Amplitude
13-17 month olds

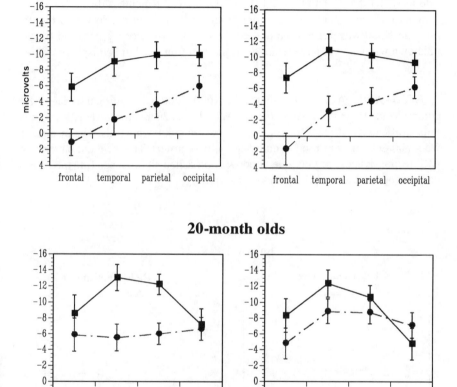

FIGURE 10   N200 peak amplitudes to comprehended and unknown words for the 13- to 17-month-old and 20-month-old infants.

20-month-olds (as noted previously), and by larger N200 responses to backward words over left anterior and right occipital regions for the 13- to 17-month-olds (Figure 11).

N375. The lateral and anterior–posterior distribution of the N350 was different for the 13- to 17-month-olds and the 20-month-olds, (Hemisphere × Electrode Site × Age; Table 12 and Figure 12). For the 13- to 17-month-olds the N350 was symmetrical and larger from posterior than from anterior regions. For the 20-month-olds the N350 was larger from anterior than from posterior regions, and for the unknown words it was larger from the right than from the left hemisphere.

N600–900. At 13 to 17 months the N600–1200 was significantly larger for comprehended than for unknown words. Whereas, at 20 months the N600–900 was not significantly different for comprehended and unknown words. The mean area from 600–900 ms was used to compare the two groups. The different patterns of ERP responsiveness in this time window approached significance (planned comparison for comprehended and unknown words).

13-20 months

Backward Words

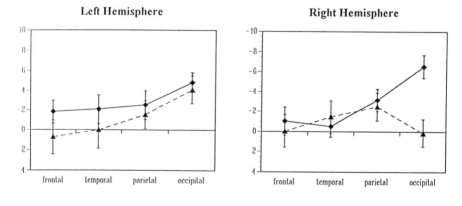

FIGURE 11   N200 mean areas to backward words for the 13- to 17-month-old and 20-month-old infants.

Summary of Age-Related Differences

The latencies of the P100, N200, and N350 were slightly earlier for the 20-month-olds than for the 13- to 17-month-olds. The duration of the late negative component was somewhat longer, by 300 ms, for the 13- to 17-months-olds than for the 20-month-olds. There also were marked age-related differences in the distribution of ERP responsiveness to the different types of words. At 13 to 17 months of age ERP differences to comprehended and unknown words were bilateral and widely distributed, whereas at 20 months these differences were limited to temporal and parietal regions of the left hemisphere. ERP differences to comprehended versus backward words were bilaterally distributed for both groups. Only the 20-month-olds showed N200 and N350 amplitude differences to unknown versus backward words.

DISCUSSION

For both the 13- to 17-month-olds and the 20-month-olds, ERPs differed as a function of word meaning within 200 ms after the onset of the word. The latencies, amplitudes, and distributions of ERPs varied as a function of age, word type, and level of language abilities. Tables 13 and 14 provide a summary of the ERP effects for the two age groups and for the 13- to 17-month-old high and low comprehenders. In the following sections we discuss the observed developmental changes in ERPs as a function of (a) the general effects of maturation, (b) the maturation of language-relevant brain systems, and (c) the development of brain systems linked to level of ability independent of chronological age. Subsequently, the implications of this research for theories of early language acquisition are discussed as they pertain to neurobiological evidence for cognitive reorganizational processes linked to changes in vocabulary size.

General Effects of Maturation

Age-related changes in the latencies, amplitudes, and distributions of ERPs that did not interact with word type or level of language abilities were interpreted as indexing maturation of auditory cortical systems not specific to language processing. The latencies of several ERP components decreased with age. This finding was consistent with other developmental ERP studies showing similar decreases in ERP latencies with increasing age (e.g., Courchesne, 1978; Holcomb et al., 1992; Kurtzberg, Stone, & Vaughn, 1986; Polich, Ladish, & Burns, 1990). However, in this study only the P100 displayed age-related latency differences that were independent of word type. Decreases in the latencies of the N200 and N350 were limited to a given word type and may therefore reflect maturation specific to language-relevant brain systems.

TABLE 13
Summary of Age-Related Event-Related Potentials Effects for Comprehended and Unknown Words

	13–17-Month-Olds (N = 28)			20-Month-Olds (N = 24)		
	P100	*N200*	*N350*	*P100*	*N200*	*N350*
Comprehended words	104 ms Symmetrical Anterior > Posterior	210 ms Right > Left Posterior > Anterior	375 ms Symmetrical Posterior > Anterior	100 ms Left > Right Anterior > Posterior	200 ms Symmetrical Largest: Temporal Parietal	350 ms Symmetrical Anterior > Posterior
Unknown words	115 ms Symmetrical Anterior > Posterior	210 ms Right > Left Posterior > Anterior	375 ms Symmetrical Posterior > Anterior	100 ms Left > Right Anterior > Posterior	200 ms Right >> Left Anterior > Posterior	350 ms Right >> Left Anterior > Posterior
Differences	No amplitude differences	Left and right	Left and right	No amplitude differences	By 150 ms	By 300 ms
Comprehended/Unknown		Frontal Temporal Parietal Occipital	Frontal Temporal Parietal Occipital		Left: Temporal Parietal	Left: Temporal Parietal

Note. P100 = positive component peaking within first 100 ms; N200 = negative deflection occurring at 200 ms; N350 = negative deflection occurring at 350 ms.

TABLE 14
Summary of 13–17-Month-Old High Versus Low Comprehenders: Event-Related Potentials Effects for Comprehended and Unknown Words

	Low Comprehenders (N = 14)			High Comprehenders (N = 14)		
	P100	*N200*	*N375*	*P100*	*N200*	*N375*
Comprehended words	104 ms	216 ms	375 ms	104 ms	197 ms	375 ms
	Symmetrical	Trend right > left	Symmetrical	Symmetrical	Right > Left	Symmetrical
	Anterior >	Posterior >	Posterior >	Anterior >	Posterior >	Posterior >
	Posterior	Anterior	Anterior	Posterior	Anterior	Anterior
Unknown words	115 ms	210 ms	375 ms	115 ms	200 ms	375 ms
	Symmetrical	Trend right > left	Symmetrical	Symmetrical	Right > Left	Symmetrical
	Anterior >	Posterior >	Posterior >	Anterior >	Posterior >	Posterior >
	Posterior	Anterior	Anterior	Posterior	Anterior	Anterior
Differences	No amplitude differences	Left and right	Left and right	No amplitude differences	Left and right	Left and right
Comprehended/Unknown		Frontal	Frontal		Frontal	Frontal
		Anterior temporal	Anterior temporal		Anterior temporal	Anterior temporal
		Temporal	Temporal		Temporal	
		Parietal	Parietal		Left parietal	
		Occipital	Occipital			

Note. P100 = positive component peaking within first 100 ms; N200 = negative deflection occurring at 200 ms; N350 = negative deflection occurring at 350 ms.

Other research has shown that after 6 months of age ERP amplitudes for both early and late components (P100, N100, N200, N400, and P300) tend to decrease with increasing age (Courchesne, 1978; Holcomb et al., 1992; Johnson, 1989; Kurtzberg et al., 1986; Mullis, Holcomb, Diner, & Dykman, 1985), although some research suggests that the amplitude of the P300 may increase with age (McIsaac & Polich, 1992; Polich, et al., 1990). Overall reductions in ERP amplitudes with increasing age were not observed in this study. These results suggest that very few of the developmental changes in ERPs observed here can be attributed solely to general maturational factors.

Age and Word Type Interactions: Maturation of Language-Relevant Brain Systems

There were several developmental changes in the latencies, amplitudes, and distribution of ERPs that interacted with word type. Age-related changes in ERPs that were specific to processing comprehended or unknown, but not backward, words were considered to index maturation of language-relevant brain systems.

Reductions in the latencies of the N200 and N350 between 13 and 20 months were observed only for the comprehended words. Moreover, N200 and N350 latencies to comprehended words were reduced with increasing language abilities when age was held constant, that is, the N200 at 13 to 17 months (with increasing receptive vocabulary size), and the N350 at 20 months (with increasing productive vocabulary size). The decreases in N200 and N350 latencies to comprehended words may index faster, or more automatic processing of word meanings as a function of increasing language comprehension and production abilities.

Developmental changes in lateralization for word comprehension. As noted earlier, there is some controversy as to whether the left-hemisphere specialization for language develops with age and experience with language or is present from birth. The results from this study suggest that different ERP components display different lateral asymmetries and may index different aspects of language processing. The P100 displays a left-greater-than-right asymmetry in the 13- to 17-month-old high producers and in the 20-month-olds. As noted in a subsequent section, the P100 is thought to index sensory processing. Here, the presence of a left asymmetry in the P100 was associated with better language abilities and may be linked to a left-hemisphere bias for processing familiar phonological stimuli.

In contrast, asymmetries observed for the later components, N200 and N350, are consistent with the position that the right hemisphere plays an important role in early language acquisition. At 13 to 17 months there was a small but reliable right-greater-than-left asymmetry in the N200 to both comprehended and unknown words. At 20 months the N200 and N350 to comprehended words were symmetri-

N350 Peak Amplitude

13-17 month olds

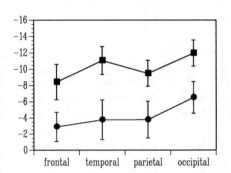 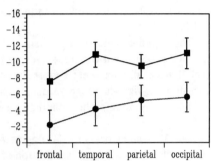

20-month olds

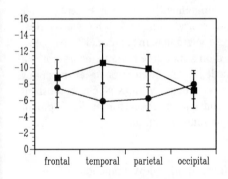 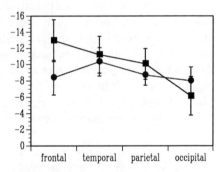

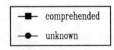

FIGURE 12 N350 peak amplitudes to comprehended and unknown words for the 13- to 17-month-old and 20-month-old infants.

cal, whereas unknown words elicited greater activity over the right hemisphere. The data showing a right-hemisphere asymmetry for both comprehended and unknown words at 13 to 17 months, but only for the unknown words at 20 months, suggested that the right hemisphere may show greater activity during the initial stages of language comprehension. Previously we speculated that the asymmetrical right-greater-than-left N200 and N350 to unknown words at 20 months may reflect right-hemisphere involvement in the processing of novel but meaningful stimuli (Mills et al., 1993).

The hypothesis that the right hemisphere is important in early language comprehension is consistent with recent results observed in infants with focal brain injury (see Bates et al., this issue; Thal et al., 1991). In those studies, 10- to 17-month-old infants with right-hemisphere damage were significantly more likely to exhibit delays in word comprehension than were children with damage to the left hemisphere.

Goldberg and Costa (1981) suggested that the right hemisphere plays a critical role in the initial stages of acquisition of a variety of cognitive abilities, including language, because the neuroanatomical organization of the right hemisphere may be better suited to processing novel stimuli, whereas the left hemisphere is superior at utilizing well-routinized codes. This raises the hypothesis that at 20 months the lack of a right-hemisphere asymmetry to comprehend words may reflect greater left-hemisphere activation and more automatic processing of familiar words. Best (1988) also proposed a right-to-left lateralization gradient in her model of neuroembryological development. Her model, based on a literature review, incorporated a three-dimensional growth vector that proceeded in a right-anterior-to-left-posterior direction and from primary sensory to tertiary association areas. She hypothesized that the morphological growth vector would have implications for the development of functional specializations preceding in the same directions.

Anterior–posterior development. In addition to developmental changes in the lateral distribution of ERPs, our results showed developmental changes in the anterior)posterior distribution of ERPs to comprehended and unknown words. At 13 to 17 months the N200 and N375 to both comprehended and unknown words were larger over posterior than over anterior regions. By 20 months of age the amplitudes of these components were reduced over the occipital regions, which has been shown to mediate processing of visual information in older children and adults. Moreover, in the 20-month-old high producers these components were largest over temporal and parietal regions, which is consistent with a more mature pattern of neural activity during auditory processing. Previously we reported that in normal 6- to 36-month-olds and adults the amplitudes of auditory ERPs over occipital areas become progressively attenuated with increasing age, whereas ERPs over temporal areas become more pronounced (Neville, 1995). Large amplitude responses to auditory stimuli over the occipital areas in the younger participants suggests less specificity and more redundant connections in auditory and visual cortex early in development. Here the reduction in the amplitudes of the N200 and N350 over the occipital areas between 13 and 20 months may reflect progressive differentiation of the auditory and visual sensory systems.

In summary, the results of this study are consistent with the position that the functional organization of language-relevant brain systems becomes progressively specialized in both the lateral and anterior–posterior dimensions during the course of development. In the next section, we further examine the extent to which the development of these specialized systems may be shaped by experience with language as indexed by increasing vocabulary size.

Development of Language-Relevant Brain Systems Linked to Level of Ability Independent of Chronological Age

Another goal of this study was to examine changes in the organization of language-relevant neural systems linked to differences in language comprehension abilities when chronological age was held constant. Significant group differences were observed for the 13- to 17-month-olds in the latency and lateral distribution of the P100; the latency of the N200; and distribution and responsiveness of the N200, N350, and N600–1200 to comprehended and unknown words. Like the results from our previous study of 20-month-olds, when group differences were observed in the latency or amplitude of ERPs, the high comprehenders tended to display ERPs that were earlier and smaller (i.e., more mature) than did the low comprehenders.

For the 13- to 17-month-olds, the latency and distribution of the P100 varied as a function of comprehension abilities. For the 13- to 17-month-old high comprehenders, like the 20-month-olds, the P100 displayed a left-greater-than-right asymmetry. For the 13- to 17-month-old low comprehenders the P100 was symmetrical. Although these results appear to suggest that the P100 asymmetry may reflect a more mature pattern, data from our studies of 20- to 42-month-old normal children and late talkers suggest that the left-greater-than-right P100 asymmetry does not develop at a particular age, and it is not linked to the attainment of a specific language milestone, rather it is correlated with a given child's percentile ranking for language abilities independent of chronological age (Mills, Thal, DiIulio, Castaneda, & Neville, 1995). That is, children at 20 months, 28 to 30 months, and 36 to 42 months who scored above the 50th percentile on the CDI for the number of words they produced showed a left-greater-than-right asymmetry for the P100 to comprehended words. Children at each of these age groups who scored below the 30th percentile for productive vocabulary showed symmetrical P100 responses to comprehended words. If the P100 indexes early sensory processing, as suggested by its latency, the results are consistent with the hypothesis that the organization of the auditory sensory system may be linked to language abilities (Tallal & Piercy, 1973). The hypothesis that an early left-hemisphere asymmetry may be linked to later language abilities also are consistent with research by Molfese and colleagues (Molfese & Betz, 1998; Molfese & Molfese, 1994) who showed that very young infants who showed ERP differences to different phonological stimuli over the left hemisphere also showed relatively better language abilities at 3 to 5 years than did infants who did not show these differences.

For the later components, N200 and N375, the results for the 13- to 17-month-olds were consistent with our previous findings from 20-month-olds. That is, when group differences were observed in the distribution of ERPs, the high comprehenders displayed more focally distributed responses than did the low producers. The hypothesis that increased specialization of neural systems subserving language may be linked to increasing language abilities has been suggested in studies of adults using a variety of techniques (Cawthon, Ojemann, & Lettich, 1991; Fedio et al., 1992; Neville et al., 1993; Ojemann, 1991; Weber-Fox & Neville, 1992, 1996). In this study, group differences were observed in the distribution of the N200 and N375 responsiveness to known and unknown words over the occipital and right parietal regions, and over the frontal and anterior temporal regions from 600–1200 ms. That is, only the low comprehenders showed ERP differences to comprehended and unknown words over these areas. A lack of ERP differences in these areas is consistent with a more mature pattern of neural activity; that is, the high comprehenders displayed a pattern of ERPs more similar to the pattern displayed by the 20-month-olds. Moreover, the 13- to 17-month-old high comprehenders showed some evidence of a left-hemisphere asymmetry, over parietal regions, in ERP differences to comprehended words, that is, again, like the 20-month-old children.

In summary, the results from this study and studies of other age groups on this paradigm (Mills et al., 1995) suggest there are marked differences in the functional significance of the P100 effects of language abilities as compared to the effects shown by the later components, the N200 and N350. The distributions and responsiveness of the N200 and N350 to different types of words changed with age and the attainment of new language milestones. In contrast, although the lateral distribution of the P100 also varied as a function of level of ability, the left asymmetry, or lack thereof, may be immutable across this period of development. It is our working hypothesis that the left asymmetry of the P100 may reflect an initial bias of the left hemisphere for making sensory or phonological discriminations, whereas changes in the distribution of the N200 and N350 may reflect development of neural systems underlying comprehension of word meaning.

ERP Indexes of Cognitive Reorganizational Processes

In the normal population, the period between 13 and 20 months is associated with dramatic changes in language comprehension and production abilities. Developmentalists studying early language acquisition have hypothesized that striking changes in vocabulary size may be attributed to some form of linguistic insight (Dore, 1978) or conceptual reorganization (e.g., Gopnik & Meltzoff, 1986). In this section we discuss neurobiological evidence that is consistent with this position.

Neurobiological   evidence   for   underlying   reorganization   of language-processing systems.   Age-related changes were observed in the lateral and anterior–posterior distribution of ERP differences to comprehended versus unknown words. At 13 to 17 months ERP differences to comprehended versus unknown words were bilateral and were distributed widely over anterior and posterior regions. By 20 months these effects were limited to temporal and parietal regions of the left hemisphere. These results raise the hypothesis that a reorganization of language-relevant neural systems occurs sometime between 13 and 20 months. It is our working hypothesis that the neurophysiological changes that give rise to the ERP effects reported here are at least in part linked to the remarkable changes in early lexical development that typically occur between 13 and 20 months.

Mount, Reznick, Kagan, Hiatt, and Szpak (1989) also found a shift from bilateral to left-lateralized neural activity in 13- to 22-month-olds during a language-processing task. In their longitudinal study, the tendency for children to look at the right member of a pair of identical pictures of familiar objects increased from 13 to 20 months and was correlated with individual differences in language production abilities. More specifically, correlations between the subjects' tendency to look to the right and their mean length of utterance were low and not significant between 13 to 15 months of age, increased linearly between 16 and 20 months, and declined between 20 and 22 months. Research on lateral eye movements in adults suggests that direction of gaze reflects hemispheric asymmetries in cognitive processing; that is, subjects tend to look to the right when processing language stimuli and to look to the left when processing spatial or musical information (Kinsbourne, 1972; Kinsbourne & Hiscock, 1983; Kocel, Galin, Ornstein, & Merrin, 1972; Schwartz, Davidson, & Maer, 1975). Mount et al. suggested that the increase in productive vocabulary observed between 16 and 20 months and the maturational changes in the central nervous system that occur during this period are associated with "a special excitatory state in the temporal cortex of the left hemisphere" (p. 406).

Developmental changes in word-processing strategies.   Developmental changes in the distribution of ERPs to comprehended and unknown words also may reflect qualitative differences in the way 13- and 20-month-olds process comprehended versus unknown words. At 20 months of age the distribution of the N200 showed distinct lateral and anterior–posterior distributions to the different types of words; that is, comprehended words elicited N200 responses that were bilateral and were most prominent over temporal and parietal regions, whereas unknown words elicited a robust right-greater-than-left asymmetry and were equipotential from anterior and posterior regions. The results indicate that at 20 months nonidentical neural systems are activated during the processing of comprehended versus unknown words. In contrast, at 13 to 17 months both comprehended and unknown words elicited N200 responses that varied in amplitude but displayed similar lateral and anterior–posterior distributions; that is, the mean areas of the N200 to both types of words were larger from the right than from the left hemisphere, and were larger from over posterior than from over anterior regions. These results suggest that at 13 to 17 months similar neural systems are activated during the processing of comprehended and unknown words, and that ERP differences to comprehended words reflect differences in the modulation of the amount of neural activity elicited to these events. Moreover, these age-related differences in the distribution of ERP responsiveness to comprehended words support the hypothesis raised in the behavioral literature that between 13 and 20 months of age there is an important reorganization in the way comprehended words are processed.

Different Brain Systems for Comprehension and Production?

Another area of interest involved the relative effects of comprehension versus production abilities on the organization of ERPs to comprehended and unknown words. We examined the contribution of production abilities by studying children who were matched for the size of their receptive vocabularies but who varied in the size of their productive vocabularies. The results suggested there were no significant differences in ERP responsiveness to the different types of words as a function of language production when comprehension was held constant. However, our paradigm employed a passive listening procedure that may activate brain systems more closely linked to word comprehension. A paradigm requiring the child to produce words or phrases may be necessary to examine developmental changes in brain activity specific to production. Previously we reported changes in brain organization linked to language production abilities in 20-month-old children (Mills et al., 1993). However, the 20-month-old high and low producers also differed on a measure of language comprehension. Further research is needed to separate the specific effects of comprehension and production on cerebral specialization for language.

CONCLUSION

The results suggest that between 13 and 20 months of age there are considerable changes in the organization of language-relevant brain systems that occur both between and within the two hemispheres. Previously (Mills et al., 1993) we suggested the working hypothesis that the N200 and N350 index neural activity elicited by processing meaningful lexical information. The results from this study support this hypothesis. Moreover, we propose that by 200 ms after word onset, ERPs to words whose meanings are comprehended by the child elicit greater negative activity than do ERPs to words whose meanings the child does not comprehend. At 13 to 17 months these ERP differences are distributed broadly over anterior and posterior regions of both the left and right hemispheres. By 20 months of age these differences are limited to temporal and parietal regions of the left hemisphere. For both age groups, unknown words elicit activity largely over the right hemisphere. However, the right-hemisphere asymmetry is more pronounced at 20 months. Backward words do not elicit N200 or N350 activity in either hemisphere at either age. In addition, the results support the hypothesis that the organization of these systems becomes progressively more specialized with both increasing chronological age and the attainment of new language milestones.

REFERENCES

Aram, D., Ekelman, B., & Whitaker, H. (1986). Spoken syntax in children with acquired unilateral hemisphere lesions. *Brain and Language, 27,* 75–100.

Aram, D., Ekelman, B., & Whitaker, H. (1987). Lexical retrieval in left- and right-brain-lesioned children. *Brain and Language, 28,* 61–87.

Barrett, M. (1995). Early lexical development. In P. Fletcher & B. MacWhinney (Eds.), *Handbook of child language* (pp. 362–392). Oxford, England: Basil Blackwell.

Basser, L. S. (1962). Hemiplegia of early onset and the faculty of speech with special reference to the effects of hemispherectomy. *Brain, 85,* 427–460.

Bates, E., Bretherton, I., & Snyder, L. (1988). *From first words to grammar: Individual differences and dissociable mechanisms.* Cambridge, MA: Cambridge University Press.

Bates, E., Thal, D., Whitesell, K., Fenson, L., & Oakes, L. (1989). *Developmental Psychology, 25,* 1004–1019.

Benedict, H. (1979). Early lexical development: Comprehension and production. *Journal of Child Language, 6,* 183–200.

Best, C. (1988). The emergence of cerebral asymmetries in early human development: A literature review and a neuroembryological model. In D. Molfese & S. J. Segalowitz (Eds.), *Brain lateralization in children* (pp. 5–34). New York: Guilford.

Bloom, L. (1973). *One word at a time: The use of single word utterances before syntax.* The Hague, Netherlands: Mouton.

Bretherton, I., McNew, S., Snyder, L., & Bates, E. (1983). Individual differences at 20 months: Analytic and holistic strategies in language acquisition. *Journal of Child Language, 10,* 293–320.

Cawthon, D. F., Ojemann, G. A., & Lettich, E. (1991). Cortical stimulation of speech in bilingual patients. *Society for Neuroscience Abstracts, 17*(Pt. 1) 21.

Courchesne, E. (1978). Neurophysiological correlates of cognitive development: Changes in long-latency event-related potentials from childhood to adulthood. *Electroencephalography and Clinical Neurophysiology, 45*, 754–766.

Dehaene-Lambertz, G., & Dehaene, S. (1994). Speed and cerebral correlates of syllable discrimination in infants. *Nature, 370*, 292–295.

Dennis, M., & Kohn, B. (1975). Comprehension of syntax in infantile hemiplegics after cerebral hemidecortication: Left-hemisphere superiority. *Brain and Language, 2*, 472–482.

Dennis, M., & Whitaker, A. (1976). Language acquisition following hemi-decoritcation: Linguistic superiority of the left over the right hemisphere. *Brain and Language, 3*, 404–433.

Dixon, W. J. (Ed.). (1992). *BMDP statistical software manual.* Berkeley: University of California Press.

Dore, J. (1978). Conditions for the acquisition of speech acts. In I. Markova (Ed.), *The social context of language* (pp. 87–111). New York: Wiley.

Dore, J. (1985). Holophrases revisited: Their "logical" development from dialogue. In M. D. Barrett (Ed.), *Children's single-word speech* (pp. 23–58), Chichester, England: Wiley.

Fedio, P., August, A., Myatt, C., Kertzman, C., Miletich, R., Snyder, P., Sato, S., & Kufta, C. (1992). Functional localization of languages in a bilingual patient with intracarotid amytol, subdural electrical stimulation, and positron emission tomography [Abstract]. *Journal of Clinical and Experimental Neuropsychology, 14*, 53.

Fenson, L., Dale, P. A., Reznick, J. S., Bates, E., & Thal, D. (1994). Variability in early communicative development. *Monographs of the Society for Research in Child Development, 59*, 5.(Serial No. 242)

Fenson, L., Dale, P. A., Reznick, J. S., Thal, D., Bates, E., Hartung, J., Pethick, S., & Reilly, J. (1993). *The MacArthur Communicative Development Inventories: User's guide and technical manual.* San Diego, CA: Singular Publishing Group.

Fenson, L., Flynne, D., Vella, D., Omens, J., Burgess, S., & Hartung, J. (1989, April). *Tools for the assessment of language in infants and toddlers by parental reports.* Paper presented at the Society for Research in Child Development, Kansas City, MO.

Goldberg, E., & Costa, L. D. (1981). Hemisphere differences in the acquisition and use of descriptive systems. *Brain and Language, 14*, 144–173.

Goldfield, B. A., & Reznick, J. S. (1990). Early lexical acquisition: Rate, content, and the vocabulary spurt. *Journal of Child Language, 17*, 171–183.

Golinkoff, R., & Hirsh-Pasek, K. (1995). Reinterpreting children's sentence comprehension: Towards a new framework. In P. Fletcher & B. MacWhinney (Eds.), *Handbook of child language* (pp. 430–461). Oxford, England: Basil Blackwell.

Gopnik, A., & Meltzoff, A. N. (1986). Words, plans, things and locations: Interactions between semantic and cognitive development in the one-word stage. In S. L. Kuczaj & M. Barrett (Eds.), *The development of word meaning* (pp. 199–223). New York: Springer-Verlag.

Hecaen, H. (1983). Acquired aphasia in children: Revisited. *Neuropsychologia, 21*, 587.

Hirsh-Pasek, K., & Golinkoff, R. M. (1993). Skeletal supports for grammatical learning: What the infant brings to the language learning task. In C. K. Rovee-Collier (Ed.), *Advances in infancy research, 10*, 299–338. Norwood, NJ: Ablex.

Holcomb, P. J., Coffey, S. A., & Neville, H. J. (1992). Auditory and visual sentence processing: A developmental analysis using event-related potentials. *Developmental Neuropsychology, 8*, 203–241.

Johnson, R. (1989). Developmental evidence for modality-dependent P300 generators: A normative study. *Psychophysiology, 26*, 651–667.

Karrer, R., & Ackles, P. (1987). Visual event-related potentials of infants during a modified oddball procedure. *Current Trends in Event-Related Potential Research 40*(EEG Suppl.), 603–608.

Kinsbourne, M. (1972). Eye and head turning indicates cerebral lateralization. *Science, 176*, 539–541.

Kinsbourne, M., & Hiscock, M. (1977). Does cerebral dominance develop? In Segalowitz and F. A. Gruber (Eds.), *Language Development and Neurological Theory* (pp. 172–191). New York: Academic Press.

Kinsbourne, M., & Hiscock, M. (1983). The normal and deviant development of functional lateralization of the brain. In M. Haith & J. Campos (Eds.), *Handbook of child psychology* (Vol. 2, pp. 157–280). New York: Wiley.

Kocel, K. M., Galin, D., Ornstein, R. E., & Merrin, E. L. (1972). Lateral eye movement and cognitive mode. *Psychometric Science, 27,* 223–224.

Kurtzberg, D. (1985, April). Late auditory evoked potentials and speech sound discrimination by infants. In R. Karrer (Chair), *Event-related potentials of the brain and perceptual/cognitive processing of infants.* Symposium conducted at the meeting of the Society for Research in Child Development, Toronto, Canada.

Kurtzberg, D., Stone, C., & Vaughn, H. (1986). Cortical responses to speech sounds in the infant. *Evoked Potentials, 3,* 513–520.

Lenneberg, E. (1967). *Biological foundations of language.* New York: Wiley.

Markman, E. M. (1991). The whole object, taxonomic and mutual exclusivity assumptions as initial constraints on word meaning. In J. P. Byrnes and S. A. Gelman (Eds.), *Perspectives on language and thought: Interrelations and development* (pp. 72–106). Cambridge, England: Cambridge University Press.

McIsaac, H., & Polich, J. (1992). Comparison of infant and adult P300 from auditory stimuli. *Journal of Experimental Child Psychology, 53,* 115–128.

McShane, J. (1979). The development of naming. *Linguistics, 17,* 879–905.

Mills, D. L., Coffey-Corina, S. A., & Neville, H. J. (1993). Language acquisition and cerebral specialization in 20-month-old infants. *Journal of Cognitive Neuroscience, 5,* 317–334.

Mills, D. L., Coffey-Corina, S. A., & Neville, H. J. (1994). Variability in cerebral organization in infancy during primary language acquisition. In G. Dawson & K. Fischer (Eds.), *Human behavior and the developing brain* (pp. 427–455). New York: Guilford.

Mills, D. L., Thal, D., DiIulio, L., Castaneda, C., & Neville, H. J. (1995). *Auditory sensory processing and language abilities in late talkers: An ERP study* (Tech. Rep. No. CND–9508). San Diego, CA: Center for Research in Language, Project in Cognitive and Neural Development.

Molfese, D. (1989). Electrophysiological correlates of word meanings in 14-month-old human infants. *Developmental Neuropsychology, 5,* 79–103.

Molfese, D. (1990). Auditory evoked responses recorded from 16-month-old human infants to words they did and did not know. *Brain and Language, 38,* 345–363.

Molfese, D., & Betz, J. (1988). Electrophysiological indices of the early development of lateralization of language and cognition, and their implication for predicting later development. In D. L. Molfese & S. J. Segalowitz (Eds.), *Brain lateralization in children: Developmental implications* (pp. 171–190). New York: Guilford.

Molfese, D., L. & Molfese, V. J. (1979). Hemisphere and stimulus differences as reflected in the cortical responses of newborn infants to speech stimuli. *Developmental Psychology, 15,* 505–511.

Molfese, D., L. & Molfese, V. J. (1994). Short-term and long-term developmental outcomes: The use of behavioral and electrophysiological measures in early infancy as predictors. In G. Dawson & K. W. Fischer (Eds.), *Human behavior and the developing brain* (pp. 493–517). New York: Guilford.

Mount, R., Reznick, J. S., Kagan, J., Hiatt, S., & Szpak, M. (1989). Direction of gaze and emergence of speech in the second year. *Brain and Language, 36,* 406–410.

Mullis, R. J., Holcomb, P. J., Diner, B. C., & Dykman, R. A. (1985). The effects of aging on the P3 component of the visual event-related potential. *Electroencephalography and Clinical Neurophysiology, 62,* 141–149.

Nelson, C., & Collins, P. F. (1991). An event-related potential and looking time analysis of infant's responses to familiar and novel events: Implications for visual recognition memory. *Developmental Psychology, 27,* 50–58.

Nelson, K. (1973). Structure and strategy in learning to talk. *Monographs of the Society for Research in Child Development, 48*(1–2, Serial No. 149).

Nelson, K. (1983). The conceptual basis for language. In T. Seiler & W. Wannemacher (Eds.), *Concept development and the development of word meaning* (pp. 173–188). Berlin: Springer-Verlag.

Neville, H. J. (1991a). Neurobiology of cognitive and language processing: Effects of early experience. In K. Gibson & A. C. Peterson (Eds.), *Brain maturation and cognitive development: Comparative and cross-cultural perspectives* (pp. 355–380). New York: Aldine-Gruyter.

Neville, H. J. (1991b). Whence the specialization of the language hemisphere? In I. Mattingly & M. Studdert-Kennedy (Eds.), *Modularity and the motor theory of speech perception* (pp. 269–294). Hillsdale, NJ: Lawrence Erlbaum Associates, Inc.

Neville, H. J. (1995). Developmental specificity in neurocognitive development in humans. In M. S. Gazzaniga (Ed.), *The cognitive neurosciences* (pp. 219–231). Cambridge, MA: MIT Press.

Neville, H. J., Coffey, S. A., Holcomb, P. J., & Tallal, P. (1993). The neurobiology of sensory and language processing in language-impaired children. *Journal of Cognitive Neuroscience, 5,* 235–253.

Neville, H. J., Corina, D., Bavelier, D., Clark, V. P., Jezzard, P., Prinster, A., Karni, A., Lalwani, A., Rauschecker, J., & Turner, R. (1994). Biological constraints and effects of experience on cortical organization for language: An fMRI study of sentence processing in English and American Sign Language (ASL) by deaf and hearing subjects. *Society for Neuroscience Abstracts, 20,* 67–83.

Neville, H. J., Corina, D., Bavelier, D., Clark, V. P., Jezzard, P., Prinster, A., Padmanabham, S., Braun, A. Rauschecker, J., & Turner, R. (1995). Effects of early experience on cerebral organization for language: An fMRI study of sentence processing in English and ASL by hearing and deaf subjects. *Proceedings of the First International Conference on Functional Human Brain Mapping,* p. 278.

Neville, H. J., Mills, D. L., & Lawson, D. S. (1992). Fractionating language: Different neural subsystems with different sensitive periods. *Cerebral Cortex, 2,* 244–258.

Neville, H. J., Nicol, J., Barss, A., Forster, K., & Garrett, M. (1991). Syntactically based sentence processing classes: Evidence from event-related brain potentials. *Journal of Cognitive Neuroscience, 3,* 150–165.

Ojemann, G. A. (1991). Cortical organization of language. *Journal of Neuroscience, 11,* 2281–2287.

Osterhout, L., & Holcomb, P. (1990). Event-related brain potentials elicited by syntactic anomaly. *Journal of Memory and Language, 31,* 785–806.

Peterson, S. E., Fox, P. T., Posner, M., Mintun, M., Raichle, M. (1989). Positron emission tomographic studies of the processing of single words. *Journal of Cognitive Neuroscience, 1,* 153–179.

Peterson, S. E., Fox, P. T., Snyder, A. Z., & Raichle, M. E. (1990). Activation of extrastriate and frontal cortical areas by visual words and word-like stimuli. *Science, 249,* 1041–1044.

Plunkett, K. (1993). Lexical segmentation and vocabulary growth in early language acquisition. *Journal of Child Language, 20,* 43–60.

Plunkett, K. (1995). Connectionist approaches to language acquisition. In P. Fletcher & B. MacWhinney (Eds.), *The handbook of child language* (pp. 37–72). Cambridge, England: Blackwell.

Polich, J., Ladish, D., & Burns, T, (1990). Normal variation of P300 in children: Age, memory span, and headsize. *International Journal of Psychophysiology, 9,* 237–248.

Posner, M. I., Peterson, S. E., Fox, P. T., & Raichle, M. E. (1988). Localization of cognitive operations in the human brain. *Science, 240,* 1627–1632.

Schafer, G., & Plunkett, K. (1996). Rapid word learning by 15-month-olds under tightly controlled conditions. *Newsletters of the Center for Research in Language, 10*(5), 1–11.

Schwartz, G., Davidson, R., & Maer, F. (1975). Right hemisphere lateralization for emotion in the human brain. *Science, 190,* 286–288.

Stromswold, K. (1995). The cognitive and neural basis of language acquisition. In M. S. Gazzaniga (Ed.), *The cognitive neurosciences* (pp. 855–870), Cambridge, MA: MIT Press.

Tallal, P., & Piercy, M. (1973). Developmental aphasia: Imparied rate of non-verbal processing as a function of sensory modality. *Neuropsychologia, 11,* 389–398.

Thal, D., & Bates, E. (1988a). Language and gesture in late talkers. *Journal of Speech and Hearing Research, 31,* 115–123.

Thal, D., Bates, E. (1988b). *Relationships between language and cognition: Evidence from linguistically precocious children.* Paper presented at the annual convention of the American Speech–Language–Hearing Association, Boston.

Thal, D., Marchman, V. A., Stiles, J., Aram, D., Trauner, D., Nass, R., & Bates, E. (1991). Early lexical development in children with focal brain injury. *Brain and Language, 40,* 491–527.

Vargha-Khadem, F., Isaacs, E. B., Papaleloudi, H., Polkey, C. E., & Wilson, J. (1991). Development of language in 6 hemispherectomized patients. *Brain, 114,* 473–495.

Vargha-Khadem, F., O'Gorman, A., & Watters, G. (1985). Aphasia and handedness in relation to hemispheric side, age at injury and severity of cerebral lesion during childhood. *Brain, 108,* 677–696.

Weber-Fox, C. M., & Neville, H. J. (1992). Maturational constraints on cerebral specializations for language processing: ERP and behavioral evidence in bilingual speakers. *Society for Neuroscience Abstracts, 18,* 331.

Weber-Fox, C. M., & Neville, H. J. (1996). Maturational constraints on functional specializations for language processing: ERP and behavioral evidence in bilingual speakers. *Journal of Cognitive Neuroscience, 8,* 231–256.

Werner, H., & Kaplan, B. (1963). *Symbol formation.* New York: Wiley.

Winer, B. J. (1962). *Statistical principles in experimental design.* New York: McGraw-Hill.

Witelson, S. F., & Pallie, W. (1973). Left hemisphere specialization for language in the newborn: Neuroanatomical evidence of asymmetry. *Brain, 96,* 641–647.

Woodward, A. L., Markman, E. M., & Fitzsimmons, C. M. (1994). Rapid word learning in 13-and 18-month-olds. *Developmental Psychology, 30,* 553–566.

DEVELOPMENTAL NEUROPSYCHOLOGY, 13(3), 447–476

Origins of Language Disorders: A Comparative Approach

Elizabeth Bates

University of California, San Diego

The five empirical articles in this special issue illustrate the value of a comparative approach to the study of normal and abnormal language development. The information presented here does not just add up; it multiplies, yielding insights that would not be available from any of the individual parts examined alone. All five articles focus on the first stages of language learning, from first signs of word comprehension to the emergence of grammar. They underscore the immense variation that can be observed in normal children, and the range of ways that language can break down or go awry in the early stages. These results place important constraints on our understanding of the origins of communication disorders. At the same time, they provide substantial hope to families of children who are not developing on a normal schedule, demonstrating there may be several different paths to the achievement of language abilities within the normal range. The human language faculty is remarkably plastic, at least within the early stages. To be sure, there are some circumstances in which this plasticity appears to be quite limited. Here too, however, there are reasons to believe that our increased knowledge of the origins of communication disorders may lead to treatments that release children from these limitations on plasticity and learning, placing them on the road to recovery.

The summary and discussion that follows is divided into four parts: (a) a brief discussion of the potential for neural and behavioral plasticity revealed by the literature on normal brain development in human and nonhuman primates, (b) a discussion of the article by Mills, Coffey-Corina, and Neville (this issue) on event-related brain potentials associated with such variations, (c) a comparison of these data with the four articles in this issue describing early language in atypical

Requests for reprints should be sent to Elizabeth Bates, Department of Psychology, University of California, San Diego, San Diego, CA 92093.

populations (Thal, Bates, Goodman, & Jahn-Samilo, on late talkers; Bates et al., on focal brain injury; Singer Harris, Bellugi, Bates, Jones, & Rossen, on Williams and Down syndromes; and Dixon, Thal, Potrykus, Bullock Dickson, & Jacoby, on infants of substance-abusing mothers), and (d) a consideration of the neural factors that may be responsible when children fail to display the kind of plasticity observed in most of our populations.

ON THE NEURAL BASES OF NORMAL LANGUAGE DEVELOPMENT

Twenty years ago, speculation about the neural bases of language development focused on the addition of new neural structures (e.g., Geschwind, 1964, 1970; Lenneberg, 1967; Parmelee & Sigman, 1983), now called *additive events.* These include (a) the birth and migration of cells to their proper sites in the cortex, (b) the growth and establishment of long-distance axonal connections (i.e., basic "wiring up"), (c) the myelination of those lines, (d) the establishment of local synaptic connections, and (e) the strengthening or weakening of those local connections. Major changes in behavior during the first years of life often have been ascribed to *maturation,* a term reserved for additive events in the first four categories; traditionally, the fifth category has been viewed as the neural consequence of experience (also called *Hebbian learning;* Hebb, 1949). In the past 20 years, this additive and unidirectional view of brain development has been replaced by a much more complex and dynamic view, a bidirectional interplay of maturation and experience achieved through a combination of additive and subtractive events (for reviews, see Bates, Thal, & Janowsky, 1992; Deacon, in press; Edelman, 1987; Elman et al., in press, chap. 5; Oyama, 1992; Quartz & Sejnowski, in press; Smith & Thelen, 1993; Thelen & Smith, 1994; Wills, 1993). Here are some reasons why the old maturational view has lost its appeal.

Among other things, we now know that additive events play a less important role in postnatal brain development than previously was believed (or, at least, a less exclusive and less direct role). In humans and other higher primates, the birth and migration of cells is essentially complete well before birth. Axonal connections are set up in the first months of postnatal life, reaching an adult configuration by approximately 9 months of age in humans. This fact may help to explain the wide range of behavioral changes that typically are observed around 8 to 10 months in humans (e.g., Diamond, 1991), but this kind of basic wiring cannot be used to explain gross changes in behavior after that point (e.g., in the period from 10 to 48 months, when most of language development takes place). By contrast, myelination of axonal connections continues for many years, a fact that makes it seem like a good first-pass candidate for a maturational account of behavioral change (Parmelee & Sigman, 1983). However, we also know that myelination is a continuous process that goes on for at least 2 decades, and that information is conducted reasonably well across axonal connections before myelination is complete. For these two reasons, it is not clear how developmental changes in the myelin sheath could be used to explain massive and apparently discontinuous changes in language ability in the first years of life.

What about synaptic growth, the fourth category of additive events? Three points are relevant here. First, it is now clear that a huge burst in synaptic branching takes place some time after birth (Rakic, 1975), reaching its peak between 9 and 24 months in humans (Huttenlocher, 1979, 1990; Huttenlocher & de Courten, 1987; Huttenlocher, de Courten, Garey, & van der Loos, 1982). In fact, synaptic density in human 2-year-olds is approximately 50% greater than the densities observed in human neonates or in human adults—which means (at least in synaptic terms) that children start to work on the language problem with a brain and a half at their disposal.

Second, it is clear that synaptic growth continues throughout life, and that the amount of growth observed in later years is affected by experience. Although synaptogenesis never occurs again on the scale observed in the first months of life, increases up to 20% or more in second- or third-order branching have been observed in some areas of the brain in older animals exposed to a radical increase in environmental stimulation (Greenough, Black, & Wallace, 1993).

Third, the patterns of synaptic connectivity established in each cortical region are affected strongly by the input to that region (e.g., Sur, Pallas, & Roe, 1990; for reviews, see Elman et al., 1996; Killackey, 1990). For example, when plugs of fetal somatosensory cortex are transplanted to visual areas, they establish patterns of connectivity appropriate for visual input; and when plugs of visual cortex are transplanted to a somatosensory zone, they take on representations appropriate to somatosensory inputs (i.e., "When in Rome, do as the Romans do"). Hence, there is remarkable plasticity at the synaptic level in the neocortex.

Putting these lines of evidence together, we may conclude that additive events play an important role in brain and behavioral development, and those additive events that take place up to age 2 are strongly constrained by genetic factors (including the burst of synaptogenesis observed between 9 and 24 months). However, the line between maturation and experience is not at all clear at the local synaptic level, and there are (to the best of our knowledge) no dramatic additive events after age 2 that could be used to explain massive, discontinuous changes that take place later on at a behavioral level.

These findings are complemented by some major discoveries in developmental neurobiology during the past 20 years, revolving around the role of *subtractive* or *regressive events,* including (a) cell death, (b) axon retraction, and (c) synaptic elimination. We now know that subtractive events play a crucial role in postnatal brain development, serving as the instrument by which experience sculpts the brain into its mature form (Chugani, Phelps, & Mazziotta, 1987; Huttenlocher et al., 1982;

Janowsky & Finlay, 1986; Rakic, 1975). The first class of subtractive events includes *programmed cell death,* a large-scale form of neural suicide that takes place in the first weeks before and after birth. It generally is assumed that the onset of programmed cell death is under strict genetic control, although the fate of individual cells has more to do with their relative success or failure (i.e., their overall level of activity and connectivity when the programmed plague begins). In a sense, programmed cell death can be viewed as a neural game of musical chairs: An arbitrary signal determines that the game is over, and those that are able to find a chair can stay. Cell death continues after this point as well, although later versions of cell death have more to do with success or failure at a local (cell by cell) level. Axon retraction is a natural consequence of cell death (i.e., dead cells lose their connections), but it is also a potential cause of cell death (i.e., cells that fail to make appropriate long-range connections are candidates for elimination).

For the most part, major changes in axonal connectivity (both additive and subtractive events) are complete within the first months of life. Under normal conditions, these axonal processes lead to species-specific, "default" forms of large-scale connectivity. However, numerous experiments in the last few years have demonstrated that alternative forms of large-scale axonal connectivity are possible if the default situation does not hold (e.g., animals that are deprived of normal visual or auditory input; Frost, 1990; Hubel & Wiesel, 1970; Killackey, 1990; Killackey, Chiaia, Bennett-Clarke, Eck, & Rhoades, 1994; Miller, Keller, & Stryker, 1989; Sur, Garraghty, & Roe, 1988; Sur et al., 1990). In particular, exuberant axons that normally would wither away can be retained into adulthood. This kind of alternative routing at the axonal level may play an important role in the forms of neural and behavioral plasticity observed in some of the clinical populations under study here, although such developments are probably restricted to the 1st year of life.

In contrast with the dramatic but time-limited events that take place at the cellular and axonal levels, a single neuron can make hundreds or even thousands of synaptic connections. Furthermore, changes at this level take place over and over again across the lifetime of a successful cell. For this reason, additive and subtractive events at the synaptic level are the most likely candidates for the neural substrates of language and cognitive development after 1 year of age. Crucial for our purposes here, these events are the direct result of neural activity and neural competition, which means that it is impossible to distinguish between maturation and learning at this level of development.

Figure 1 (from Bates et al., 1992) illustrates the developmental course of synaptic growth and synaptic elimination from birth to adulthood in the human brain. According to Huttenlocher's (1979) cross-sectional analysis of human brains, synaptic density reaches a peak in the posterior cortex (especially the visual areas) around 9 to 12 months of age, whereas the corresponding peak in the frontal cortex is not observed until approximately 24 months. Rakic, Bourgeois, Eckenhoff,

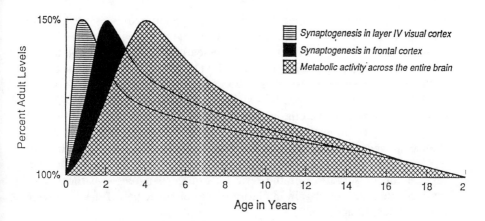

FIGURE 1 Successive "peaks" in brain development for synaptogenesis and metabolic activity from birth to adolescence. (Reprinted from Bates et al., *Early Language Development and its Neural Correlates,* 1992, pp. 69–110, with kind permission from Elsevier Science - NL, Sara Burgerhartstraat 25, 1055 KV Amsterdam, The Netherlands.)

Zecevic, & Goldman-Rakic (1986) disputed this point, arguing instead that synaptogenesis reaches its peak simultaneously in all areas of the cortex. Because Rakic et al.'s results are based on monkey data, it is difficult to be precise about the temporal location of the corresponding peak in human brains; but if they are correct, the most likely point would be somewhere around 24 months. Figure 1 also includes metabolic results from Chugani et al.'s (1987) positron emission tomography studies of human infants and children. Although the peak in brain metabolism observed in Chugani's studies appears approximately 1 to 2 years downstream from Huttenlocher's data for synaptogenesis, the shape of all three curves in Figure 1 is quite similar: a huge burst between 9 and 48 months of age, followed by a long, slow decline that reaches asymptote somewhere in the 2nd decade of life.

The functional consequences of Figure 1 are quite dramatic for our understanding of the relation between brain and language development. Language typically starts around 8 to 9 months (with first signs of word comprehension) and stabilizes around 4 years of age (when most normal children have acquired the fundamental structures of their native grammar). This means that normal language development takes place during a neural firestorm, when synapses are coming and going at an astronomical rate. This is the period in which the child has an enormous number of potential connections (i.e., maximum capacity), which in turn means the child has an enormous number of possible outcomes (i.e., maximum plasticity).

We should note there are two opposing ways to interpret the data in Figure 1. We propose these events form the basis for a highly interactive, bidirectional theory of brain and behavioral development. By contrast, Piatelli-Palmarini (1989) argued for a radical nativist interpretation of the same facts. In particular, he suggested the infant brain contains a large set of innately specific, domain-specific patterns of connectivity, available prior to any form of learning or experience. Brain development after birth constitutes nothing more than a process of selection from this stock of innate possibilities. Hence, the gradual process of synaptic elimination illustrated in Figure 1 could be viewed as the elimination of innate options that will not be used (referred to in the linguistic literature as *parameter setting*). Indeed, Piatelli-Palmarini went on to suggest that learning itself is an illusion; everything of any importance is already there at the beginning: "I, for one, see no advantage in the preservation of the term 'learning.' I agree with those who maintain that we would gain in clarity if the scientific use of the term were simply discontinued" (p. 2).

Although this radical nativist scenario is logically possible, it is not borne out by modern research in developmental neurobiology. As noted earlier, a growing body of evidence on plasticity and development at the cortical level shows that fine-grained patterns of cortical connectivity are not laid out in advance, at least not at the synaptic level (see Elman et al., 1996, chap. 5, for a detailed review). Neurons are not born knowing what kinds of patterns they have to establish with their near neighbors. Instead, brain development in mammals appears to be based on a process of synaptic exuberance (i.e., more connections than the animal will need), followed by a process of elimination through competition—what Edelman (1987) called "neural Darwinism" (p. 19). The huge burst in connectivity illustrated in Figure 1 thus can be viewed (metaphorically) as a large block of marble delivered to the artist's studio. The sculpting process that follows is a bidirectional event, reflecting the joint constraints of structure and experience, maturation and learning. It is probably no accident that language development takes place in this period of maximum capacity and maximum plasticity.

VARIATION IN NORMAL LANGUAGE DEVELOPMENT

As Thal and Reilly note in the introduction to this issue, recent large-sample studies of early language development using the MacArthur Communicative Development Inventories (CDI) (Fenson et al., 1993, 1994) provide evidence for massive individual differences in onset time and rate of development for all major milestones—differences large enough to challenge the very concept of "normality." However, this variation is quite orderly, and systematic relations have been observed between the pace of language development (independent of age) and brain activity associated with linguistic stimuli. Studies using variants of the MacArthur CDI in other languages confirmed that similar means and similar ranges of variability can be observed in languages as diverse as English, Spanish, Italian, Japanese, Swedish, Icelandic, and American Sign Language (ASL).

Among other things, these findings raise a red flag for cross-linguistic studies based on small longitudinal samples—a common methodology in the child language literature (cf. Slobin, 1985, 1992). If we were to select at random one child from each of the languages we are interested in, we might find huge differences that have little or nothing to do with language input per se. If we were unlikely enough to choose children from opposite extremes (e.g., a slow Italian child and a precocious ASL child), we might be tempted to conclude that these variations are caused by differences in the structure, the processing, or both the structure and the processing of Italian and ASL. It is much more likely, however, that these differences are based on chance variation (i.e., the putative cross-linguistic difference is a false positive). Within a given language, case studies can be a rich source of information about patterns that are *possible* (e.g., interesting error types, cross-language variations in the sequence of development), but they should not be used to draw inferences about those patterns that are *probable* or *typical* within that language environment.

At the same time, cross-linguistic studies of normal children also demonstrate that a certain amount of variation is *inevitable,* regardless of the language to which children are exposed. So, from where does all this variation come? Some of this variation undoubtedly is due to differences in the amount and quality of parental input (although Fenson et al., 1994, noted that correlations with crude environmental measures such as birth order and social class are relatively low in the original norming sample). Some of it may come from natural variations in the rate of maturation (e.g., in the additive and subtractive events illustrated in Figure 1); if this is the case, it would help to explain why equivalent variability is observed in dramatically different language types. Some of it also may come from characteristics of the child that are related only indirectly to language itself. These might include temperamental differences (e.g., shyness, risk taking, and sociability), cognitive differences in rate and style of learning that cut across linguistic and nonlinguistic domains, differences in perceptual acuity, auditory short-term memory, and so forth (for a discussion, see Bates, Dale, & Thal, 1995). For our purposes, the point is that large individual differences are present across the normal range in every language community studied to date, from first signs of word comprehension to the mastery of grammar. Hence, the word *normal* applies to a very broad range of performance at any given point in development—a fact that must be kept in mind when we undertake studies of the origins of communication disorders in clinical populations.

Fortunately, evidence suggests that this variation is neither random nor chaotic. In particular, the article by Mills et al. (this issue) demonstrates that individual differences in the rate of language development during the 2nd year of life are linked to observable changes in brain activity. Several findings from Mills et al. are worthy of note.

First, Mills et al. (this issue) uncover distinct patterns of electrical activity over the scalp in response to (a) familiar words (as established for each child by parental report and laboratory testing), (b) real English words that are unfamiliar to the child, and (c) backwards speech (auditory stimuli that are unrecognizable as English words but are equivalent in complexity). This methodological contribution has great theoretical and empirical consequences. Comprehension is notoriously difficult to measure in this age range. Parent report measures of comprehension have proven to be valid and reliable up to, but not beyond, 16 to 18 months of age (at least for children who are developing at an average or greater-than-average rate). Laboratory measures are quite unreliable before this point because they require a degree of cooperation that is difficult to obtain in children under 18 months of age. Mills, Coffey, and Neville (1991) demonstrated that electrophysiological techniques can be used to measure word recognition across this age range, starting as early as 10 months and continuing through the preschool years and beyond. To be sure, some cooperation is required (e.g., the child must be willing to wear the electrode cap and sit still long enough to register single word stimuli without movement artifacts), but the degree of cooperation is far less than usually is required for picture-pointing or acting-out tasks. The authors also show that these event-related potentials (ERP) measures correlate with parent report and behavioral indexes of word comprehension, concurrently and longitudinally (over periods as long as 12 to 36 months in some cases; see also Molfese, 1989, 1990). This finding constitutes yet another cross-validation of ERP, laboratory, and parent report measures (for reviews of validity studies, see Bates, Bretherton, & Snyder, 1988; Fenson et al., 1993). More important still, it provides us with another way to uncover risk for language impairment before 2 years of age (Thal et al., this issue; see discussion later in this article).

Second, Mills et al. (this issue) demonstrate a consistent developmental pattern in the neural activity associated with familiar words. In the first stages (when a difference between known and unknown words first appears), this activity is distributed broadly over the two hemispheres and is (if anything) slightly larger on the right. Later on in the 2nd year, brain response to familiar words is larger on the left and more focally distributed over the frontotemporal cortex. As is discussed in more detail later, this kind of dynamic change in brain activity is compatible with studies of language ability in children with focal brain injury (Bates et al., this issue).

Finally, the Mills et al. (this issue) article clearly shows that language ability is a better predictor of these developmental changes than is chronological age. This finding is compatible with theories of brain development that emphasize the bidirectional relation between maturation and experience. In fact, the left-anterior shift in brain activity observed by Mills et al. may be the product of linguistic experience rather than its cause. This finding also suggests that the wide range of individual differences seen across the many languages now sampled using variants of the MacArthur CDI (e.g., Caselli & Casadio, 1995; Jackson-Maldonado,

Marchman, Thal, Bates, & Gutierrez-Clellen, 1993; Ogura, Tamashita, Murase, & Dale, 1993; Reilly, Provine, & Anderson, 1996) have clear and measurable neural correlates, opening up promising avenues for future research on normal language development.

DEVELOPMENT, DEVIANCE, AND DELAY IN ATYPICAL POPULATIONS

The four articles in this issue on early language development in atypical populations provide a wealth of detailed information that is difficult to summarize. I concentrate here on highlights that are particularly relevant for the issues of variation and plasticity.

Late and Early Talkers

Thal and her colleagues have spent many years seeking early indicators of risk for language delay. The article by Thal et al. in this issue focuses on short-term predictors at both the group and the individual levels. Three studies are presented using the MacArthur CDI (Fenson et al., 1993), identifying children in the top and bottom 10th percentiles for expressive vocabulary at various points in time (i.e., early talkers and late talkers). The first two studies present new information from a 6-month longitudinal follow-up of children who participated in the original MacArthur norming study (Fenson et al., 1994). The third study represents a first round of results from an intensive, month-by-month longitudinal study of 30 children from 8 to 30 months of age (Goodman & Bauman, 1995).

Demographic factors such as sex, birth order, ethnicity, and social class did not have any reliable predictive value in any of their analyses, but measures of language and communication did show continuity over time at the group level. In the two short-term longitudinal studies, late and early talkers both had a higher-than-chance probability of retaining their extreme-group status across a 6-month period. In the period between approximately 13 and 20 months, Time 1 word comprehension, gesture, and word production (including the percentage of comprehended words that also are produced) all made significant and independent contributions to later status. It is interesting to note, however, that the pattern of predictors was different for early versus later talkers. For late talkers at 20 months, the best 13-month predictors were gesture and the percentage of comprehended words that also are produced (both significantly lower in children who later were destined to end up in the bottom 10th percentile for expressive vocabulary). For early talkers at 20 months, the only predictor that made a significant independent contribution was total vocabulary size when the children were just 1 year of age. Results from their third study, with more finely grained longitudinal data, confirm this picture: Late talkers lagged consistently throughout the study in comprehension and gesture as well as in expressive vocabulary, but early talkers differed from average children only on the expressive language measures by which they were defined. The differential predictive value of these 13-month measures is interesting when the Thal et al. (this issue) results for late and early talkers are compared with the Bates et al. (this issue) results for differential breakdown of comprehension, gesture, and production in children with focal brain injury. In the period between approximately 20 and 26 months, the single best predictor of either late- or early-talker status at Time 2 was total expressive vocabulary at Time 1. There was no compelling evidence that grammar and vocabulary dissociate or make differential predictions within this age range. That is, 20-month vocabulary is a solid predictor of both precocity and delay at 26 months in both vocabulary and grammar. As is discussed in more detail later, this apparent inseparability of lexical and grammatical development also is compatible with the Bates et al. results for children with unilateral brain damage.

These findings at the group level are intriguing, but Thal et al. (this issue) conclude that it still is difficult to predict the outcome for individual children within these groups. Some late talkers stay delayed, others burst upward to the median and beyond. Unfortunately, none of the variables examined by these authors can distinguish those who "catch up" from those who stay behind. These findings can be viewed from three different points of view.

At a clinical level, these results are discouraging, that is, we do not have a litmus test that can be used before 2 years of age to identify children who need services. The litmus test approach is often used in educational circles to identify children who require special services for learning disabilities (broadly defined). In recent writings, Thal and others (Thal & Katich, in press; Whitehurst & Fischel, 1994) have suggested that we abandon this approach to the early identification of risk for language impairment and turn instead to a risk factor model of the sort that commonly is used in medical research and practice. For example, we know that a number of different risk factors contribute to the likelihood that an individual will develop breast or colon cancer (e.g., positive family history and dietary patterns). However, responsible physicians use this information with great caution when dealing with individual patients. Risk factors are assessed, advice is given where warranted, and patients with a high risk index are carefully monitored; but probabilistic information of this sort never is used to say to an individual patient "You are in trouble." Instead, patients are given all the available information, including a list of options that they may want to follow while their progress is monitored. This is the approach that Thal and her colleagues (this issue) recommend for the assessment of language delay before 3 years of age (see also Paul, 1991; Rescorla et al., 1995; Whitehurst, Fischel, Arnold, & Lonigan, 1992).

At a more personal level, the Thal et al. (this issue) results provide a message of hope for worried families. Parents are right to be concerned and vigilant if their children are delayed in the attainment of language milestones. Under the risk factor model recommended by Thal et al., parents should be encouraged to bring their concerns to the attention of physicians and other practitioners as soon as they think there might be a problem, and to insist (if necessary) that someone take a closer look. Indeed, a host of robust and positive results using the MacArthur CDI proves that parent report is a valid index of current language abilities, with considerable predictive validity as well. Parents know a lot about their children's progress, and their concerns should be taken seriously. At the same time, the dramatically different growth trajectories displayed by individual children in the Thal et al. article can be a source of comfort for parents who have undertaken this course of action. A slow start does not preclude a brilliant finish.

At a scientific level, these results for late and early talkers provide a substantial challenge. There clearly is evidence for continuity in the rate and style of development (see also Bates et al., 1988), but there also is substantial evidence for plasticity. Children who start out at the same level can reach very different endpoints, and children can move toward the same endpoint from very different positions. The mechanisms responsible for continuity versus plasticity are virtually unknown, and they constitute an important direction for future research. In this respect, the electrophysiological methods described by Mills and her colleagues (this issue) for normally developing children may prove very useful in assessing alternative pathways from first words to grammar. Our efforts to understand the mechanisms responsible for behavioral plasticity also will profit from investigations of both behavioral and neural plasticity in other clinical populations—which brings us to results for children with focal brain injury.

Children With Focal Brain Injury

Bates et al. (this issue) summarize more than 8 years of research in three large cities that looked at the course of early language development for 53 children with unilateral brain injuries incurred some time before 6 months of age (i.e., before the point at which language acquisition normally begins). These results were compared with findings in another article (Reilly, Bates, & Marchman, in press) that looked at language and discourse abilities between 3.5 and 12 years of age for a partially overlapping group of children with the same etiology. In total, the results discussed by Bates et al. are based on a sample of 72 children. Although results still are tentative (and must be viewed as working hypotheses for future research), it is worth noting that this is the largest and most homogeneous sample of children with early focal brain injury ever studied across this age range. A brief summary of these complex results includes the following highlights:

1. Although children with early brain lesions are (as a group) behind their normal age mates, individual differences within the focal-lesion population span the full range of variability, from under the 5th percentile to above the 90th percentile at every point in development and on every measure of language and communication.

2. Deficits in comprehension and gesture in the earliest stages of language development are more common in children with right-hemisphere damage. This directly contradicts findings for brain-injured adults (for whom deficits in comprehension, communicative gesture, and pantomime are more common following left-hemisphere damage), but it is compatible with dissociations observed in normal infants.

3. There is no evidence whatsoever for a dissociation between vocabulary and grammar during the first stages of language development (i.e., the passage from first words to grammar, from 8 to 30 months). This result contrasts sharply with claims made in the literature on adult aphasia, but it is compatible with the close association between lexical and grammatical development observed in cross-sectional and longitudinal studies of normal infants.

4. Deficits in expressive vocabulary and grammar are more likely in children with left-temporal injuries throughout the period from 10 to 60 months. None of the infants with left-temporal damage in our sample showed delays in comprehension, and none of them displayed the kind of fluent but empty speech associated with damage to the left-temporal cortex in an adult (i.e., no developmental cases of Wernicke's aphasia). In other words, injury to the region that includes Wernicke's area leads to a "Broca-like" pattern of deficits in very young children.

5. Frontal damage increases the risk for expressive language delay, but only within a narrow time window from 19 to 30 months, and it occurs with both left- and right-frontal damage; there is no evidence that left-frontal tissue is "special" at any point from first words through the acquisition of grammar. One possible interpretation of this finding is that the localization of key language functions in and around Broca's area is the product, rather than the cause, of normal language development.

6. None of these site-specific effects are observed in the Reilly et al. (in press) study of older focal-lesion children with the same early-onset etiology. After some point between 5 and 7 years of age, focal-lesion children, as a group, perform within the normal range but significantly below a matched sample of normal controls on most language measures—which means that some kind of price has been paid for reorganization in response to early injury. However, there are no longer any significant effects of size or site of lesion, suggesting that reorganization for language in the focal-lesion population takes place within the period from 0 to 5 years of age.

These findings underscore the important role of neural plasticity during the infant and preschool years. In contrast with old claims about equipotentiality (e.g., Lenneberg, 1967), lesion site does matter, even in children whose lesions are acquired at or shortly after birth. However, the lesion-symptom mappings observed in young children are qualitatively and quantitatively different from those observed in adults with homologous injuries. Among other things, this suggests that "the regions responsible for language learning are not necessarily the same as the regions responsible for use and maintenance of language in the adult" (Thal et al., 1991, p. 499). At the same time, these findings prove that alternative forms of brain organization for language are possible, and that these alternatives probably emerge at some point between 0 and 5 years of age.

Although these results are quite surprising from the point of view of lesion-symptom mapping in adults, they are compatible with other studies of children with focal brain injury (see Bates et al., this issue, for a list), and they are compatible with results by Mills et al. (this issue; see also Mills, Coffey-Corina, & Neville, 1993, 1994, in press) on the normal development of language-related brain activity. As noted, Mills et al. showed that the electrophysiological response to familiar words is broadly distributed and (if anything) somewhat larger on the right during the first stages of language learning. This finding complements the Bates et al. finding for word comprehension from 10 to 17 months, that is, a small but reliable disadvantage for children with right-hemisphere damage, suggesting that the right hemisphere may play a more important role (or, at least, an equally important role) during the period in which children break the code connecting sound and meaning. Later in the 2nd year for normal children (sooner for children who are developing at a rapid rate), Mills et al. observe a progressive left-anterior shift in the ERP to familiar words, suggesting that left-temporal areas are taking on a more important role in the mediation of meaningful speech. This developmental pattern may reflect the emergence of default organization in children without brain injury. It remains to be seen what kind of pattern would emerge at a comparable point in the development of children with left-temporal injuries. Mills is now conducting collaborative studies with the San Diego focal-lesion team, using ERP technology to observe the emergence of alternative forms of brain organization for language in the focal-lesion population.

But why is the left-temporal cortex so important? On the one hand, the Mills et al. (this issue) finding for normal children is compatible with 100 years of research on normal and brain-injured adults suggesting that the perisylvian areas of the left hemisphere play a critical role in language processing. On the other hand, research on infants with focal brain injury contradicts the adult findings in two important respects: (a) In the short run, left temporal lesions have a greater effect on production than on comprehension; and (b) in the long run, left-temporal lesions do not result in a permanent aphasia. Bates et al. (this issue) propose that this contradiction can be resolved if we assume the default pattern of brain organization for language emerges out of initial biases in style of computation that are related only indirectly to the final state. In the infant brain there are no "innate language centers." Instead, there are regional differences in information-processing capacity (i.e., what Elman et al., 1996, called "architectural contraints" rather than "representational constraints," p. 27).

Comparing their results for language to those of Stiles and colleagues (Stiles & Thal, 1993) for visuospatial cognition in children with focal brain injury, Bates et al. (this issue) suggest the left-temporal cortex is particularly well suited for the extraction of detailed perceptual information (both spatial and temporal), a capacity that is especially important during language learning. Ironically, the ability to perceive fine-grained details may be more important for production than it is for comprehension because children have to conduct a detailed perceptual analysis to create their first motor templates for familiar words. Under default conditions, the left-temporal cortex is recruited for this function via a competitive process (not unlike the process by which tall and agile children end up on the basketball team). However, if the left-temporal cortex is injured in some way, other areas are able to take over the task. They may not perform quite as well, but they are perfectly adequate for the job.

Williams Syndrome and Down Syndrome

The article by Singer Harris et al. (this issue) compares the first stages of language development in populations of children with two forms of mental retardation: Williams syndrome and Down syndrome. Both are genetically based disorders, and in both cases the cognitive disorder is accompanied by a host of other physical and behavioral markers. Hence, we would not expect (and we did not find) any simple mapping from genes to language (for a more detailed discussion of this point, see Elman et al., 1996). The crucial point for our purposes is that adults and adolescents with Williams syndrome display a remarkable sparing of language, compared with the severe delays and disabilities that they display in many other cognitive domains (Bellugi, Wang, & Jernigan, 1994; Giannotti & Vicari, 1994; Wang & Bellugi, 1994). By contrast, adults and adolescents with Down syndrome often display language abilities below their mental age, including a marked deficit in the production of grammatical morphemes (Chapman, 1995). To be sure, this apparent double dissociation between grammar and cognition must be interpreted with caution. First, there is substantial variability in both groups, and many children who do not display the "signature profile." Second, both groups display uneven patterns of sparing and impairment within language and within nonverbal cognition (including a remarkable sparing of face perception in children with Williams syndrome, who are otherwise quite impaired in visuospatial cognition). Nevertheless, the degree of dissociation observed in older children and adults provides a substantial challenge to theories that presuppose a tight link between linguistic and cognitive abilities.

How serious is this challenge? Suppose we can show that a retarded 16-year-old with an IQ of 50 has mastered English grammar? Is this is a surprise? Not necessarily. Roughly speaking, a 16-year-old with an IQ of 50 has a mental age equivalent to that of a normal 6- to 8-year-old. Because most normal 6-year-olds have mastered their grammar, we should not be surprised to find that a retarded adolescent with a 6-year-old mind has managed the same feat (particularly when we take into account the fact that this adolescent has been 6 years old for a very long time). For this reason, a better test of the link between language and cognition would come from the study of much younger children. When do children with Williams and Down syndromes diverge? Are their contrasting profiles evident from the very beginning, or do they emerge at a later point in development? If language is an independent cognitive system, or *module,* as some authors have proposed (Curtiss, 1988; Pinker, 1991, 1994; Roeper, 1988), it should be possible for language to develop well before the point at which putative cognitive prerequisites are in place. However, if language development depends on the prior attainment of certain key cognitive abilities, it should not be possible for children to acquire grammar until those abilities are in place (Bates & Thal, 1991; Bates, Thal, & Marchman, 1991; A. Gopnik & Meltzoff, 1987).

The article by Singer Harris et al. (this issue) resolves a number of important points in this regard. First, their results clearly indicate that both groups of children are delayed massively in the attainment of early language milestones, approximately 2 years behind normal controls on virtually every aspect of language and communication. Second, the two groups are delayed equally in expressive vocabulary across the period covered by this cross-sectional study (i.e., from 1 to 6 years of age). Third, there appear to be qualitative differences between the two groups in the relations observed among word comprehension, word production, gesture, and grammar. In the first stages (equivalent to normal development from 8 to 16 months), children with Down syndrome have a marked advantage in the use of gesture compared with children with Williams syndrome and with younger normal controls at the same levels of word comprehension or production). In the later stages (equivalent to normal development from 16 to 30 months), children with Down syndrome also have a significant disadvantage in the production of grammar (compared with children with Williams syndrome and with younger normal controls at the same level of expressive vocabulary). In contrast with the very uneven profile displayed by children with Down syndrome, the Williams syndrome sample shows a relatively normal profile of cross-domain relations—except, of course, that this "normal" profile is shifted downstream by approximately 2 years.

What can we conclude from these findings? The global delays in language development displayed by both groups are compatible with the claim that language is dependent on the attainment of certain minimum cognitive/conceptual abilities (i.e., "cognitive infrastructures"; Bates et al., 1995, p. 146). On the other hand, the two groups display markedly different patterns of development across domains. In particular, children with Down syndrome manifest a selective deficit in grammatical production from the very beginning, a deficit that cannot be explained by their cognitive levels or by the lack of progress in expressive or receptive vocabulary. This finding suggests that cognitive, lexical, or both cognitive and lexical abilities are necessary, but not sufficient, for grammar to emerge, but it does not tell us anything about the "missing ingredient." There are at least two possibilities: (a) Grammar is selectively delayed in children with Down syndrome because these children lack a language-specific ability revolving around the analysis and acquisition of grammatical morphemes, or (b) grammar is selectively delayed in children with Down syndrome because grammatical morphemes make a greater demand on perceptual abilities that are selectively impaired in this group.

Support for the second hypothesis comes from several quarters. First, it has been established independently that children with Williams syndrome tend to have remarkably acute hearing (i.e., *hyperacusis;* Klein, Armstrong, Greer, & Brown, 1990; Martin, Snodgrass, & Cohen, 1984; Morris, Demsey, Leonard, Dilts, & Blackburn, 1988), and there is also some evidence to suggest that their visual processing is disturbed (Morris et al., 1988). These two facts could lead indirectly to a relatively greater reliance on linguistic communication. Second, the selective advantage in gesture and the selective disadvantage in grammar displayed by children with Down syndrome are both compatible with a profile in which vision outstrips audition. This idea received support from a study by Wang and Bellugi (1994), who reported a double dissociation between visual and auditory short-term memory in adults and adolescents with Williams and Down syndromes (i.e., visual > auditory in Down syndrome; auditory > visual in Williams syndrome). Finally, studies of word and sentence processing in normal adults have demonstrated that the perception and use of grammatical morphemes can be selectively impaired when normal adults are tested under adverse processing conditions. If children with Williams and Down syndromes differ in their ability to perceive, encode, and remember phonologically weak morphemes, we might expect different profiles of grammatical development even though both groups are impaired equally at a semantic/conceptual level.

Do we know anything about differences between individuals with Williams and Down syndromes at the neural level that could be used to interpret these behavioral contrasts? Detailed neuroanatomical and neurophysiological comparisons have been conducted (Galaburda, Wang, Bellugi, & Rossen, 1994; Jernigan & Bellugi, 1990, 1994; Jernigan, Bellugi, & Hesselink, 1989; Jernigan, Bellugi, Sowell, Doherty, & Hesselink, 1993), but they raise more questions than they answer. Based on the behavioral contrasts observed in adults with Williams and Down syndromes, one might predict a difference along the left–right axis (e.g., left-hemisphere abnormalities in Down syndrome, right-hemisphere abnormalities in Williams). However, magnetic resonance imaging studies yield no evidence whatsoever for a left–right difference between these two populations. Instead, a range of significant differences is observed along the rostral–caudal axis (e.g., hyperfrontal presentation in Williams syndrome, hypofrontal in Down syndrome, controlling for overall cerebral volume, which is smaller than normal in both groups). In addition, the two groups show surprising differences in the shape and size of the cerebellum. This structure is about the right size in individuals with Down syndrome (controlling for overall brain size), but it is abnormally large in individuals with Williams syndrome. Furthermore, an area within the cerebellum called the vermis is also disproportionally large in individuals with Williams syndrome. This last finding is particularly interesting in view of reports by Courchesne and colleagues (Courchesne, 1991; Courchesne, Hesselink, Jernigan, & Yeung-Courchesne, 1987; Courchesne, Yeung-Courchesne, Press, Hesselink, & Jernigan, 1988) suggesting that the neocerebellum may be disproportionately small in individuals with autism. Finally, electrophysiological studies suggest that the relative sparing of language displayed by older individuals with Williams syndrome may be mediated by an unusual form of brain organization for language, including unexpected evidence for greater activity over right-anterior regions during sentence processing (Neville, Mills, & Bellugi, 1994). In other words, the spared language of individuals with Williams syndrome may not be based on the neural mechanisms that normally are used to mediate language processing.

Infants of Substance-Abusing Mothers

As Dixon et al. (this issue) note in their article on early language development in children of substance-abusing mothers (CSAMs), the use of stimulant drugs has reached record levels among pregnant women, now estimated to occur in 5% to 12% of all pregnancies nationwide. Because many of these drugs can cross the placental barrier to alter the course of prenatal brain development, it is imperative that we learn more about the effect of prenatal drug exposure on language, cognition, and social development in this growing population of children at risk. This is no easy task because of the many environmental and biomedical confounds that plague any study of development in CSAMs.

Dixon et al. (this issue) focus on the early stages of language development in infants and toddlers with prenatal exposure to cocaine, methamphetamine, or both. Sixty children were studied, including a sample who had been removed from their birth homes and placed in foster care. Using a combination of laboratory measures and parental report (the MacArthur CDI), Dixon et al. report that CSAMs, as a group, performed below normal controls on several different measures of language and communication. In fact, 5 times as many children as would be expected by chance fell into the 5th percentile on one or more language measures in the period between 8 and 30 months. Although this finding is discouraging, it is not surprising because it is consistent with a growing literature on early development in CSAMs. However, some of their other findings were quite unexpected.

First, children raised in foster care appear to be at greater risk than children who are in their home environment. This is surprising if we assume that foster parents provide better care than do biological mothers with a history of substance abuse. However, as Dixon et al. (this issue) note, this finding is subject to a number of confounds (e.g., mothers who lose or abandon their children to foster care may have had more serious problems, including, but not restricted to, a more serious drug habit).

Second, it looks like things may be getting worse instead of better for a substantial number of children. In fact, the lowest levels of performance in this study are observed in children between 25 and 30 months. Grammatical abilities, which emerge in this phase of development, were particularly at risk. Among the possibilities they entertain to explain this downward shift, Dixon et al. (this issue) underscore the growth of the frontal cortex that normally takes place around 24 months of age (e.g., the synaptic peak in the frontal cortex, illustrated in Figure 1). Recall that Bates et al. (this issue) found evidence that children with injuries to the left-frontal or right-frontal cortex perform especially poorly in the period from 19 to 31 months. As Dixon et al. note, there is some reason to believe that prenatal exposure to cocaine and methamphetamine has particularly deleterious consequences for dopaminergic areas on the frontal cortex. In fact, at least one study uncovered visible evidence of bilateral structural damage in the frontal cortex for a subset of the CSAMs population (Dixon & Bejar, 1989). Hence, the linguistic drop from 25 to 30 months may be a "sleeper effect," reflecting specific damage to frontal areas that takes on special importance at this point in development (see Goldman-Rakic, Isseroff, Schwartz, & Bugbee, 1983, for an animal model of this delayed frontal effect).

A third result in the Dixon et al. (this issue) article brings us back to the themes of variation and plasticity. Although some of the CSAMs in this study are at serious risk for language impairment (falling below the 5th percentile on several measures), others are doing surprisingly well. In fact, the mean percentile scores in Dixon et al.'s Study 1 range from 33% to 49% for expressive language, with standard deviations of more than 20 percentile points. Why are some children protected from the effect of prenatal drug exposure? Some of this apparent sparing may have to do with the biomedical and demographic confounds that plague this research area. Other factors may include timing and the amount of drug exposure, with consequences for the presence or absence of bilateral cortical damage. Another factor that we must keep in mind is the immense variation that also is observed in normal children growing up in healthy environments. Prenatal drug exposure occurs in children who might fall anywhere within the broad range of normal development. Hence, some of the sparing or impairment that we see in drug-exposed children may reflect individual differences that are independent of drug use (Bates & Appelbaum, 1994).

WHEN PLASTICITY FAILS: A FINAL COMMENT

The articles in this special issue underscore a vast range of variation in the early stages of language development, in normal children and in several different clinical populations. When the brain is damaged in some fashion during the early stages of development (due to accidents of nature or nurture), this damage is superimposed on a dynamic landscape of individual differences. Drawing on a growing literature in developmental neurobiology, I argue here that human brain development involves intricate, bidirectional interactions between maturation and experience. Mechanisms of plasticity and learning that are crucial to normal development come to play an even more important role when areas of the brain are injured early on. In a complex, nonlinear system of this kind, brain injury may serve to augment some forms of variation and to dampen others. It also may result in qualitatively different forms of brain organization for language and other higher cognitive processes.

Evidence for alternative forms of organization comes from the focal-lesion findings described by Bates et al. (this issue), and from the behavioral and neural findings for individuals with Williams and Down syndromes described by Singer Harris et al. (this issue). It is less clear how recovery from delay or resistance to damage are achieved by those late talkers and drug-exposed children who catch up with their age mates. However, there are good reasons to believe that the same additive and subtractive events that underlie normal brain development also are responsible for all these alternative patterns, for example, exuberant growth, competition, elimination of unsuccessful connections, and retention of those that work.

Although these "alternative brain plans" all are sufficient to support the acquisition of language, some of them are more successful than others. For example, some of the late talkers studied by Thal and her colleagues (this issue) went on to qualify for a diagnosis of specific language impairment (SLI). Like the children with Down syndrome described by Singer Harris et al. (this issue), children with SLI eventually acquire their grammar (see also Chapman, 1995), but they often display (among other things) sporadic, residual deficits in the production of grammatical morphemes (Johnston & Kamhi, 1984; Marchman, Wulfeck, & Weismer, 1995; Rice, 1996). Does this mean some children suffer from selective and irreparable damage to an autonomous "language organ" (Chomsky, 1980; M. Gopnik & Crago, 1991; Pinker, 1994)? And if this is the case, where is the language organ located in the brain? Why is plasticity for language blocked or limited in some clinical groups when children with extensive left-hemisphere damage are able to acquire language within the normal range?

SLI is particularly relevant to this argument. SLI has been under study for more than 30 years (West, 1962). It usually is defined as a syndrome in which expressive and (perhaps) receptive language abilities are 1 *SD* or more below the mean, and below the same child's performance IQ, in the absence of evidence for mental retardation, frank neurological impairment, abnormal hearing, socioemotional disorders, or sociodemographic conditions that could explain the disparity between language and other cognitive functions (Bishop, 1992; Bishop & Rosenbloom, 1987). Hence, by definition, SLI is supposed to represent an impairment that affects language and nothing else. Furthermore, it has been demonstrated repeatedly that grammatical morphology is particularly vulnerable in children with SLI (Johnston & Kamhi, 1984; Leonard, 1992), albeit with little evidence for the claim that regular morphemes are more vulnerable than are irregular morphemes (see Marchman et al., 1995, for a discussion of this point). Perhaps most important for our purposes, a number of studies have shown that SLI and associated disorders (especially dyslexia) tend to run in families (Bishop, 1992; Bishop & Rosenbloom, 1987; Pennington, 1991; Tallal, Ross, & Curtiss, 1989; Tallal, Townsend, Curtiss, & Wulfeck, 1991).

At face value, this looks like evidence for a specific and genetically based language organ, one that cannot be replaced if it is damaged early on. However, detailed studies of children with SLI have shown that the syndrome is not restricted to language, and it certainly is not restricted to grammar. For instance, Tallal and her colleagues (Tallal, 1988; Tallal, Stark, & Mellits, 1985) amassed a large and compelling body of evidence suggesting that children with SLI suffer from a deficit in the processing of rapid temporal sequences of auditory and (perhaps) visual stimuli. Other specific nonlinguistic deficits implicated in SLI include symbolic play in younger children (Rescorla & Goossens, 1992; Thal et al., 1991), aspects of spatial imagery in older children (Johnston, 1994), specific aspects of nonverbal attention (Townsend, Wulfeck, Nichols, & Koch, 1995), and a wide range of neurological soft signs (e.g., Trauner, Wulfeck, Tallal, & Hesselink, 1995). Particularly informative in this regard is a study by Tallal et al. (1991) of a very large sample of children with SLI comparing children with and without a family history of language disorders. There were no differences whatsoever between the two groups in the nature or extent of their language impairment (i.e., they were equally impaired, with specific pockets of vulnerability in the same areas); however, the subgroup with a family history of language disorders appeared to have a less specific disorder, with greater impairments on nonlanguage tasks, including a test of auditory temporal processing. At this writing, the nonlinguistic correlates of SLI have accumulated to the point where the original definition of the syndrome is at risk. For example, Bishop (1992) and Locke (1995) argued that children with SLI suffer from subtle but diffuse neurological impairments that have particularly cruel implications for language but which are in no way specific to it.

Although SLI is not as specific as we once believed, it is still the case that grammatical morphology is a highly vulnerable domain in SLI and in other disorders with an attested or suspected genetic base. As we just noted, a variant of the SLI pattern is frequently reported for children with Down syndrome. Although Singer Harris et al. (this issue) do not find a selective deficit in grammar in young children with Williams syndrome, other investigators have reported specific problems with grammatical morphology in older children with Williams syndrome. For example, Karmiloff-Smith and Grant (1993) reported that French-speaking adolescents with Williams syndrome have difficulty extracting and generalizing information about grammatical gender; and Volterra, Sabbadini, Capirci, Pezzini, and Osella (1995) reported that Italian-speaking children with Williams syndrome make a broad range of substitution errors in grammatical morphology, including many errors that are never observed in Italian children with Down syndrome, Italian children with SLI, or in normally developing Italian children at any stage of grammatical development. So we find grammatical impairments in several different genetically based syndromes. Could there be a gene for grammar that sits in close proximity to other genetically based functions, so close that these functions are felled by the same developmental axe?

Perhaps such a gene exists, but it has been demonstrated that grammatical morphology is selectively vulnerable in populations for whom genetic arguments are not viable. For example, problems with expressive grammar have been observed in both fluent and nonfluent aphasia (Bates, 1991; Pick, 1913/1973). They also have been observed in spoken and written language among neurologically intact individuals who are congenitally deaf (Caselli, Maragna, Pagliarini-Rampelli, & Volterra, 1994; Volterra & Bates, 1989). Problems with the receptive processing of grammatical morphemes have been observed in an even wider range of populations, including anomic aphasics who displayed no grammatical deficits in their spoken language (Bates et al., 1994; Devescovi et al., 1997) and a subset of elderly patients hospitalized for nonneurological disorders (Bates, Friederici, & Wulfeck, 1987). In fact, receptive agrammatism was induced in college students who were forced to process sentences under stress (e.g., perceptual degradation, cognitive overload, or both; Bates et al., 1994; Blackwell & Bates, 1995; Kilborn, 1991; Miyake, Carpenter, & Just, 1994). It appears that grammatical morphology is selectively vulnerable under a wide range of conditions, genetic and environmental. A parsimonious account of all these findings would be that grammatical morphology is a weak link in the processing chain, one that is highly likely to fall apart when things go awry.

That leaves us with a problem: Some children continue to suffer from communication disorders into adolescence and adulthood, whereas others recover and move into the normal range. Whether or not the grammatical deficits displayed in SLI and other syndromes are specific to language, their persistence cannot be denied. Why are children with unilateral left-hemisphere injuries able to overcome their initial deficits and find a workable solution, whereas populations of children with no apparent lesions to the classical brain region have persistent problems (e.g., SLI, Down syndrome, autism, and a number of other groups)? What factors might account for the failure of plasticity in these populations? At least three possibilities come to mind.

One possibility might be that some children with persistent deficits do have damage to the classical language zones, but this damage is so subtle that other regions of the brain do not come to the rescue (Galaburda, Menard, & Rosen, 1994). In other words, they keep trying to solve the language problem with functional but inefficient parts. In this regard, consider the data in Figure 2, taken from Irle's (1990) review of more than 200 primate lesion studies. The dotted line in Figure 2 represents findings from Lashley's (1950) classic article, In Search of the Engram, which showed the effect of lesion size on subsequent learning ability in adult rats. These data indicate that learning ability is a linear function of lesion size, a finding that is virtually independent of lesion location. These are, of course, the findings that led Lashley to propose his famous principles of mass action and equipotentiality. By contrast, the full line in Figure 2 represents findings from Irle's meta-analysis of lesion size and learning ability in primates. This function is noteworthy in two key respects: (a) Primates are a lot smarter than rats (performing very well with less than half a brain), and (b) lesion size has a nonlinear, U-shaped effect on learning ability. That is, the worst performance is observed in primates with midsized lesions; animals with very small or very large lesions perform much better. Obviously, this nonlinear function cannot be extrapolated very far ("Gee, if I can do so well with half a brain, imagine how well I could do if they took the whole thing out!"). Nevertheless, Irle's findings for lesions in the middle range demand an explanation.

Irle's (1990) explanation for this U-shaped function is based on what I would call the "fresh start hypothesis." That is, primates with very large lesions are forced to adopt a completely new learning strategy, based on the remaining healthy tissue (i.e., a fresh start). By contrast, animals with midsized lesions persist in their efforts to learn with familiar strategies, based on damaged and inefficient neural mechanisms. Similar accounts have been offered to explain why some epileptic children improve markedly on linguistic tasks following a left hemispherectomy (e.g., the right hemisphere is finally released for service without interference from the left hemisphere (F. Vargha-Khadem, personal communication, July 1995). In the same vein, it is possible that some populations of children with communication disorders are working with functional but inefficient neural tools, preventing them from taking a fresh start with one of the alternative brain plans adopted by children with frank lesions to the left-perisylvian cortex.

A second possibility may be that children with persistent language impairments suffer from bilaterally distributed cortical microlesions, too small to be detected in most magnetic resonance imaging studies, but serious enough to deter and delay

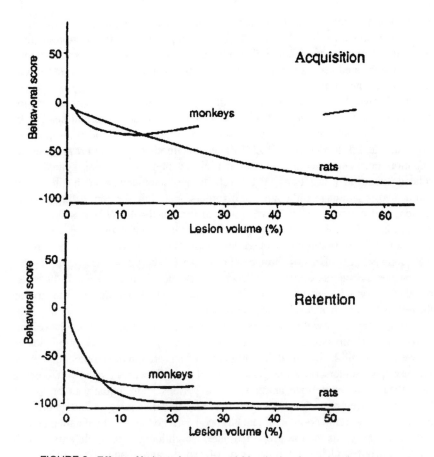

FIGURE 2   Effects of lesion volume on acquisition (top) and retention (bottom) of a new skill. There is a linear relation between lesion volume and loss of new learning in rats, whereas monkeys maintain relatively high levels of learning even after 40% to 50% of the cortex is lesioned (Reprinted from *Brain Research Review, 15,* by E. Irle, "An Analysis of the Correlation of Lesion Size, Location, and Behavioral Effects in 283 Published Studies of Cortical and Subcortical Lesions in Old-World Monkeys," pp. 181–213, 1990, with kind permission from Elsevier Science - NL, Sara Burgerhartstraat 25, 1055 KV Amsterdam, The Netherlands.)

language learning. In other words, these children do not arrive at an alternative organization for language because there simply is not enough healthy cortical tissue available to support a new brain plan. Some evidence for this view comes from autopsy studies of dyslexic individuals by Galaburda and his colleagues (Galaburda, 1994; Galaburda & Livingstone, 1993; Galaburda et al., 1994), who reported a high incidence of ectopias (literally "brain warts") and other abnormalities in both cerebral hemispheres. Galaburda insisted that these abnormalities are more common in the left hemisphere, but their diffuse and unpredictable distribution suggests to me that a more pervasive and diffuse defect may be present across the cerebral cortex (for related results in magnetic resonance imaging studies of children with SLI, see Trauner et al., 1995).

Finally, we should consider the possibility that the neural deficits underlying persistent language impairment are caused not by cortical abnormalities but by some kind of abnormality at a subcortical level that affects the learning process. For example, Eisele and Aram (1995) argued that linguistic deficits are more severe and more persistent in children with focal injuries involving the basal ganglia and related subcortical structures. The cerebellum is another region that has been implicated in language and cognitive disorders, including the contrasting patterns in neo- and paleocerebellar areas described previously for Williams syndrome. Another candidate might be the thalamus, a critical input station that is known to play a major role in the establishment of cortical maps. The major point for our purposes is that language learning in the child and maintenance and the use of language in the adult are not the same thing. Lesions that affect early learning may have no discernible effect on adult performance, and vice versa. We may have to look outside the cortex to find the neural culprit when developmental plasticity fails.

We do not yet know the answer to these and related questions about the origins of communication disorders. However, there are many reasons to be optimistic that answers soon will be obtained. Twenty years of research in developmental neurobiology have underscored the plastic and activity-dependent nature of cortical specialization in vertebrate animals. These lessons apply equally to brain and behavioral development in human beings. Our understanding of the nature and etiology of communication disorders has been enriched greatly by detailed behavioral studies such as the ones reported here, which identify these deficits at their point of origin and lay out trajectories of growth and change from infancy to adolescence. New technologies have made it possible to complement these behavioral studies with structural and functional studies of the developing brain. The message that has emerged from these studies to date supports a dynamic, bidirectional theory of brain and behavioral development, a perspective that gives great cause for hope to parents and scientists alike.

ACKNOWLEDGMENTS

This research was supported by National Institutes of Health/National Institute on Deafness and Other Communication Disorders Program Project P50 DC01289–0351, Origins of Communicative Disorders, to Elizabeth Bates, and by a grant from the John D. and Catherine T. MacArthur Foundation.

REFERENCES

Bates, E. (Ed.). (1991). Cross-linguistic studies of aphasia [Special issue]. *Brain and Language, 41*(2).

Bates, E., & Appelbaum, M. (1994). Methods of studying small samples: Issues and examples. In S. Broman & J. Grafman (Eds.), *Atypical cognitive deficits in developmental disorders: Implications for brain function* (pp. 245–280). Hillsdale, NJ: Lawrence Erlbaum Associates, Inc.

Bates, E., Bretherton, I., & Snyder, L. (1988). *From first words to grammar: Individual differences and dissociable mechanisms.* New York: Cambridge University Press.

Bates, E., Dale, P. S., & Thal, D. (1995). Individual differences and their implications for theories of language development. In P. Fletcher & B. MacWhinney (Eds.), *Handbook of child language* (pp. 96–151). Oxford, England: Basil Blackwell.

Bates, E., Devescovi, A., Dronkers, N., Pizzamiglio, L., Wulfeck, B., Hernandez, A., Juarez, L., & Marangolo, P. (1994). Grammatical deficits in patients without agrammatism: Sentence interpretation under stress in English and Italian. *Brain and Language, 47,* 400–402.

Bates, E., Friederici, A., & Wulfeck, B. (1987). Comprehension in aphasia: A crosslinguistic study. *Brain and Language, 32,* 19–67.

Bates, E., & Thal, D. (1991). Associations and dissociations in child language development. In J. Miller (Ed.), *Research on child language disorders: A decade of progress* (pp. 145–168). Austin, TX: Pro-Ed.

Bates, E., Thal, D., & Janowsky, J. (1992). Early language development and its neural correlates. In I. Rapin & S. Segalowitz (Eds.), *Handbook of neuropsychology: Vol. 7. Child neuropsychology* (pp. 69–110). Amsterdam: Elsevier.

Bates, E., Thal, D., & Marchman, V. (1991). Symbols and syntax: A Darwinian approach to language development. In N. Krasnegor, D. Rumbaugh, R. Schiefelbusch, & M. Studdert-Kennedy (Eds.), *Biological and behavioral determinants of language development* (pp. 29–65). Hillsdale, NJ: Lawrence Erlbaum Associates, Inc.

Bellugi, U., Wang, P. P., & Jernigan, T. L. (1994). Williams syndrome: An unusual neuropsychological profile. In S. Broman & J. Grafman (Eds.), *Atypical cognitive deficits in developmental disorders: Implications for brain function* (pp. 23–56). Hillsdale, NJ: Lawrence Erlbaum Associates, Inc.

Bishop, D. V. M. (1992). The underlying nature of specific language impairment. *Journal of Child Psychology and Psychiatry, 33,* 3–66.

Bishop, D. V. M., & Rosenbloom, L. (1987). Childhood language disorders: Classification and overview. In W. Yule & M. Rutter (Eds.), *Language development and disorders.* Oxford, England: Blackwell.

Blackwell, A., & Bates, E. (1995). Inducing agrammatic profiles in normals: Evidence for the selective vulnerability of morphology under cognitive resource limitation. *Journal of Cognitive Neuroscience, 7,* 228–257.

Caselli, M. C., & Casadio, P. (1995). *Il primo vocabulario del bambino* [Children's first words]. Milan: FrancoAngeli.

Caselli, M. C., Maragna, S., Pagliarini-Rampelli, L., & Volterra, V. (1994). *Linguaggio e sordità: Parole e segni nell'educazione dei sordi* [Language and deafness: Words and signs in the education of the deaf]. Florence, Italy: La Nuova Italia.

Chapman, R. S. (1995). Language development in children and adolescents with Down syndrome. In P. Fletcher & B. MacWhinney (Eds.), *The handbook of child language* (pp. 641–663). Oxford, England: Basil Blackwell.

Chomsky, N. (1980). *Rules and representations.* New York: Columbia University Press.

Chugani, H. T., Phelps, M. E., & Mazziotta, J. C. (1987). Positron emission tomography study of human brain functional development. *Annals of Neurology, 22,* 487–497.

Courchesne, E. (1991). Neuroanatomic imaging in autism. *Pediatrics, 87,* 781–790.

Courchesne, E., Hesselink, J. R., Jernigan, T. L., & Yeung-Courchesne, R. (1987). Abnormal neuroanatomy in a nonretarded person with autism: Unusual findings with magnetic resonance imaging. *Archives of Neurology, 44,* 335–341.

Courchesne, E., Yeung-Courchesne, R., Press, G., Hesselink, J. R., & Jernigan, T. L. (1988). Hypoplasia of cerebellar vermal lobules V and VI in infantile autism. *New England Journal of Medicine, 318,* 1349–1354.

Curtiss, S. (1988). Abnormal language acquisition and the modularity of language. In F. J. Newmeyer (Ed.), *Linguistics: The Cambridge survey: Vol. 2. Linguistic theory: Extensions and implications* (pp. 96–116). Cambridge, England: Cambridge University Press.

Deacon, T. (in press). *The symbolizing brain.* New York: Norton.

Devescovi, A., Bates, E., D'Amico, S., Hernandez, A., Marangolo, P., Pizzamiglio, L., & Razzano, C. (1997). An on-line study of grammaticality judgment in normal and aphasic speakers of Italian. *Aphasiology, 11,* 543–579.

Diamond, A. (1991). Neuropsychological insights into the meaning of object permanence. In S. Carey & R. Gelman (Eds.), *The epigenesis of mind: Essays on biology and cognition* (pp. 67–110). Hillsdale, NJ: Lawrence Erlbaum Associates, Inc.

Dixon, S. D., & Bejar, R. (1989). Echoencephalographic findings in neonates associated with maternal cocaine and methamphetamine use: Incidence and clinical correlates. *Journal of Pediatrics, 115,* 770–778.

Edelman, G. M. (1987). *Neural Darwinism: The theory of neuronal group selection.* New York: Basic Books.

Eisele, J., & Aram, D. (1995). Lexical and grammatical development in children with early hemisphere damage: A cross-sectional view from birth to adolescence. In P. Fletcher & B. MacWhinney (Eds.), *The handbook of child language* (pp. 664–689). Oxford, England: Basil Blackwell.

Elman, J., Bates, E., Johnson, M., Karmiloff-Smith, A., Parisi, D., & Plunkett, K. (1996). *Rethinking innateness: A connectionist perspective on development.* Cambridge, MA: MIT Press/Bradford Books.

Fenson, L., Dale, P. A., Reznick, J. S., Bates, E., Thal, D., & Pethick, S. J. (1994). Variability in early communicative development. *Monographs of the Society for Research in Child Development, 59*(5, Serial No. 242).

Fenson, L., Dale, P., Reznick, J. S., Thal, D., Bates, E., Hartung, J., Pethick, S., & Reilly, J. (1993). *The MacArthur Communicative Development Inventories: User's guide and technical manual.* San Diego, CA: Singular Publishing Group.

Frost, D. O. (1990). Sensory processing by novel, experimentally induced cross-modal circuits. *Annals of the New York Academy of Sciences, 608,* 92–112.

Galaburda, A. M. (1994). Language areas, lateralization and the innateness of language. *Discussions in Neuroscience, 10*(1–2), 118–124.

Galaburda, A. M., & Livingstone, M. (1993). Evidence for a magnocellular defect in neurodevelopmental dyslexia. *Annals of the New York Academy of Sciences, 682,* 70–82.

Galaburda, A. M., Menard, M. T., & Rosen, G. D. (1994). Evidence for aberrant auditory anatomy in developmental dyslexia. *Proceedings of the National Academy of Sciences USA, 91,* 8010–8013.

Galaburda, A. M., Wang, P. P., Bellugi, U., & Rossen, M. (1994). Cytoarchitectonic anomalies in a genetically based disorder: Williams syndrome. *Neuroreport, 5,* 753–757.

Geschwind, N. (1964). The development of the brain and the evolution of language. *Monograph Series of Languages and Linguistics, 17,* 155–169.

Geschwind, N. (1970). The organization of language and the brain. *Science, 170,* 940–944.

Giannotti, A., & Vicari, S. (Eds.). (1994). *Il bambino con sindrome di Williams* [The child with Williams syndrome]. Milan: FrancoAngeli.

Goldman-Rakic, P. S., Isseroff, A., Schwartz, M. L., & Bugbee, N. M. (1983). The neurobiology of cognitive development. In P. H. Mussen (Ed.), *Handbook of child psychology* (pp. 281–344). New York: Wiley.

Goodman, J. C., & Bauman, A. (1995). Group uniformity and individual differences in the rate and shape of language development. *Society for Research in Child Development Abstracts, 10,* 112.

Gopnik, A., & Meltzoff, A. (1987). The development of categorization in the second year and its relation to other cognitive and linguistic developments. *Child Development, 58,* 1523–1531.

Gopnik, M., & Crago, M. B. (1991). Familial aggregation of a developmental language disorder. *Cognition, 39,* 1–50.

Greenough, W. T., Black, J. E., & Wallace, C. S. (1993). Experience and brain development. In M. Johnson (Ed.), *Brain development and cognition: A reader* (pp. 290–322). Oxford, England: Blackwell.

Hebb, D. O. (1949). *The organization of behavior: A neuropsychological theory.* New York: Wiley.

Hubel, D. H., & Wiesel, T. N. (1970). The period of susceptibility to the physiological effects of unilateral eye closure in kittens. *Journal of Physiology, 206,* 419–436.

Huttenlocher, P. R. (1979). Synaptic density in human frontal cortex: Developmental changes and effects of aging. *Brain Research, 163,* 195–205.

Huttenlocher, P. R. (1990). Morphometric study of human cerebral cortex development. *Neuropsychologia, 28,* 517–527.

Huttenlocher, P. R., & de Courten, C. (1987). The development of synapses in striate cortex of man. *Human Neurobiology, 6,* 1–9.

Huttenlocher, P. R., de Courten, C., Garey, L., & van der Loos, H. (1982). Synaptogenesis in human visual cortex synapse elimination during normal development. *Neuroscience Letters, 33,* 247–252.

Irle, E. (1990). An analysis of the correlation of lesion size, localization and behavioral effects in 283 published studies of cortical and subcortical lesions in old-world monkeys. *Brain Research Review, 15,* 181–213.

Jackson-Maldonado, D., Marchman, V., Thal, D., Bates, E., & Gutierrez-Clellen, V. (1993). Early lexical development in Spanish-speaking infants and toddlers. *Journal of Child Language, 20,* 523–550.

Janowsky, J. S., & Finlay, B. L. (1986). The outcome of perinatal brain damage: The role of normal neuron loss and axon retraction. *Developmental Medicine, 28,* 375–389.

Jernigan, T. L., & Bellugi, U. (1990). Anomalous brain morphology on magnetic resonance images in Williams syndrome and Down syndrome. *Archives of Neurology, 47,* 429–533.

Jernigan, T. L., & Bellugi, U. (1994). Neuroanatomical distinctions between Williams and Down syndromes. In S. Broman & J. Grafman (Eds.), *Atypical cognitive deficits in developmental disorders: Implications for brain function* (pp. 57–66). Hillsdale, NJ: Lawrence Erlbaum Associates, Inc.

Jernigan, T. L., Bellugi, U., & Hesselink, J. (1989). Structural differences on magnetic resonance imaging between Williams and Down syndrome. *Neurology, 39*(Suppl. 1), 277.

Jernigan, T. L., Bellugi, U., Sowell, E., Doherty, S., & Hesselink, J. R. (1993). Cerebral morphological distinctions between Williams and Down syndromes. *Archives of Neurology, 50,* 186–191.

Johnston, J. R. (1994). Cognitive abilities of language-impaired children. In R. Watkins & M. Rice (Eds.), *Specific language impairments in children: Current directions in research and intervention* (pp. 107–122). Baltimore: Paul Brookes.

Johnston, J. R., & Kamhi, A. G. (1984). Syntactic and semantic aspects of the utterances of language-impaired children: The same can be less. *Merrill–Palmer Quarterly, 30,* 65–85.

Karmiloff-Smith, A., & Grant, J. (1993, March). *Within-domain dissociations in Williams syndrome: A window on the normal mind.* Poster session presented at the 60th annual meeting of the Society for Research in Child Development, New Orleans, LA.

Kilborn, K. (1991). Selective impairment of grammatical morphology due to induced stress in normal listeners: Implications for aphasia. *Brain and Language, 41,* 275–288.

Killackey, H. P. (1990). Neocortical expansion: An attempt toward relating phylogeny and ontogeny. *Journal of Cognitive Neuroscience, 2,* 1–17.

Killackey, H. P., Chiaia, N. L., Bennett-Clarke, C. A., Eck, M., & Rhoades, R. (1994). Peripheral influences on the size and organization of somatotopic representations in the fetal rat cortex. *Journal of Neuroscience, 14,* 1496–1506.

Klein, A. J., Armstrong, B. L., Greer, M. K., & Brown, F. R. (1990). Hyperacusis and otitis media in individuals with Williams syndrome. *Journal of Speech and Hearing Disorders, 55,* 339–344.

Lashley, K. S. (1950). In search of the engram. In *Symposia of the Society for Experimental Biology: No. 4. Physiological mechanisms and animal behaviour* (pp. 454–482). New York: Academic.

Lenneberg, E. H. (1967). *Biological foundations of language.* New York: Wiley.

Leonard, L. B. (1992). The use of morphology by children with specific language impairment: Evidence from three languages. In R. S. Chapman (Ed.), *Processes in language acquisition and disorders* (pp. 186–201). St. Louis, MO: Mosby Year Book.

Locke, J. L. (1995). More than words can say. *New Scientist, 145*(1969), 30–33.

Marchman, V., Wulfeck, B., & Weismer, S. E. (1995). *Productive use of English past-tense morphology in children with SLI and normal language* (Tech. Rep. No. CND–9514). La Jolla: University of California, San Diego, Center for Research in Language, Project in Cognitive and Neural Development.

Martin, N. D. T., Snodgrass, G. J. A. I., & Cohen, R. D. (1984). Idiopathic infantile hypercalcaemia: A continuing enigma. *Archives of Disease in Childhood, 59,* 605–613.

Miller, K. D., Keller, J. B., & Stryker, M. P. (1989). Ocular dominance column development: Analysis and simulation. *Science, 245,* 605–615.

Mills, D. L., Coffey, S. A., & Neville, H. J. (1991). Language abilities and cerebral specializations in 10-20-month-olds. *Society for Research in Child Development Abstracts.*

Mills, D. L., Coffey-Corina, S. A, & Neville, H. J. (1993). Language acquisition and cerebral specialization in 20-month-old infants. *Journal of Cognitive Neuroscience, 5,* 317–334.

Mills, D. L., Coffey-Corina, S. A., & Neville, H. J. (1994). Variability in cerebral organization during primary language acquisition. In G. Dawson & K. Fischer (Eds.), *Human behavior and the developing brain* (pp. 427–455). New York: Guilford.

Mills, D. L., Coffey-Corina, S. A., & Neville, H. J. (in press). The development of neural subsystems for open- and closed-class words in children from 13 months to three years of age. *Developmental Neuropsychology.*

Miyake, A., Carpenter, P. A., & Just, M. A. (1994). A capacity approach to syntactic comprehension disorders: Making normal adults perform like aphasic patients. *Cognitive Neuropsychology, 11,* 671–717.

Molfese, D. (1989). Electrophysiological correlates of word meanings in 14-month-old human infants. *Developmental Neuropsychology, 5,* 70–103.

Molfese, D. (1990). Auditory evoked responses recorded from 16-month-old human infants to words they did and did not know. *Brain and Language, 38,* 345–363.

Morris, C. A., Demsey, S. A., Leonard, C. O., Dilts, C., & Blackburn, B. L. (1988). National history of Williams syndrome: Physical characteristics. *Journal of Pediatrics, 113,* 318–326.

Neville, H. J., Mills, D., & Bellugi, U. (1994). Effects of altered auditory sensitivity and age of language acquisition on the development of language-relevant neural systems: Preliminary studies of Williams syndrome. In S. Broman & J. Grafman (Eds.), *Atypical cognitive deficits in developmental disorders: Implications for brain function* (pp. 67–83). Hillsdale, NJ: Lawrence Erlbaum Associates, Inc.

Ogura, T., Yamashita, Y., Murase, T., & Dale, P. S. (1993). Some findings from the Japanese Early Communicative Development Inventory. *Memoirs of the Faculty of Education,* Shimane University, Matsue, Japan, 29(1).

Oyama, S. (1992). The problem of change. In M. Johnson (Ed.), *Brain development and cognition: A reader* (pp. 19–30). Oxford, England: Blackwell.

Parmelee, A. H., & Sigman, M. D. (1983). Perinatal brain development and behavior. In M. M. Haith & J. Campos (Eds.), *Infancy and the biology of development: Vol. 2. Handbook of child psychology* (pp. 95–155). New York: Wiley .

Paul, R. (1991). Profiles of toddlers with slow expressive language development. *Topics in Language Disorders, 11*(4), 1–13.

Pennington, B. F. (1991). Genetic and neurological influences on reading disability: An overview. *Reading and Writing, 3, 191–201.*

Piatelli-Palmarini, M. (1989). Evolution, selection and cognition: From "learning" to parameter setting in biology and the study of language. *Cognition, 31,* 1–44.

Pick, A. (1973). *Aphasia.* (J. Brown, Trans.) Springfield, IL: Charles C. Thomas. (Original work published 1913)

Pinker, S. (1991). Rules of language. *Science, 253,* 530–535.

Pinker, S. (1994). *The language instinct: How the mind creates language.* New York: Morrow.

Quartz, S. R., & Sejnowski, T. J. (in press). The neural basis of cognitive development: A constructivist manifesto. *Brain and Behavioral Sciences.*

Rakic, P. (1975). Timing of major ontogenetic events in the visual cortex of true rhesus monkey. In N. Buchwald & M. Brazier (Eds.), *Brain mechanisms in mental retardation* (pp. 3–40). New York: Academic.

Rakic, P., Bourgeois, J. P., Eckenhoff, M. F., Zecevic, N., & Goldman-Rakic, P. S. (1986). Concurrent overproduction of synapses in diverse regions of the primate cerebral cortex. *Science, 232,* 232–235.

Reilly, J., Bates, E., & Marchman, V. (in press). Narrative discourse in children with early focal brain injury. In M. Dennis (Ed.), *Special Issue, Discourse in Children with Anomalous Brain Development or Acquired Brain Injury, Brain and Language.*

Reilly, J. S., Provine, K., & Bellugi, U. (1993). *Does modality influence lexical development: Parent report data on the emergence of American sign language.* Paper presented at the Sixth International Congress for the Study of Child Language, Trieste, Italy.

Rescorla, L., & Goossens, M. (1992). Symbolic play development in toddlers with specific expressive language impairment. *Journal of Speech and Hearing Research, 35,* 1290–1302.

Rescorla, L., Ratner, N. B., Pharr, A., Pavluk, D., Torgerson, D., & Skripak, J. (1995). Phonetic profiles of toddlers with specific expressive language delay (SELD). *Society for Research in Child Development Abstracts, 10,* 645.

Rice, M. (Ed.). (1996). *Towards a genetics of language.* Hillsdale, NJ: Lawrence Erlbaum Associates, Inc.

Roeper, T. (1988). Grammatical principles of first language acquisition: Theory and evidence. In F. J. Newmeyer (Ed.), *Linguistics: The Cambridge survey: Vol. 2. Linguistic theory: Extensions and implications* (pp. 35–52). Cambridge, England: Cambridge University Press.

Slobin, D. (Ed.). (1985). *The crosslinguistic study of language acquisition* (Vols. 1 & 2). Hillsdale, NJ: Lawrence Erlbaum Associates, Inc.

Slobin, D. (Ed.). (1992). *The crosslinguistic study of language acquisition* (Vol. 3). Hillsdale, NJ: Lawrence Erlbaum Associates, Inc.

Smith, L. B., & Thelen, E. (Eds.). (1993). *A dynamic systems approach to development: Applications.* Cambridge, MA: MIT Press.

Stiles, J., & Thal, D. (1993). Linguistic and spatial cognitive development following early focal brain injury: Patterns of deficit and recovery. In M. Johnson (Ed.), *Brain development and cognition: A reader* (pp. 643–664). Oxford: Blackwell Publishers.

Sur, M., Garraghty, P. E., & Roe, A. W. (1988). Experimentally induced visual projections into auditory thalamus and cortex. *Science, 242,* 1437–1441.

Sur, M., Pallas, S. L., & Roe, A. W. (1990). Cross-modal plasticity in cortical development: Differentiation and specification of sensory neocortex. *Trends in Neuroscience, 13,* 227–233.

Tallal, P. (1988). Developmental language disorders. In J. F. Kavanagh & T. J. Truss, Jr. (Eds.), *Learning disabilities: Proceedings of the national conference* (pp. 181–272). Parkton, MD: York.

Tallal, P., Ross, R., & Curtiss, S. (1989). Familial aggregation in specific language impairment. *Journal of Speech and Hearing Disorders, 54,* 157–173.

Tallal, P., Stark, R., & Mellits, D. (1985). Identification of language-impaired children on the basis of rapid perception and production skills. *Brain and Language, 25,* 314–322.

Tallal, P., Townsend, J., Curtiss, S., & Wulfeck, B. (1991). Phenotypic profiles of language-impaired children based on genetic/family history. *Brain and Language, 41,* 81–95.

Thal, D. & Katich, J. (in press). Early identification of risk for language impairment: Are there any robust measures. In K. Cole, P. Dale, & D. Thal (Eds.), *Advances in the assessment of communication and language.* Baltimore: Paul Brookes.

Thal, D., Marchman, V., Stiles, J., Aram, D., Trauner, D., Nass, R., & Bates, E. (1991). Early lexical development in children with focal brain injury. *Brain and Language, 40,* 491–527.

Thelen, E., & Smith, L. B. (1994). *A dynamic systems approach to the development of cognition and action.* Cambridge, MA: MIT Press.

Townsend, J, Wulfeck, B., Nichols, S., & Koch, L. (1995). *Attentional deficits in children with developmental language disorder* (Tech. Rep. No. CND–9503). La Jolla: University of California, San Diego, Center for Research in Language, Project in Cognitive and Neural Development.

Trauner, D., Wulfeck, B., Tallal, P., & Hesselink, J. (1995). *Neurologic and MRI profiles of language-impaired children* (Tech. Rep. No. CND–9513). La Jolla: University of California, San Diego, Center for Research in Language, Project in Cognitive and Neural Development.

Volterra, V., & Bates, E. (1989). Selective impairment of Italian grammatical morphology in the congenitally deaf: A case study. *Cognitive Neuropsychology, 6,* 273–308.

Volterra, V., Sabbadini, L., Capirci, O., Pezzini, G., & Osella, T. (1995). Language development in Italian children with Williams syndrome. *Journal of Genetic Counseling, 6,* 137–138.

Wang, P. P., & Bellugi, U. (1994). Evidence from two genetic syndromes for a dissociation between verbal and visual–spatial short-term memory. *Journal of Clinical and Experimental Neuropsychology, 16,* 317–322.

West, R. (Ed.). (1962). Childhood Aphasia. *Proceedings of the Institute on Childhood Aphasia* (1960, Stanford University School of Medicine). San Francisco: California Society for Crippled Children.

Whitehurst, G., & Fischel, J. (1994). Early developmental language delay: What, if anything, should the clinician do about it? *Journal of Child Psychology and Psychiatry, 35,* 613–648.

Whitehurst, G., Fischel, J., Arnold, D., & Lonigan, C. (1992). Evaluating outcomes with children with expressive language delay. In S. Warren & J. Reichle (Eds.), *Causes and effects in communication and language intervention* (pp. 277–324). Baltimore: Paul Brookes.

Wills, C. (1993). *The runaway brain.* New York: Basic Books.

Subscription Order Form

Please ❑ enter ❑ renew my subscription to

DEVELOPMENTAL
NEUROPSYCHOLOGY
Volume 13, 1997, Quarterly

Subscription prices per volume:

Individual: ❑ $49.50 (US/Canada) ❑ $79.50 (All Other Countries)

Institution: ❑ $295.00 (US/Canada) ❑ $330.00 (All Other Countries)

Subscriptions are entered on a calendar-year basis only and must be prepaid in US currency -- check, money order, or credit card. **Offer expires 12/31/97. NOTE: Institutions must pay institutional rates.** Any institution paying for an individual subscription will be invoiced for the balance of the institutional subscription rate.

❑ Payment Enclosed

Total Amount Enclosed $_____

❑ Charge My Credit Card

   ❑ VISA   ❑ MasterCard   ❑ AMEX   ❑ Discover

   Exp. Date_____

   Card Number _____

   Signature _____
   (Credit card orders cannot be processed without your signature.)

Please print clearly to ensure proper delivery.

Name _____

Address _____

_____

City _____ State _____ Zip+4 _____
Prices are subject to change without notice.

Lawrence Erlbaum Associates, Inc.
Journal Subscription Department
10 Industrial Avenue, Mahwah, NJ 07430
(201) 236-9500   FAX (201) 236-0072

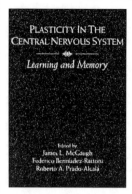

PLASTICITY IN THE CENTRAL NERVOUS SYSTEM
LEARNING and MEMORY

edited by

James L. McGaugh
University of California, Irvine
Federico Bermúdez-Rattoni
Universidad Nacional Autónoma de México
Roberto A. Prado-Alcala
Universidad Nacional Autónoma de México

Catalyzed by the development of new neurobiological and behavioral techniques as well as new conceptual and theoretical approaches to the study of the relationship between brain and behavior, research exploring brain functions enabling learning and memory has greatly accelerated in recent years. The chapters in this book reflect current theoretical approaches to the study of brain and memory and provide new insights concerning the cellular bases of memory and the differential involvement of brain systems in different forms of memory. By presenting up-to-date summaries of research investigating brain mechanisms underlying learning and memory, these chapters help to place current findings in appropriate theoretical context, and further stimulate research inquiry attempting to understand how the brain makes memory.

Divided into three sections, coverage in this volume includes:
- ❖ a discussion of pharmacological approaches to the study of brain and memory;
- ❖ a review of experiments using a variety of techniques, including brain lesions, brain grafting, and electrophysiological recording to investigate the role of different brain regions in learning and memory; and
- ❖ an examination of molecular analyses of events associated with memory formation.

Contents: Preface. **J. Garcia,** Brain and Behavior: Bridging the Barranca. **J.L. McGaugh, L. Cahill, M.B. Parent, M.H. Mesches, K. Coleman-Mesches, J.A. Salinas,** Involvement of the Amygdala in the Regulation of Memory Storage. **I. Izquierdo,** Role of the Hippocampus, Amygdala and Entorhinal Cortex in Memory Storage and Expression. **R.A. Prado-Alcalá,** Serial and Parallel Processing During Memory Consolidation. **F. Bermúdez-Rattoni, C.E. Ormsby, M.L. Escobar, E. Hernández-Echeagaray,** The Role of the Insular Cortex in the Acquisition and Long Lasting Memory for Aversively Motivated Behavior. **F.H. Gage, M. Kawaja, K. Eagle, G. Chalmers, J. Ray, L.J. Fisher,** Somatic Gene Transfer to the Brain: A Tool to Study the Necessary and Sufficient Structure/Function Requirements for Learning and Memory. **J. Bures,** Reversible Lesions Reveal Hidden Stages of Learning. **R.F. Thompson,** Cerebellar Localization of a Memory Trace. **H. Eichenbaum, B. Young, M. Bunsey,** Persisting Questions About Hippocampal Function in Memory. **J.M. Fuster,** Frontal Cortex and the Cognitive Support of Behavior. **Y. Dudai, K. Rosenblum, N. Meiri, R. Miskin, R. Schul,** Correlates of Taste- and Taste-Aversion Learning in the Rodent Brain. **S.P.R. Rose,** Time-dependent Biochemical and Cellular Processes in Memory Formation.

0-8058-1573-2 [cloth] /1995 / 216pp. / $39.95
Special Prepaid Offer! $22.50
No further discounts apply.

Prices subject to
change without notice.

Lawrence Erlbaum Associates, Inc.
10 Industrial Avenue, Mahwah, NJ 07430
201/236-9500   FAX 201/236-0072

Call toll-free to order: 1-800-9-BOOKS-9...9am to 5pm EST only.
e-mail to: orders@erlbaum.com
visit LEA's web site at http://www.erlbaum.com

NEUROBEHAVIORAL PLASTICITY
Learning, Development, and Response to Brain Insults

edited by
Norman E. Spear
Linda P. Spear
State University of New York, Binghamton
Michael L. Woodruff
East Tennessee State University

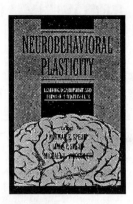

"This book is one of the most integrated and informative texts that have appeared within the general domain of neurobehavioral plasticity. Although there are 23 chapters written primarily by multiple authors, the style, content, and rich theoretical and empirical contributions are remarkably homogeneous."
-- Contemporary Psychology

This book describes a unique combination of research programs based on a striking variety of hypotheses and procedures directed toward understanding the sources and consequences of neurobehavioral plasticity. This remarkable attribute of the nervous system — to be pliable and capable of being shaped or formed by natural or artificial sources toward adaptation or maladaptation — is considered in terms of the neurochemical forces and neuroanatomical structure that has been found to be pivotal for this function. The impetus for this volume was a symposium held to honor Robert L. Isaacson for his scientific and pedagogical achievements as well as his contributions to behavioral neuroscience.

Corresponding to his three major research interests, the book is divided into three sections as follows:

- the first explores the relationship between the limbic system and behavior, with an emphasis on learning and memory;
- the second considers — through a wide range of approaches — issues of plasticity in behavior and brain; and
- the third deals with neural and chemical determinants of normal and abnormal behavior.

This volume is not only a fitting tribute to Isaacson, but also an unusual collection of new evidence, procedures, and theories destined to have significant influence on behavioral neuroscience.
0-8058-1425-6 [cloth] / 1995 / 488pp. / $99.95
Special Prepaid Offer! $45.00
No further discounts apply.

Lawrence Erlbaum Associates, Inc.

10 Industrial Avenue, Mahwah, NJ 07430

Prices subject to
change without notice.

201/236-9500   FAX 201/236-0072

Call toll-free to order: 1-800-9-BOOKS-9...9am to 5pm EST only.
e-mail to: orders@erlbaum.com
visit LEA's web site at http://www.erlbaum.com

RECOVERY AFTER TRAUMATIC BRAIN INJURY

edited by

Barbara P. Uzzell
Memorial Neurological Association

Henry H. Stonnington
Memorial Rehabilitation Center

A VOLUME IN THE INSTITUTE FOR RESEARCH IN BEHAVIORAL NEUROSCIENCE SERIES

Emotions, behaviors, thoughts, creations, planning, daily physical activities, and routines are programmed within our brains. To acquire these capacities, the brain takes time to fully develop — a process that may take the first 20 years of life. Disruptions of the brain involving neurons, axons, dendrites, synapses, neurotransmitters or brain infrastructure produce profound changes in development and functions of the one organ that makes us unique. To understand the functions and development of the brain is difficult enough, but to reverse the consequences of trauma and repair the damage is even more challenging. To meet this challenge and increase understanding, a host of disciplines working and communicating together are required.

The International Association for the Study of Traumatic Brain Injury tried to correct this limitation during its meetings of international clinicians, researchers, and scientists from many fields. It was felt that many of the outstanding thoughts and ideas from the most recent meeting and from others working in the field of traumatic brain injury (TBI) should be shared in written communication. Hence, this book was conceived not as proceedings of the conference, but as a collection of knowledge for those working in the acute and chronic recovery aspects of head injury.

This book reflects the importance of the team treating patients with TBI in that the chapter authors come from a diverse array of disciplines — basic science, neurosurgery, neurology, radiology, psychology, neuropsychology, and legal, consumer, and speech/language science. Their contributions provide the most current research and the latest ways of managing a variety of aspects of TBI.

Contents: B.P. Uzzell, H.H. Stonnington, Introduction. **Part I:** *Diagnoses and Management.* **J.D. Lewine, W.W. Orrison, J.T. Davis, B. Hart, J. Spar, P.W. Kodituwakku, D. Hill, S. Chang, V.A. Waldorf, P. Shaw, C. Edgar, J.H. Stone,** Neuromagnetic Evaluation of Brain Dysfunction in Postconcussive Syndromes Associated with Mild Head Trauma. **J.T.L. Wilson, D.M. Hadley, L.C. Scott, A. Harper,** Neuropsychological Significance of Contusional Lesions Identified by MRI. **J.L. Dowling, R.G. Dacey, Jr.,** Factors Affecting Brain Injury in Subarachnoid Hemorrhage. **Y. Katayama, A. Yoshino, T. Kawamata, T. Tsubokawa,** Role of Excitatory Amino Acids in Neuronal and Glial Responses to Trauma Brain Injury. **W.D. Dietrich,** Light and Electron Microscopic Studies of Fluid Percussion Brain Injury in Rats: Posttraumatic Considerations. **T. Tsubokawa,** Chronic Brain Simulation as a Restorative Treatment for Brain Damage. **W.E. Lux,** Pharmacological Strategies in the Management of Cognition and Behavior Following Traumatic Brain Injury. **Part II:** *Clinical States.* **B. Johnstone, T.S. Callahan,** Neuropsychological Evaluation of Traumatic Brain Injury in the United StatesL A Critical Analysis. **J.D. Corrigan,** Assessment of Agitation During the Acute Phase of Recovery. **J.D. Corrigan,** The Incidence and Impact of Substance Abuse Following Traumatic Brain Injury. **Z. Kalisky, B.P. Uzzell,** Florid Confabulation Following Brain Injury. **B.E. Murdoch,** Physiological Rehabilitation of Disordered Speech Following Closed Head Injury. **N.D. Zasler,** Vegetative State: Challenges, Controversies, and Caveats. A Physiatric Perspective. **Part III:** *Timing and Outcomes.* **B. Kolb,** Brain Plasticity and Behavior During Development. **J.L. Ponsford, J.H. Olver, C. Curran,** Outcome Following Traumatic Brain Injury: An Australian Study. **A-L. Christensen, C. Caetano, G. Rasmussen,** Psychosocial Outcome After an Intensive, Neuropsychologically Oriented Day Program: Contributing Program Variables. **M.J. Fuhrer, J.S. Richards,** Medical Rehabilitation Outcomes for Persons with Traumatic Brain Injury: Some Recommended Directions for Research. **P. Wehman,** Traumatic Brain Injury: Work Outcome and Supported Employment. **Part IV:** *Family and Community.* **J.E. Farmer, R. Stucky-Ropp,** Family Transactions and Traumatic Brain Injury. **F. Krause,** The Development of Grassroots Support for Research and Services in Brain Injury. **D.N. Cope,** A Databased Managed Care System of Catastrophic Neurologic Injury Rehabilitation. **J.S. Taylor,** Neurolaw: Medicolegal Aspects of Traumatic Brain Injury. **B.P. Uzzell, H.H. Stonnington,** Speculations for the Future.

0-8058-1823-5 [cloth] / 1996 / 360pp. / $69.95
0-8058-1824-3 [paper] / 1996 / 360pp. / $34.50

Prices subject to
change without notice.

Lawrence Erlbaum Associates, Inc.
10 Industrial Avenue, Mahwah, NJ 07430
201/236-9500   FAX 201/236-0072

Call toll-free to order: 1-800-9-BOOKS-9...9am to 5pm EST only.
e-mail to: orders@erlbaum.com
visit LEA's web site at http://www.erlbaum.com

LEA